THE NURSE'S LIABILITY
FOR MALPRACTICE
A Programmed Course

THE NURSE'S LIABILITY FOR MALPRACTICE
A Programmed Course

Fourth Edition

Eli P. Bernzweig, J.D.
Member of the New York Bar

McGraw-Hill Book Co.

*New York   St. Louis   San Francisco   Auckland   Bogotá   Hamburg
Johannesburg   London   Madrid   Mexico   Milan   Montreal   New Delhi   Panama
Paris   São Paulo   Singapore   Sydney   Tokyo   Toronto*

NOTICE

As new medical and nursing research and clinical experience
broaden our knowledge, changes in treatment and drug
therapy are required. The editors and the publisher of this
work have made every effort to ensure that the drug dosage
schedules herein are accurate and in accord with the
standards accepted at the time of publication. Readers are
advised, however, to check the product information sheet
included in the package of each drug they plan to administer
to be certain that changes have not been made in the
recommended dose or in the contraindications for
administration. This recommendation is of particular
importance in regard to new or infrequently used drugs.

THE NURSE'S LIABILITY FOR MALPRACTICE
A PROGRAMMED COURSE

1 2 3 4 5 6 7 8 9 0 DOCDOC 8 9 4 3 2 1 0 9 8 7 6

ISBN 0-07-005066-X

Library of Congress Cataloging-in-Publication Data

Bernzweig, Eli P.
   The nurses's liability for malpractice.

   Includes bibliographies and index.
   1. Nurses—Malpractice—United States—Programmed
instruction.   I. Title.   [DNLM: 1. Malpractice—
programmed instruction.   2. Nursing—programmed
instruction.   WY 18 B531n]

KF2915.N83B4 1987	346.7303'32	86-12510
ISBN 0-07-005066-X	346.306332	

This book was set in Times Roman by Better Graphics, Inc.
The editor was Sally J. Barhydt;
the cover was designed by Jane Moorman;
the production supervisors were Phil Galea and Fred Schulte.
Project supervision was done by The Total Book.
R. R. Donnelley & Sons Company was printer and binder.

3. Identify patients who are more likely to be suit-prone and take the steps necessary in caring for such patients to forestall the possibility of later malpractice claims.

4. Employ the terminology of malpractice law in a meaningful way when discussing specific legal problems with nursing supervisors, hospital administrators, lawyers, or others.

How to Proceed

A programmed course builds a structure of information in systematically arranged steps, each of which is referred to as a frame. This particular program utilizes the multiple-choice type of frame, which requires the learner to check the correct response or responses to each question. Programmed instruction is an active teaching process, which requires active responding on the part of the learner. *Checking the appropriate box or boxes, therefore, is a vital and necessary part of the program.* The choice made should be compared with the correct response set at the bottom of the page. The learner should not look at the answer until she has indicated what she believes to be the appropriate response. It may be helpful to cover the answer with the provided mask while reading the text.

The questions presented throughout the program are not intended to be deceptive or unusually difficult. The purpose is to teach, not to confuse or confound. The learner who reads carefully and pays close attention to the instructional material should get correct responses to the questions posed in all or nearly all the frames.

Test questions that appear at the end of the program may be used both for pretest and posttest purposes.

INTRODUCTION

This self-instructional course is intended to teach nurses in understandable terms about their legal liability for acts of malpractice. Some nurses may have only the vaguest idea what the terms *liability* and *malpractice* even mean, but by the time this course is completed, the learner will not only know what these words mean but will begin to appreciate the fact that many of the routine nursing functions performed each day have important legal consequences.

Knowledge precedes meaningful action, and nurses who know the legal consequences of daily patient care activities will soon begin to think and act preventively; that is, they will consciously conduct themselves in a manner designed to prevent unwanted suits from ever arising. This conscious behavior on the part of the nurse will save the embarrassment, loss of prestige, and worry that accompany every lawsuit, and it is bound to result in better patient care.

Throughout this course (except where specifically indicated) no attempt has been made to distinguish between the liability of the registered nurse, the practical nurse, and the nursing student since the courts themselves have generally made little distinction in this respect. In the final analysis, the same body of legal principles is equally applicable to all classes of nurses. This fact emphasizes the need for all nurses to become familiar with the information taught in this course.

Statement of Behavioral Objectives

The purpose of this program is not to make lawyers out of nurses or even to teach nurses how to solve specific legal problems. That role is best played by the medicolegal specialist, and the intelligent nurse will always consult such a person when in need of legal advice concerning a particular aspect of this complex field of law. The prime objective of this course is to give the learner a grounding in the fundamental principles of malpractice law and then to show how these fundamental principles are applied in specific fact situations. Upon completion of the program, the learner should be able to do the following:

1. Analyze a fact situation involving a particular aspect of nursing care, identify the principles of malpractice law that apply, and determine with reasonable certainty the legal consequences (if any) for her or him in the given situation.

2. Determine his/her malpractice-liability potential in carrying out various types of nursing functions and make appropriate changes in behavior to assure not only conformity with the applicable legal standards of care but higher quality care for all her patients.

ABOUT THE AUTHOR

ELI P. BERNZWEIG is a consultant, writer, and frequent speaker on professional liability issues and is widely recognized as one of the top authorities on medical malpractice in the country. During his 20-year tenure as a government attorney, he was chief legal advisor to the U.S. Public Health Service hospital system, where he was responsible for reviewing all malpractice claims against the Public Health Service. From 1971 through 1973, he held the post of Executive Director of the H.E.W. Secretary's Commission on Medical Malpractice, the first national body to explore the basic causes and consequences of the medical malpractice problem.

In addition to his government service, Bernzweig served two years as vice president of one of the country's largest medical malpractice insurance carriers and later spent two years as a guest scholar at the Brookings Institution in Washington, D.C., analyzing and critiquing our various injury compensation systems.

Bernzweig has his law degree from the Rutgers University Law School and is a member of the New York and U.S. Supreme Court bars. He is a frequent lecturer and the author of three books and numerous articles on professional liability issues. He is a regular contributor to *RN* Magazine and other publications on the legal liability of nurses.

To the loving memory of my parents

ABRAHAM AND FANNIE BERNZWEIG

CONTENTS

Preface   *xi*
Introduction   *xiii*

Part 1 GENERAL PRINCIPLES

Types and Sources of Law   3
Concept of Negligence   20
Concept of Malpractice   24
The Nurse-Patient Relationship   31
Duty to Give Emergency Care   39
The Hospital Emergency Department   41
Good Samaritan Statutes   46
The Nurse's Legal Standard of Care   49
Standard of Care of the Nurse-Specialist   55
Standard of Care of the Nursing Student   57
Determining Negligent Conduct   62
Violation of Statutes   70
Other Applicable Standards of Care   72
Selected References   74

Part 2 SPECIAL RULES OF LIABILITY

Rule of Personal Liability   82
Supervisor's Liability for the Acts of Subordinates   84
Assignment Problems Faced by Supervisory Nurses   86
Doctrine of *Respondeat Superior*   88
Hospital Liability under *Respondeat Superior*   97
The "Borrowed Servant" Doctrine   99
The "Captain of the Ship" Doctrine   103
Doctrine of Charitable Immunity   104
Doctrine of Governmental Immunity   106
Governmental Immunity from Torts Suits   107
Liability of the School Nurse   108
Liability of Federal Government Nurses   113
Liability of the Occupational Health Nurse   115

Special Problems Arising Out of Home Health Care   117
Selected References   121

Part 3   SPECIFIC TYPES OF NEGLIGENT CONDUCT

Patient Safety Errors   128
Following Physicians' Orders   136
Physicians' Assistants and Nurses   141
Observation and Diagnosis Errors   146
Failure to Communicate   152
Improper Supervision   154
Supervisors and the Making of Float Assignments   158
Medication Errors   160
Negligence in Caring for Mentally Ill Patients   164
Selected References   170

**Part 4   INTENTIONAL WRONGS AND CONSENT
           TO TREATMENT**

Assault and Battery   178
The Concept of Consent to Treatment   182
Consent in Emergency Situations   187
Consent for Treating Minors and Mental Incompetents   190
Treating Mature Minors   191
Informed Consent   196
The Nurse's Role in Obtaining the Patient's Consent   201
Consent to Abortion, Sterilization, Receipt of Birth
Control Information, and Treatment of Venereal Disease   206
     Abortion   206
     Sterilization   207
     Birth Control Information   208
     Treatment of Venereal Disease   208
False Imprisonment   209
Selected References   214

**Part 5   REGULATION OF NURSING AND
           SCOPE OF NURSING PRACTICE**

Regulation of the Practice of Nursing   222
Scope of Nursing Practice   224
The Expanded Role of Nurses: *Sermchief* v. *Gonzalez*   230
Selected References   232

Part 6 PROVING THE NURSE'S LIABILITY

Who Can Sue and Be Sued   236
Elements of a Malpractice Suit   238
Questions of Fact and Law   243
Legal Precedents   246
Judicial Notice   247
Burden of Proof   250
Contributory Negligence   258
Comparative Negligence versus Contributory Negligence 261
Assumption of Risk   262
Emergency   264
Directed Verdicts   267
Need for Expert Testimony   268
Doctrine of *Res Ipsa Loquitur*   271
Selected References   276

Part 7 PRINCIPLES OF MALPRACTICE CLAIMS PREVENTION

Malpractice Claims Prevention   282
Causes of Malpractice Suits   284
Psychological Aspects of Patient Care   297
The Suit-Prone Patient   302
The Suit-Prone Nurse   312
Risk Management in the Hospital   316
Selected References   318

Part 8 MISCELLANEOUS LEGAL MATTERS

Medical Records   324
    Contents   324
    Alteration of Records   324
    Countersigning   325
    Confidential Nature of Medical Information   326
    Disclosure of Medical Information   326
    Use of Medical Records in Court   327
Invasion of Privacy   328
Reporting Child Abuse   329
Reporting of Elder and Spouse Abuse   330
Witnessing Wills   330
    Preparing versus Witnessing   331
    Legalities Associated with Wills   331

Living Wills—Right to Die Statutes   333
Durable Powers of Attorney   334
Malpractice Insurance for Nurses   336
    Is Malpractice Insurance Necessary?   336
    Protection Afforded   339
Selected References   340

Test Questions   *343*
Answers to Test Questions   *378*
Glossary   *385*
Index   *391*

PREFACE

The entire health care field has undergone important changes within the recent past, most notably in the areas of cost containment, the proliferation of walk-in emergency and surgery centers, the vast increase in home health care, the aging of the population, and dramatic increases in the use of high technology equipment. In one way or another, all of these have legal significance for nurses. Take cost containment, for example. The federal government's implementation of the program for payment by Diagnosis Related Groups (DRGs) as a mechanism for reducing hospital costs necessarily brings into focus quality of care issues related to the early (and perhaps premature) discharge of patients. The obvious alternative treatment sites will be extended care facilities, rehabilitation facilities, and patients' homes. Clearly, the nurse who provides care in these locations will be required to make many critical nursing assessments and judgments without the more sophisticated medical and nursing backup available in the hospital setting, thereby increasing the potential for making errors and her consequent legal liability.

Perhaps more than anything else, however, the aging of the population and the providing of health services in the patient's home is likely to affect nurses and nursing care substantially in the years ahead. By 1990, according to Census Bureau estimates, more than a quarter of the population in the United States will be 65 or over. With DRGs mandating the early discharge of acute care patients, many of the elderly will have to be treated in their homes by nurses who will have to assume much greater responsibilities for total case management of these patients. In addition to the usual nursing services, the home health nurse will be responsible for teaching, coordinating other services, and working with teams of physical and respiratory therapists, speech pathologists, nutritionists, social workers, and home health aides. On top of all this, nurses will be responsible for using and monitoring the performance of a wide array of high-tech equipment that can cause serious injury or death if it is not working properly. All this merely increases the chances of things going wrong in the home environment, thereby compounding the already-existing liability woes facing today's nurses.

The growing number of court cases against nurses bears out earlier predictions regarding the targeting of nurses as defendants in medical malpractice litigation and further emphasizes the importance of understanding the legal standards and principles by which nurses are judged. New responsibilities inevitably bring with them greater accountability and added liabilities, a fact that has not gone unnoticed either by attorneys representing injured patients or by the courts.

And at least one major legal decision, *Sermchief* v. *Gonzales*, 660 S.W. 2d 683 (Mo. 1983), has officially recognized the expanded role of nurses into areas traditionally held to be the sole province of the physician.

This fourth edition of The Nurse's Liability for Malpractice has been revised and expanded fairly extensively. It contains new or updated material on such issues as the mechanisms that regulate nurses and nursing practice, emergency care, informed consent to treatment, consents for minors, liability of supervisors, Good Samaritan statutes, liability of nursing students, charitable and governmental immunity, home health nursing, living wills and durable powers of attorney, liability of nurse-specialists, reporting of elder abuse, risk management principles, dealing with physicians' assistants, and the importance of malpractice insurance. These are legal areas of great concern to today's practitioners and have been addressed with that in mind. This fourth edition also inaugurates something entirely new—authoritative, up-to-date Selected References at the end of each part. These references have been included to enable the nurse who wants more detailed information to locate source materials and get an even better understanding of the legal concepts and principles set forth in this work.

More than ever, the ability of the modern nurse to function effectively requires something beyond the mere acquisition of basic nursing knowledge and skills. Fundamental concern for the patient's welfare and safety, always a prime focus of nurses, calls for a heightened awareness of the legal parameters within which they are expected to fulfill their customary nursing duties. This programmed course is geared to meeting that objective, and it is hoped that nurses who complete this material will be better prepared to serve patients as well as to protect themselves against the legal hazards in modern nursing practice.

Eli P. Bernzweig

Part One
General Principles

Types and Sources of Law

1-1   Throughout this course we will have occasion to refer to the words "law," "common law," "civil law," and "statutory law," so it is important for you to have a reasonably clear understanding of the meaning of these words and the distinctions between them.

The word "law" has many different meanings and is used in many different ways, depending upon the subject under discussion. For example, we refer to physical laws (such as the law of gravity), economic laws (such as Gresham's law), and psychological laws (such as the law of operant conditioning), and although all these have an effect on human beings in one way or another, none of them have any *legal significance*.

"Law," in the sense we will be using the term in this course, refers to those rules made by humans which regulate social conduct in a formally prescribed and legally binding manner.

Without knowing the exact context in which the word law was being used, a person

☐ could   ☐ could not   be sure of the specific sense in which the word was intended.

1-2   Human beings are affected by various types of laws. We will be discussing in this course only those types of laws which

☐   determine human behavior and psychological motivation

☐   regulate human social conduct in a legally binding manner

☐   determine and influence physical environment

1-1 *could not*	**1-2** *regulate human social conduct in a legally binding manner*

1-3   Check each of the laws listed below that has legal significance in the sense that it regulates human social conduct in a legally binding manner.

☐   law of gravity

☐   law of diminishing returns

☐   Indiana Nursing Practice Act

☐   Federal Drug Abuse Control Act

☐   Murphy's Law

☐   Florida Motor Vehicle Law

☐   law of economic cycles

1-4   Laws that regulate human social conduct are derived from two basic sources. One source of law finds expression in formal legislative enactments, generally referred to as "statutes." When law is formally expressed in a statute, we refer to it as statutory law. A law passed by Congress or a state or a provincial legislative body would be an example of statutory law.

The *distinguishing* feature of statutory law is that it

☐   regulates human social conduct

☐   is one of two basic kinds of law

☐   is derived from formal legislative enactments

1-3   ☐   If you are not sure of the dis-
           ☐   tinction between laws that do
           ☑   and laws that do not regulate
           ☑   human social conduct, turn to
           ☐   p. 8, Note A.
           ☑
           ☐

1-4   *is derived from formal legisla-tive enactments*

The other two items are also features, but neither of them is the *distinguishing* feature of statutory law.

> NOTE: While all statutes are the result of formal legislative enactments, a statute enacted by the legislative body of one jurisdiction would have no legal effect outside that jurisdiction. Thus, the Nursing Practice Act of the Province of Ontario would not apply to nurses in the State of New York or the Province of Manitoba.

1-5   Legislative bodies cannot possibly enact statutes to cover all types of human conduct, and thus there are gaps in the law that must be filled in another way. The second source of law that regulates human social conduct is expressed in judicial decisions that interpret legal issues raised in disputes taken to court. This judge-made law is referred to as common law to distinguish it from the more formal type of law expressed in legislative enactments. Although common law and statutory law are derived from different sources, they are both of equal importance and legal effect.

How does common law differ from statutory law?

☐   Common law is not the result of a legislative enactment.

☐   Common law is less important than statutory law.

☐   Common law does not have the legal effect of statutory law.

1-6   Statutory law and common law have the following features in common (select one):

☐   They both represent the formal expression of law by a legislative (lawmaking) body.

☐   They both regulate the conduct of human beings in a legally binding manner.

☐   They both result from legal disputes between individuals.

1-5   *Common law is not the result of a legislative enactment.*

1-6   ☐   Only statutory law has to be
          ☑   enacted by a legislative body,
          ☐   and only common law is derived from court decisions. However, they *both* regulate human social conduct.

1-7   As mentioned before, both statutory law and common law are of equal importance and legal effect, and it is possible for both types of law to be involved in a single lawsuit.

Consider the following example:

In a malpractice suit filed against a licensed practical nurse, the complaining party introduces into evidence the state Practical Nursing Practice Act. The complainant does this to prove that the nurse attempted (unsuccessfully) to perform a function that should have been performed only by a registered nurse. After carefully reading the act, the trial judge rules that the nurse was legally permitted to perform the particular nursing function and that the only question to be resolved by the jury is whether the nurse performed it in a safe and proper manner.

The Practical Nursing Practice Act in this case is an example of

☐ common law   ☐ statutory law   because

☐   it was introduced into evidence in a court of law

☐   it represents a specific legislative enactment or statute applicable in that jurisdiction

---

1-8   The trial judge's ruling in this case is an example of   ☐ common law
☐ statutory law   because

☐   it relates to a specific legislative enactment

☐   it laid down a legal principle that will be binding on other courts in future similar cases

---

1-7   *statutory law*

*it represents a specific legis-
lative enactment . . .*

1-8   *common law*

*it laid down a legal principle
that will be binding on other
courts . . .*

1-9   A statute that deals with a particular aspect of nursing practice would have

☐   greater legal effect than

☐   the same legal effect as

☐   less legal effect than

a judicial decision that deals with the identical subject matter.

NOTE: In the material just presented, our primary concern has been to clarify the distinction between statutory and common law. It should be pointed out, however, that many of the nurse's day-to-day professional activities are governed by the nurse practice act of the state in which he or she practices. This statute customarily delegates to the state Board of Nursing the authority to lay down admission standards as well as to grant, suspend, or revoke licenses, establish minimum continuing education standards, and so forth. The statute also grants the board authority to issue rules and regulations, which have the same legal effect as a statute. We will have occasion to refer again to the legal role played by state nurse practice acts later in this chapter.

1-10   Now that you know the kind of law we will be talking about and its two basic sources, let us see where the particular branch of law known as malpractice law fits into the picture. To do this we must first understand how the entire body of statutory and common law is classified. Although the law is classified in many different ways, for our purposes it is sufficient if we distinguish between two major classifications: criminal law and civil law.

Criminal law relates solely to conduct that is considered an offense against the general public because it is detrimental to the welfare of society as a whole. Criminal conduct includes such public offenses as murder, robbery, burglary, larceny, embezzlement, and assault.

Which of the following statements *best* expresses the role and function of criminal law?

☐   Criminal law deals with violent conduct.

☐   Criminal law deals with conduct that offends one or more individuals in society.

☐   Criminal law deals with conduct considered offensive to society as a whole.

1-9   *the same legal effect as*

If you selected the wrong answer, turn to p. 8, Note B.

1-10   *Criminal law deals with conduct considered offensive to society as a whole.*

EXPLANATORY NOTES

Note A   (from Frame 1-3)

All the laws that are listed have *some* effect on human beings, but not all of them *regulate* the conduct or behavior of human beings in a formal, legal manner. To illustrate, the law of gravity clearly affects all of us in that it determines the force of our attraction downward toward the center of the earth, but it is not the kind of law that guides us in our social conduct as members of society. The key, then, to the type of law or laws we will be talking about in this course is the word "regulate." Unless a particular law *regulates* our social conduct in a formal, legal manner, it is not the type of law we will be concerned with.

Proceed to Frame 1-4.

Note B   (from Frame 1-9)

The correct answer is that a statute that deals with a particular aspect of nursing practice would have the *same* legal effect as a judicial decision that deals with the same subject matter. The particular source of law has no bearing on the importance or legal effect of either type of law. Thus, the court's decision in a nursing malpractice suit would be just as binding and controlling with respect to the nursing function in question as a statute that announces a specific rule or standard of conduct applicable to that same nursing function.

The key points to remember are: (1) Both statutory law and common law regulate human social conduct in a formal manner, and (2) both have the same legal significance.

Proceed to Frame 1-10.

1-11   Although we ordinarily associate criminal conduct with violent behavior, this need not be the case. As long as the conduct is expressly prohibited under the common law or by a specific statute, it is considered a crime. And even though the prohibited act is directed against a particular person or the person's property (with or without his or her knowledge), legally it is viewed as an offense against society as a whole.

Indicate whether the following statements are true or false:

True	False	
☐	☐	All violent behavior is considered criminal conduct.
☐	☐	Some acts may be considered crimes even though perpetrated entirely without the knowledge of the victim.
☐	☐	To be considered a crime, a person's conduct must be directed against a specific person.

1-12   Criminal actions cannot be prosecuted by private citizens since they are considered offenses against the general public. Accordingly, they are prosecuted by the controlling government authority (Federal, state, or provincial), and if found guilty, the accused may be punished by being fined, imprisoned, or both.

A and B are neighbors who do not like each other. One day, in a heated argument over the placement of a boundary fence, A attacks and seriously wounds B with a kitchen knife.

Since A and B know each other and since no one else was involved in the incident, A's conduct would be considered noncriminal.

True	False
☐	☐

1-13   In the previous example, who could institute a criminal action against A?

☐ only B

☐ B or B's spouse

☐ only the controlling governmental authority

☐ any offended onlooker

1-11	*True*	*False*	**1-12** *False*	**1-13**	
	☐	☑	Assaulting another per-	☐	If the correct an-
	☑	☐	son with a deadly	☐	swer seems con-
	☐	☑	weapon is considered a	☑	fusing to you, turn
			criminal act in all civi-	☐	to p. 16, Note A.
			lized societies.		

1-14   If A is found guilty in a criminal action arising out of the incident described in Frame 1-12, which of the following would be the likely consequence thereof?

☐   A will be fined, sentenced to prison, or placed on probation.

☐   A will be required to pay all B's medical expenses arising out of the wounds inflicted.

☐   A will have to publicly apologize to B for such violent conduct.

1-15   The second major class of law, civil law, is concerned with the legal rights and duties of private persons (or combinations of persons, such as corporations). It is in contrast with criminal law, which is concerned solely with public rights and public authority to punish for unlawful conduct. Thus, the unsuccessful party in a civil suit is usually required to pay a sum of money to the successful party in the suit, but is not imprisoned or fined, as in a criminal case.

In what significant respect does civil law differ from criminal law?

☐   Civil law is concerned with less important matters.

☐   Civil law is concerned with conduct that violates the rights of all members of society.

☐   Civil law is concerned with the legal rights and relationships that exist between private persons.

1-14 *A will be fined, sentenced to prison, or placed on probation.*

1-15 *Civil law is concerned with the legal rights and relationships that exist between private persons.*

1-16   Which two of the following statements correctly describe the characteristics of civil law?

☐   The successful party in a civil suit is usually awarded a sum of money.

☐   Civil law does not deal with public offenses or conduct that is deemed detrimental to society as a whole.

☐   Civil law deals only with financial rights and interests of private persons.

1-17   Although criminal law is concerned only with the public interest and civil law is concerned only with private interests, *both* classes of law frequently involve the interpretation of statutes.

Keeping in mind the differences in the legal interests concerned, indicate which of the following statutes relate to criminal law and which relate to civil law.

Criminal	*Civil*	
☐	☐	"It shall be unlawful for any person to practice any of the healing arts in this state without first having obtained a license from the State Board of Regents."
☐	☐	"If either party to a contract agrees thereto by reason of fraud, there is no legal agreement and said contract shall be unenforceable in this state."
☐	☐	"No will shall be admitted to probate in this state unless the instrument shows on its face that it has been duly witnessed by at least two persons."
☐	☐	"It shall be unlawful for any licensed physician or nurse to fail to report the existence of a contagious or communicable disease to the local health authorities immediately upon discovery."

1-16   ☑   If you checked the 3d box,
         ☑   turn to p. 16, Note B.
         ☐

1-17   *Criminal*   *Civil*
              ☑   ☐
              ☐   ☑
              ☐   ☑
              ☑   ☐

POINTS TO REMEMBER

1. While many types of laws affect human beings, not all of them have legal significance.

2. In this course the term "law" refers to those rules made by humans that regulate social conduct in a formal and legally binding manner.

3. Law is derived from legislative enactments (statutory law) and from judicial decisions (common law).

4. Both statutory and common law are of equal importance and legal effect.

5. Criminal law and civil law are two of the major classifications of law.

6. Criminal law deals with offenses against society as a whole, and criminal actions are accordingly brought by the appropriate governmental authorities.

7. Criminal conduct may be associated with violent behavior, but this is not always the case. To be criminal, the conduct need only be an offense against society prohibited under the common law or, as is usually the case, by statute.

8. If found guilty, the accused in a criminal action is punished.

9. Civil law deals with private legal rights and interests, and the unsuccessful party in a civil action is usually (but not always) required to pay money to the successful party.

1-18   Some nursing activities, if performed in an unlawful manner, can constitute criminal conduct, so a brief explanation of how criminal law relates to nursing practice may be of value at this point.

Consider the following situation:

State S has a statute that provides: "Only a physician or dentist may prescribe, administer, and dispense narcotic drugs, or he may cause the same to be administered by a nurse or intern under his direction and supervision. . . . Violation of this statute is made a crime, punishable by fine or imprisonment, or both."

Doctor D orders Nurse N to administer a specific quantity of a pain-killing narcotic drug to a patient, and Nurse N administers the drug as directed. Later that evening the patient again complains of severe pain. Nurse N is unable to reach the doctor. Nurse N then obtains and administers a second dose of the narcotic drug, which relieves the patient's pain immediately.

What is the legal effect of Nurse N's conduct?

☐ Nurse N can be held criminally liable for violating the state's narcotic drug statute.

☐ Nurse N can be sued for money damages in a civil suit brought by the patient.

☐ Nurse N's conduct is of no legal effect since no harm resulted to the patient.

1-19   Nurse N violated the state statute by

☐ administering a narcotic drug to a patient

☐ failing to call a second physician for advice

☐ prescribing a narcotic drug for a patient

1-18 ☑
☐
☐

1-19 *prescribing a narcotic drug for a patient*

1-20   Based on the given example, which of the following conclusions is the most accurate?

- ☐ Nurses will be held criminally liable whenever they administer narcotic drugs to patients outside a prescribing doctor's presence.

- ☐ Nurses cannot be held criminally liable for prescribing narcotic drugs if a doctor gives them permission to do so.

- ☐ Nurses may be held criminally liable whenever they prescribe narcotic drugs.

1-21   State and federal laws mandating the reporting of suspected child abuse (including child neglect and sexual exploitation) are directly applicable to nurses as well as to other health care practitioners. Under most of the state laws, the *good faith* reporting of such cases to the proper authorities—meaning the nurse has reasonable cause to believe the child's injuries were not accidental—will protect the nurse against liability in any lawsuit that might be brought for defamation of character or invasion of privacy. On the other hand, these laws make the *failure* to report such cases the basis for imposing criminal penalties, including fines and jail sentences.

Which of the following statements best expresses the nurse's criminal liability under child abuse reporting laws?

- ☐ A nurse can be held criminally liable for failure to report in good faith all cases of suspected child abuse.

- ☐ A nurse cannot be held criminally liable as long as the nurse reports under the child abuse statute every instance of serious injury or trauma to a child.

- ☐ A nurse cannot be held criminally liable for failing to report any suspected child abuse case where the nurse is not certain who is responsible for abusing the child.

1-20   ☐   If you checked the 2d box,   **1-21**   ☑
            ☐   turn to p. 16, Note C.   ☐
            ☑   ☐

1-22   Based on the foregoing, it is clear that a nurse   ☐ can   ☐ cannot   be held criminally liable both for taking action and for failing to take action under a particular statute.

1-23   We have just touched upon two ways in which a nurse, in the course of her normal duties, may become involved in criminal conduct. It is important that you understand the relationship of criminal law to nursing activities. We return now, however, to the prime subject of this course, the nurse's liability for malpractice, which falls within the general classification of civil law.

The nurse's legal liability for malpractice is more important than the nurse's liability for criminal acts.

True   *False*
☐   ☐

1-24   We have thus far discussed:

1. What we mean by "law"

2. Two basic sources of law

3. Two major classifications of law

Now we will get more specific and see just how malpractice law is related to other kinds of law. Civil law, which deals with the legal rights and relationships existing between private persons, includes many different categories, each dealing with a different subject matter.

The general category of civil law with which we are concerned is called the law of torts. A "tort" is a legal wrong committed by one person against the person or property of another. To compensate for such a private legal wrong, the law permits the harmed person to bring a civil action (a lawsuit) against the wrongdoer to recover a sum of money.

Civil law consists of

☐   a single, comprehensive body of law

☐   two fundamental categories of law

☐   many different categories of law

1-22 *can*	**1-23** *False* If you are at all uncertain about this point, turn to p. 16, Note D.	**1-24** *many different categories of law*

EXPLANATORY NOTES

Note A   (from Frame 1-13)

Criminal actions are legal processes that can be initiated only by the controlling governmental authority. This does not mean that the victim of a criminal act (such as B in the given example) will not be *involved* in the criminal prosecution. In fact, B will be the principal witness for the state (or province); without B's testimony, A could not be convicted. It should be noted that the fact that B cannot institute a *criminal* action against A does not affect B's right to institute a *civil* action arising out of the incident. This point is discussed more fully later in Part 1.

Proceed to Frame 1-14.

Note B   (from Frame 1-16)

While it is true that civil law is concerned with private legal interests and that payment of a sum of money is the *usual* way in which these private legal interests are vindicated, there are other private legal interests that do not involve an award of money. Examples are the granting of a divorce, the granting of an injunction or restraining order against some specific type of offensive conduct, and a declaratory judgment establishing the ownership of property. Accordingly, one cannot categorically state that *all* civil actions involve purely financial interests.

Proceed to Frame 1-17.

Note C   (from Frame 1-20)

Getting the doctor's permission to perform an unlawful act (prescribing a narcotic drug) will not help the nurse escape criminal liability. It will simply make the doctor an accessory to the crime. Because the administering of narcotic drugs is a common nursing function, all nurses should become thoroughly familiar with the pertinent statutes governing their use in the state or province in which they practice. These statutes must be followed *strictly* if criminal consequences are to be avoided.

Proceed to Frame 1-21.

Note D   (from Frame 1-23)

Many aspects of criminal law are of special interest and importance to practicing nurses, and since their criminal liability can conceivably result in a fine or imprisonment, as well as the loss of their license to practice, it would be foolish to say that their criminal liability is less important than their civil liability. However, the subject of criminal law is so extensive that it really warrants a separate study in itself. For that reason, *and that reason alone,* we will not be discussing the nurse's criminal liability any further in this course.

Proceed to Frame 1-24.

1-25   The particular branch of civil law that deals with private legal wrongs (i.e., wrongs committed by and against private persons) is called

    ☐ the law of torts

    ☐ the law of private interests

    ☐ the law of compensation

1-26   A tort may be either an *intentional* wrong, such as assault, battery, false imprisonment, libel, or invasion of privacy, or an *unintentional* wrong, such as negligence. The one thing all torts have in common, however, is that the person or persons who have been wronged have the legal right to institute a civil action (i.e., a lawsuit) against the person (or legal combination of persons) who caused the wrong.

    Which of the following statements is correct?

    ☐ Private legal wrongs (torts) may result from conduct that the wrongdoer never intended.

    ☐ All private legal wrongs (torts) arise out of intentional willful behavior.

    ☐ An intentional private legal wrong (tort) will subject the wrongdoer to a criminal action.

1-27   Which of the following involves unintentional conduct?

    ☐ false imprisonment

    ☐ invasion of privacy

    ☐ negligence

1-25 ☑ ☐ ☐	1-26 ☑ ☐ ☐	1-27 *negligence*

1-28   A tort action can be brought by

□   a single individual only

□   one or more private persons

□   local governmental units only

1-29   The common element of all torts is that they concern

□   intentional conduct

□   private wrongs

□   unintentional conduct

1-30   Some *intentional* torts represent antisocial behavior of a sort that is also punishable under the criminal law. Examples are the torts of assault and battery. If A assaults B and is brought to trial on a charge of *criminal* assault, B would still be legally entitled to bring a civil action against A for the tort of *civil* assault.

Which of the following statements accurately summarizes the foregoing?

□   An act that constitutes a tort may also constitute a crime.

□   An act must be either a tort or a crime, but cannot be both.

□   An assaulted person can bring both a tort action and a criminal action against the wrongdoer.

NOTE: From this point on all references to torts will be limited to their civil-law aspect only. We will discuss several intentional torts later in the course.

1-28 *one or more private persons*	**1-29** *private wrongs*	**1-30** ☑ If you would like further clarification of this point, turn to p. 23, Note A.

1-31   There are many types of torts, but the one that relates most directly to the basic subject of this course is the tort of negligence. Negligence law is a broad field of law that includes many types of negligent conduct in carrying out one's legal responsibilities to others. It embraces the area commonly referred to as malpractice law and includes the negligent conduct of physicians, dentists, nurses, pharmacists, engineers, lawyers, architects, and other professionally trained persons.

The law of negligence is a subcategory of

☐   the law of contracts

☐   the law of torts

☐   the law of malpractice

1-32   The circles below symbolically represent the fields of tort law, negligence law, and malpractice law. Place the letter of each circle in the box beside the field of law it represents.

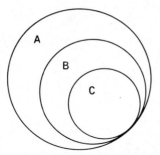

☐   Tort law

☐   Malpractice law

☐   Negligence law

1-31 *the law of torts*	1-32 Ⓐ
	Ⓒ
	Ⓑ

1-33   Malpractice law is concerned with

☐   all types of negligent conduct

☐   the negligent conduct of all professional persons

☐   the negligent conduct of professional medical personnel only

---

Concept of Negligence

1-34   Now that you have some idea of the general relationship between tort law, negligence law, and malpractice law, let us analyze the concept of negligence in more detail.

At law *every* person is always responsible for behaving in a reasonable and prudent manner, whether a layperson or a professional and whether engaged in the simplest or most complex type of activity. When persons fail to conduct themselves in this required manner and thereby do harm to others, we say they are legally "negligent."

Insofar as the law is concerned, persons are expected to conduct themselves in a reasonable and prudent manner

☐   at all times

☐   only when engaged in professional activities

☐   only when performing simple functions

☐   only if they are professional persons

1-33 *the negligent conduct of all professional persons*

1-34 *at all times*

1-35   Persons are expected to conduct themselves in this manner

□   whether they are professionals or laypersons

□   only if they are professionals

□   only if they are laypersons

1-36
as being   The law characterizes a person who fails to act in a reasonable and prudent manner

□   imprudent

□   unreasonable

□   negligent

1-37   A person whose negligence causes harm or injury to the person or property of another may be legally required to pay a sum of money to that person. This type of remedy, as you will recall, is what distinguishes civil law from criminal law.

The law provides that if injury results to a person because of negligent conduct on the part of another, the one whose negligence caused the injury

□   can avoid liability by showing that he or she is a professional

□   may be required to pay a sum of money to the injured person

□   will be subject to a criminal action

1-35 *whether they are professionals or laypersons*	1-36 *negligent*	1-37 *may be required to pay a sum of money to the injured person*

1-38   In general, the term "negligence" as used in malpractice law has the same meaning as the term "carelessness." Thus, conduct that is careless is usually negligent. But a person might be held negligent in the eyes of the law even if he or she acts carefully *from a personal point of view*. Here is a simple illustration: If a nurse attempts a nursing procedure for which he has had no prior training and does it as carefully as he knows how, his conduct may nevertheless be deemed negligent if, *judged by objective standards,* his conduct was careless and caused harm to the patient. To begin with, he should not have attempted the procedure at all without previous training or experience. The fact that he was as careful as possible, in his subjective opinion, is considered immaterial from the legal standpoint.

Indicate whether the following statements are true or false:

True	*False*	
☐	☐	In malpractice law the terms negligence and carelessness generally have the same meaning.
☐	☐	A nurse who fails to meet the required standard of care in a given situation may be deemed legally negligent even though he acts as carefully as he knows how.
☐	☐	When a nurse's carelessness in carrying out his professional duties causes harm to his patient, the nurse probably will be found legally negligent.
☐	☐	Harm resulting from the performance of an act that is beyond a nurse's training and experience may be the basis for holding the nurse legally negligent.

1-38   *True*   *False*
       ☑   ☐   If you missed any of these,
       ☑   ☐   see p. 23, Note B.
       ☑   ☐
       ☑   ☐

EXPLANATORY NOTES

Note A   (from Frame 1-30)

Many find this concept somewhat difficult to understand, so a little further explanation may be helpful. To begin with, a tort is usually defined as a wrongful act done by one person to the injury of another for which the injured party may demand legal redress (usually money damages) in a civil suit. But a *wrongful* act under tort law does not necessarily mean an act that is morally wrong or intentionally harmful. Thus, a man erroneously believing himself to be the owner of certain real property may be sued by the true landowner for the tort of trespass without regard to any question of morality or harmful intent involved.

On the other hand, *some* wrongful acts that fall into the category of tortious conduct, and thereby give rise to civil suits for damages, are simultaneously considered violations of public rights (i.e., crimes) since they strike at the very being of society. In the case of assault, the private right violated is the right of every individual that one's bodily safety shall be respected; and for the wrong done to this right, the sufferer is entitled to legal damages. But the act of violence is likewise viewed as a menace to the safety of society in general and will therefore be punished by the state. So it is not such a far-fetched idea, after all, for one and the same act to constitute both a tort and a crime.

Proceed to Frame 1-31.

Note B   (from Frame 1-38)

This is not an easy concept to grasp, so do not feel disappointed if you missed one or more of these true-false choices. The point being made is that a nurse's *careful* conduct may still be *legally negligent* if what the nurse does (even though with great care) is not what other prudent nurses would have done in the same circumstances. This statement assumes, of course, that some harm results from the nurse's act, for without any harm resulting, no legal wrong (tort) has been committed. In the overwhelming majority of cases, careful conduct will *not* give rise to a charge of negligence. The exceptional situation was outlined in Frame 1-38 only to explain how the rule might apply to an act of nursing practice.

Proceed to Frame 1-39.

Concept of Malpractice

1-39   The word "liability" appears in the title of this book, and you will see the words "liable" and "liability" used repeatedly throughout the course. Since these words have a specific, technical meaning in the law, now would be a good time to make their legal meaning as clear as possible.

When we say that an individual is legally liable to another person because of negligent conduct, we mean the individual can be held *legally responsible* for the harm caused the other person. "Liability" refers to the state of being held legally liable. In a malpractice action (as in most other civil actions) liability is assessed in monetary terms, commonly referred to as either "money damages" or simply "damages."

Which one of the following comes *closest* to the meaning of the phrase "legal liability"?

- ☐   legal indebtedness

- ☐   legal impediment

- ☐   legal responsibility

1-40

P, a former patient, sues Nurse N in a malpractice action in which P claims N's negligent conduct caused him serious injury. Nurse N is found legally liable for the harm caused P.

What is the *most likely* legal effect this ruling will have on Nurse N?

- ☐   Nurse N's license to practice as a nurse will be revoked.

- ☐   Nurse N will be obligated to reimburse P for the financial loss P sustained as a result of his injuries.

- ☐   Nurse N will have to stand trial on a criminal charge for the harm she caused P.

1-39 *Legal responsibility*	**1-40**	☐ If you checked the 1st or 3d
		☑ box, turn to p. 29, Note A.
		☐

1-41   As you have already learned, at law all persons are held legally responsible for conducting themselves in a reasonable and prudent manner, and can be held legally liable for failure to act as other reasonably prudent persons would act in the same situation.

The term "malpractice" is used to refer to the negligent acts of persons engaged in professions or occupations in which highly technical or professional skills are employed. *Negligence* is the general term embracing all negligent acts, while *malpractice* is the specific term used in referring to negligent conduct in the rendering of professional services by a person with professional education and training.

Indicate whether the following statements are true or false:

True	*False*	
☐	☐	Not every act of negligence can be classified as an act of malpractice, but every act of malpractice involves some type of negligent conduct.
☐	☐	Malpractice and negligence are totally unrelated concepts.
☐	☐	Negligent conduct may or may not be considered malpractice depending on the background of the individual in question.

1-41   *True*

False

True

1-42   Assume that each of the following persons failed to act in a reasonable and prudent manner in carrying out some aspect of his or her normal work duties. Which of them could be held liable for malpractice, and which of them could be held liable only for negligence?

Malpractice	Negligence	
☐	☐	Veterinarian
☐	☐	Ambulance driver
☐	☐	Pharmacist
☐	☐	Medical secretary
☐	☐	Public health nurse
☐	☐	Licensed practical nurse

1-43   A negligent act committed by a professional person constitutes malpractice only if it involves negligence in the carrying out of his or her professional duties.

A physician fails to exercise caution in driving her automobile into the hospital parking lot and her vehicle causes injury to a patient being moved in a wheelchair between two wings of the hospital.

Under these circumstances which of the following is true?

☐   The physician can be held liable for negligence, but not malpractice.

☐   The physician can be held liable only for malpractice.

☐   The physician can be held liable both for negligence and for malpractice.

1-42   *Malpractice   Negligence*

☑	☐
☐	☑
☑	☐
☐	☑
☑	☐
☑	☐

1-43   *The physician can be held liable for negligence, but not malpractice.*

1-44   Under appropriate circumstances, even a layperson could be held liable for malpractice.

                                        True   *False*
                                          ☐   ☐

1-45   Since the concept of malpractice is limited to those situations in which persons with specialized professional training are negligent in carrying out some phase of their professional duties, in which of the following instances might the person in question be held liable for malpractice?

   ☐   A consulting engineer miscalculates the tensile strength of certain structural materials, resulting in the collapse of a building.

   ☐   A hospital orderly negligently mops a hallway, causing a patient on crutches to slip and fall on a wet spot and thereby sustain further serious injury.

   ☐   A nurse-anesthetist's negligence in administering an anesthetic agent during a surgical procedure causes the patient's face to be seriously burned.

   ☐   A lawyer's negligence in failing to file suit on behalf of a client before a certain date results in the client's claim being barred by the statute of limitations.

   ☐   A medical ward nurse negligently mishandles a patient's dentures and they cannot be found.

NOTE: Medical malpractice is that type of malpractice that relates specifically to the acts of professional medical personnel when they are carrying out their normal patient care responsibilities. In other words, medical malpractice is simply negligence in some aspect of medical care and treatment. The legal standards of care reflect the distinction between ordinary negligence and malpractice. This point is covered more fully later in Part 1.

1-44 *False*	1-45 ☑
	☐
	☑
	☑
	☐

1-46   Which of the following types of negligent conduct would fall within the broad category of medical malpractice?

☐ A physician injures a patient with a sharp instrument while conducting a routine physical examination.

☐ A hospital pharmacist erroneously dispenses a drug in a form which is double the strength ordered by the physician, causing harm to the patient.

☐ A nurse knocks over an IV stand in a patient's room. The stand strikes the ankle of the patient's husband, causing a serious fracture.

☐ An intern neglects to check a patient's chart, which clearly shows a hypersensitivity to penicillin. The intern prescribes the drug for the patient, who suffers a severe reaction.

1-47   You have now been exposed to a whole series of terms and concepts that are related to the course you are studying. These words and concepts, and their meanings, are listed below in random order. Match the letter of each word or concept with its meaning.

A. Negligence

The state of being held legally responsible to another for some harm caused that person.   ☐

B. Tort

Negligent conduct by professional medical personnel   ☐

C. Malpractice

A legal wrong committed against the person or property of another   ☐

D. Legal liability

Failure to act in a reasonable and prudent manner   ☐

E. Medical malpractice

Negligent conduct in the performance of professional duties   ☐

1-46   ☑   If you checked the 3d box,
            ☑   turn to p. 29, Note B.
            ☐
            ☑

1-47   D
            E
            B
            A
            C

EXPLANATORY NOTES

Note A   (from Frame 1-40)

Negligent conduct—or malpractice—on the part of a nurse rarely involves the willful intent to harm another, but if such intent *could* be shown, the nurse could be guilty of criminal behavior. In such event, the nurse's license to practice might well be revoked upon conviction for the crime in question. Under ordinary circumstances, however, negligent conduct would not give rise to such drastic action, and the likelihood of criminal action is too remote to warrant serious consideration in this context.

Proceed to Frame 1-41.

Note B   (from Frame 1-46)

The nurse who knocked over the IV stand in the third example undoubtedly would be held liable for the harm caused the patient's husband, but for ordinary *negligence* rather than *malpractice*. The nurse was legally required to exercise reasonable care to see that no harm would come to the patient's husband (or any other visitor, for that matter), and failure to do so would constitute negligence. "Malpractice" is a term we use only when referring to negligent conduct on the part of professional persons in carrying out their professional duties on behalf of someone to whom they owe a special duty of care, such as a nurse's duty to a patient. (This latter point is covered more fully in the material that immediately follows.)

Turning the situation around, if the stand had fallen upon the patient, the nurse *could* be held liable for malpractice since (1) the safety and welfare of the patient is one of the nurse's fundamental responsibilities and (2) the proper positioning of an IV stand is a function the nurse would normally be expected to perform with care to assure the patient's safety and welfare.

Proceed to Frame 1-47.

POINTS TO REMEMBER

1. Tort law is that branch of civil law that deals with legal wrongs committed by one person against the person or property of another.

2. Torts (legal wrongs) may be intentional or unintentional.

3. Negligence is an unintentional tort that involves harm resulting from the failure of persons to conduct themselves in a reasonable and prudent manner.

4. Negligence and carelessness are not synonymous. One can be careful and yet be considered legally negligent for failure to act as other reasonably prudent persons would have acted in the particular circumstances.

5. Malpractice refers to the negligent acts of persons with specialized professional training and education.

6. An act constituting malpractice necessarily reflects negligence, but not all negligent acts constitute malpractice.

7. When persons are held legally responsible for their negligent conduct, we say they are legally liable.

8. A person held legally liable in a civil suit for harm caused another is required to pay money damages to the latter.

9. Medical malpractice refers to the negligent acts of health professionals in carrying out their professional responsibilities.

NOTE: When an act of nursing malpractice occurs, the law holds the nurse legally liable to the patient because of the particular legal relationship that exists between them—the nurse-patient relationship. In the material that follows we will see how this relationship is created and some of the legal consequences thereof.

The Nurse-Patient Relationship

1-48   The nurse-patient relationship is a legal status that is created the moment a nurse actually provides nursing care to another person. This relationship is important because of the legal duties and responsibilities that are attached. Once a nurse-patient relationship is established, the nurse legally owes a *special duty of care* to the patient that is greater than the *general duty of care* the nurse owes to other persons generally. As we shall see a little later, it is the failure to meet this special duty of care owed to their patients that forms the heart of all malpractice suits against nurses.

An act of nursing malpractice will give rise to legal liability only if a

☐ sociological   ☐ legal   ☐ moral   relationship exists between the parties.

1-49   The particular legal status or relationship in question is called the

☐ nurse-patient   ☐ nurse-litigant   ☐ nurse-liability   relationship.

1-48 *legal*

1-49 *nurse-patient*

1-50   Which of the following statements correctly explains the difference between the nurse's legal responsibilities to one who is his or her patient and to the public generally?

- ☐ Because of their professional training, nurses owe a greater duty of care than others to members of the general public as well as to their patients.

- ☐ A nurse's legal duty of care to his or her patient is neither greater nor lesser than his or her legal duty of care to members of the general public.

- ☐ As ordinary citizens, nurses owe members of the general public a general duty of care, but as nurses they owe their patients a greater duty of care.

1-51   What must the nurse and the patient do or say to create the nurse-patient relationship? No special words, agreement, or contract is required. The only thing that *is* required is the actual providing of nursing services. The fact that the recipient (the patient) may not have requested such services, or may even resent them, has no bearing on the legal effect or consequences of the nurse's actions. In either case a nurse-patient relationship will come into being as soon as the nurse undertakes to provide nursing care.

The essence of the nurse-patient relationship is

- ☐ a verbal or written agreement to provide nursing care to the patient
- ☐ a good therapeutic relationship with the patient
- ☐ the actual furnishing of nursing care to the patient

1-50 *As ordinary citizens, nurses owe members of the general public . . .*

1-51 *the actual furnishing of nursing care to the patient*

1-52   The patient's consent to enter into a nurse-patient relationship   ☐ is
☐   is not   necessary.

1-53   Could a nurse-patient relationship be established with an unconscious person?

Yes   *No*
☐   ☐

1-54   The manner in which nurses are employed, by whom they are employed, or whether they are technically employed at all is of no legal significance with respect to their legal liability for malpractice. Insofar as the law is concerned, the crucial factor is whether a nurse-patient relationship existed.

Typically, general-duty nurses do not enter into a series of contracts to provide nursing care to selected persons but enter into single contracts of employment with a hospital, an industrial firm, a public health department, a school, or the like. The important thing to note is that, although their contracts may be with particular employers, *the law holds them legally responsible to all persons to whom they actually provide nursing services.*

From the standpoint of legal liability for nursing malpractice, the manner in which a nurse's professional services are engaged   ☐ is   ☐ is not   a matter of legal significance.

1-55   The legal consequences of a nurse's performance of nursing services are primarily based on

☐   formal legal arrangements made with specific patients

☐   the manner in which the nurse renders those services

☐   the nature of the nurse's specific nursing assignments

1-52 *is not*	**1-53** *Yes*	**1-54** *is not*	**1-55** *the manner in which the nurse renders those services*

1-56

The nurse for an industrial firm is informed of an injury to an employee of a neighboring firm that has no nurse. The nurse rushes next door to give the necessary emergency care but negligently injures the employee while in the process.

Under these circumstances which of the following is true?

- [ ] The nurse can be held liable for malpractice because the act of giving emergency care created a nurse-patient relationship.

- [ ] The nurse cannot be held liable for malpractice but only for negligence because no nurse-patient relationship could have been created with an employee of a firm by whom the nurse was not employed.

- [ ] The nurse cannot be held liable for malpractice because the giving of emergency care does not create a nurse-patient relationship.

1-57

A former hospital patient sues a hospital nurse for malpractice that occurred while he was a patient at the hospital. Before he is permitted to offer proof of the nurse's negligence, he must first establish the fact that a nurse-patient relationship was in existence between himself and the nurse.

Which *one* of the following offers of proof by the patient would most effectively establish this fact?

- [ ] proof that he was over 21 years of age and could legally enter into a contractual relationship

- [ ] proof that the nurse was employed as a full-time staff nurse at the hospital

- [ ] proof that the nurse provided nursing care to him while he was a patient at the hospital

---

1-56 ☑ If you checked the wrong an-
       □ swer, turn to p. 37, Note A.
       □

1-57 *proof that the nurse provided nursing care to him while he was a patient at the hospital*

1-58   Consider the following situation:

Operating room Nurse N, while on a coffee break, strikes up a conversation in the hallway with Patient P while the latter is waiting to undergo a diagnostic test for stomach pain. N tells P that he definitely needs surgery, and suggests that he do so promptly. P decides to take the advice. When P's surgery turns out poorly, P sues N along with the operating surgeon.

What is the court most likely to say about the inclusion of N as a defendant in this case?

☐ N is a proper defendant because, even though P was not N's patient, N's advice had a direct bearing on P's decision to undergo surgery, which led to the poor result.

☐ N should be dismissed as a defendant because N was under no obligation to treat P and, hence, there was no nurse-patient relationship between N and P.

☐ N should be dismissed as a defendant because a nurse could not be held responsible for advising a patient on a medical matter so clearly beyond the scope of normal nursing care.

1-58   *N should be dismissed as a defendant because
N was under no obligation to treat P and,
hence, there was no nurse-patient relationship
between N and P.*

1-59   In contrast to general-duty hospital nurses who normally are expected to provide nursing care to all assigned hospital patients, private-duty nurses are considered free agents and may decide for themselves whether they wish to accept employment by any particular person. Their refusal to accept an offer of private employment will not subject them to any legal liability because no nurse-patient relationship has come into being.

Consider the following situation:

The family of a hospitalized patient hires a private-duty nurse through a local nurses' registry. When the nurse arrives at the patient's room, she recognizes him as the same disagreeable, uncooperative patient she had attended during a prior illness. The nurse tells the family member present that she will not accept the assignment and will arrange for the registry to send another nurse immediately. She then leaves, and on her way out arranges with the regular nursing staff to provide necessary nursing care until her replacement arrives.

Indicate whether each of the following statements is true or false:

True   *False*
☐   ☐   The nurse had a legal right to refuse the assignment.

☐   ☐   The moment the nurses' registry made the assignment a nurse-patient relationship came into being.

☐   ☐   The nurse's reasons for not wishing to accept the assignment are unimportant in determining whether a nurse-patient relationship came into being.

☐   ☐   The nurse had no legal right to refuse the assignment.

1-59   *True*   *False*
            ☑   ☐   For more information about
            ☐   ☑   the employment of private-
            ☑   ☐   duty nurses, turn to p. 37,
            ☐   ☑   Note B.

EXPLANATORY NOTES

Note A   (from Frame 1-56)

It was pointed out before that a nurse-patient relationship can come into being in a number of ways, and the precise manner in which this occurs is not really important. Moreover, whether or not a nurse-patient relationship exists does not depend on the nurse's employment status. As stated earlier, the *manner* in which a nurse is employed, *by whom* the nurse is employed, or *whether* the nurse is technically employed at all has no bearing on the creation of a nurse-patient relationship. The only thing that counts (in the legal sense) is the nurse's *actual providing of nursing care*.

The industrial nurse in this example may have had no contractual duty to give care to the injured employee for the neighboring firm, and indeed could have declined to give any help whatsoever. (We will discuss this point in detail very shortly.) But the fact is that the nurse *did* undertake to give care to the injured person, and that in itself is sufficient to create a nurse-patient relationship.

As you have already learned, whenever a nurse commits a negligent act while performing professional (i.e., nursing) duties, the nurse will be held liable for malpractice, and not ordinary negligence. That liability may be excused, however, under state Good Samaritan laws, which will be discussed shortly.

Proceed to Frame 1-57.

Note B   (from Frame 1-59)

Private-duty nurses are hired by the patient or patient's family to perform nursing services for that patient only. They receive their compensation directly from the patient or family, and are considered independent contractors, not employees of the hospital. For this reason, independent legal liability attaches to their negligent conduct in treating their employer-patients.

When a private-duty nurse is requested by a patient, but selected and paid for by the hospital, some courts have held the nurse to be an employee of the hospital. This is particularly true where the nurse has been given certain administrative functions to perform for the hospital in addition to the private-duty nursing. The hospital's liability for the nurse's negligent conduct in this situation is discussed in Part 2 of this course.

Proceed to Frame 1-60.

1-60   If, while leaving the hospital, the private-duty nurse discussed in the previous frame had gone to the assistance of another patient and committed an act of malpractice while so doing, would the law consider that a nurse-patient relationship had come into being?

Yes   No
□   □

1-61   Would the fact that the private-duty nurse was not employed either by the hospital or the patient have any bearing on the establishment of a nurse-patient relationship?

Yes   No
□   □

1-62   The nurse-patient relationship is not an exclusive legal status, and several nurses may have a nurse-patient relationship with a particular patient at the same time.

Consider the following situation:

A private-duty nurse engaged to care for an elderly hospitalized patient leaves the patient's bedside for 10 minutes to make some personal telephone calls. During the nurse's absence the patient suffers an acute coronary episode, and a nurse from the pediatric unit, on the way to lunch, rushes to the patient's aid. Because of limited experience with geriatric patients, the pediatric nurse makes a serious error of professional judgment in assisting the patient, causing him further harm.

Under these facts, which of the following statements is correct?

□   Since the patient already had a specially assigned (private-duty) nurse, it was legally impossible for a new nurse-patient relationship to come into being with the pediatric nurse.

□   Although the private-duty nurse had a valid nurse-patient relationship with the patient, as soon as the pediatric nurse went to the patient's assistance this relationship was temporarily suspended.

□   Upon going to the patient's assistance, the pediatric nurse established a new nurse-patient relationship with him.

1-60 *Yes*	**1-61** *No*	**1-62** □ □ ☑

1-63   In the previous example, who do you think would be held liable for the harm that resulted to the patient?

      ☐ the private-duty nurse only

      ☐ the pediatric nurse only

      ☐ both nurses

NOTE: Private-duty nursing has taken on added significance as more patients are being discharged earlier from hospitals in accordance with government regulations under Medicare and Medicaid. The present discussion relates only to the creation of the nurse-patient relationship. The broader legal aspects of home health nursing are discussed in greater detail in Part 2.

The Duty to Give Emergency Care

1-64   You have just seen how an emergency situation may be the stimulus for the establishment of a nurse-patient relationship. We will now discuss the nurse's legal obligation to give emergency care.

As the last example illustrated, an emergency that occurs in the normal hospital setting may call for immediate action on the part of a nurse to provide care to a patient even though the patient may not be assigned to the nurse. This is so because a general-duty nurse employed by a hospital assumes a duty of care to all patients for whose benefit that nurse's professional services are engaged. The same may be said for nurses who are employed by school systems, industrial plants, public health departments, and the like.

A general-duty nurse employed by a hospital would be legally responsible for providing emergency care

      ☐ only to those patients to which the nurse is specifically assigned

      ☐ to any patient in the hospital in need of such care

      ☐ both to patients in the hospital and to members of the general public in need of such care

---

1-63   ☐ If you checked either the 1st
       ☐ or 2d box, turn to p. 44, Note
       ☑ A.

1-64   *to any patient in the hospital in need of such care*

1-65

A secondary school in Toronto, Canada, plays host to a visiting group of school children from the United States of America. Several of the American visitors are injured in a minor bus accident on the school property, and the Canadian school nurse deliberates whether she is legally obligated to give them treatment.

Which of the following statements correctly states her responsibility?

☐ A Canadian nurse is under no legal obligation to treat nonresidents of Canada.

☐ Since the injured children are not enrolled in the school where she is employed, the nurse has no legal obligation to give them emergency care.

☐ The duties of the school nurse include the legal responsibility to furnish emergency care to all persons in need of such care while on the school property where she is employed, and this would include the injured children in question.

NOTE: The same rule would apply if the injured children were Canadians visiting an American school. The choice of a Toronto school was made simply to show that the general legal principles concerning establishment of the nurse-patient relationship and the duty to give emergency care are the same both in Canada and the United States.

1-65   ☐
       ☐
       ☑

THE HOSPITAL EMERGENCY DEPARTMENT

In recent years, the hospital emergency department has become the entry point into the health-care system for growing numbers of persons. As a consequence, emergency room personnel (and nurses in particular) are responsible for making many key decisions regarding treatment priorities and initiating the necessary care. For this reason, it is essential that the nurse assigned to work in the hospital emergency department be able to demonstrate superior diagnostic skills and judgment. Even though government regulations under the Medicare program require that adequate medical personnel be available in the emergency department, with very few exceptions emergency departments have constant staffing problems. This makes the emergency department nurse's work that much more difficult and greatly increases the chances for making errors and consequent exposure to malpractice suits.

What are the standards of care applicable to nurses who provide care to patients in the emergency room? First and foremost, emergency department nurses must be capable of acting swiftly, basing their actions often as much on instinct as on pure technical knowledge. One of the first things the nurse must do is evaluate the patient's condition, often with little opportunity to obtain a complete history, and make an initial decision regarding the degree of urgency of treatment and the need to summon a physician. This process is called *triage* ("sorting out"), and because patients' lives often are at stake, the margin for error is exceedingly slim. Nurses customarily perform triage in accordance with guidelines developed by the American Hospital Association, appropriately adapted to each hospital's needs and made a part of its own protocols and standing orders.

Most courts have ruled that the applicable standard of care in these situations is a nursing standard—what would a reasonably prudent emergency department nurse do under the given circumstances?—but at least one court has held the nurse working in the emergency room to the standard of a physician [*Fein* v. *Permanente Medical Group*, 175 Cal. Rptr. 177 (Cal. 1981)]. This result is not in accord with the majority of decisions dealing with emergency department care and is probably distinguishable from other cases in that the nurse in question was a duly certified nurse-practitioner working under the immediate and direct supervision of a physician. *Fein* has been appealed to the California Supreme Court, which is expected to clarify the standard of care applicable to ER nurse practitioners.

Certainly, the emergency department is no place for the inexperienced nurse; since emergency department care calls for such a high level of diagnostic and treatment skills, it is possible that nurses in the future may have to qualify as clinical specialists in emergency care before being assigned to hospital emergency department duty. Some 10,000 nurses already have been certified as specialists in emergency nursing.

We resume our discussion of the nurse's duty to provide emergency care in the nonhospital setting, but the reader should bear in mind the distinction between the provision of nursing care within the hospital and elsewhere.

1-66   The nurse's legal responsibility to provide emergency care to persons within a normal employment setting is quite different from the nurse's legal responsibility under other circumstances. In a noncontractual and nontherapeutic setting nurses have no *legal* obligation to render emergency care to someone in need, even though they may have a *moral* and *ethical* obligation to render such care.* Thus, a nurse ordinarily cannot be held legally liable for refusing to offer emergency care to the victim of a highway accident or other similar occurrence, no matter how life-threatening the circumstances.

In the hospitals, schools, or industrial plants where they are employed, the obligation of nurses to provide emergency nursing care to persons noted to be in physical or mental

distress is   ☐ greater than   ☐ the same as   ☐ less than   their obligation to provide

such care to persons in distress outside such environment.

* This general rule of the common law has a few statutory exceptions, discussed more fully on p. 47.

1-67   A nurse's legal obligation to go to the aid of someone in need of emergency care normally extends

☐   to all persons in need of such care (i.e., the general public)

☐   only to those persons encompassed within the terms of the contract of employment

☐   to no one

1-66   *greater than*

1-67   *only to those persons encompassed within the terms of the contract of employment*

1-68   The reason a nurse ordinarily is not required to aid someone who is the victim of a highway accident or other similar emergency is that

☐   the nurse has no way of being assured of payment for the services

☐   the nurse has no opportunity to ascertain the patient's medical history

☐   the nurse stands in no special relationship to such person and therefore owes him no special duty of care

---

1-69

A general-duty nurse coming home from work at the local hospital stops briefly to watch a holiday parade. Just as the nurse approaches the parade grounds a grandstand collapses, causing injury to many persons. A local physician watching the parade immediately begins giving emergency aid to the injured. Noticing the nurse (still in uniform), the physician beckons for assistance with the injured. However, because of a strong personal dislike of the physician, the nurse ignores the request and refuses to render any help to the injured.

Under the given facts:

	Yes	No
Has the nurse violated any legal duty to render care to the injured persons?	☐	☐
Will the injured persons, or their legal representatives, have a legal basis for suing the nurse for her conduct?	☐	☐
Do you think the nurse exercised good judgment in refusing to offer help for the stated reason?	☐	☐

1-68   *the nurse stands in no special relationship to such person . . .*

1-69   Yes   No

☐   ☑

☐   ☑

☐   ☐   ←*You decide. See p. 44, Note B.*

EXPLANATORY NOTES

Note A   (from Frame 1-63)

Both nurses would be held liable, but each for a different reason. The pediatric nurse's "error of professional judgment" is just another way of saying "malpractice," and the nurse will be held legally responsible for such an error of judgment. However, limited experience with geriatric patients and the emergency circumstances that prompted the nurse's assistance in the first place would be important factors in assessing the *extent* of liability, that is, how much money damages the nurse will be required to pay.

The private-duty nurse, on the other hand, clearly would be held liable, along with the pediatric nurse, for the harm that resulted to the patient since it was her neglect of the patient that necessitated the emergency care by the pediatric nurse. The private-duty nurse cannot escape liability for neglect by claiming sole responsibility for the patient and that the nurse-patient relationship with the patient was interfered with when the pediatric nurse went to the patient's assistance. As you have been informed, it is perfectly possible for more than one nurse-patient relationship to exist with respect to the same patient at any one time and, as this example clearly illustrates, it is the act of *giving* professional nursing care—not what prompted such care—that brings the nurse-patient relationship into existence, with all its legal consequences.

Proceed to Frame 1-64.

Note B   (from Frame 1-69)

Most members of the nursing profession would say that the nurse exercised very poor judgment in this case. There is no doubt that the nurse had a legal right to refuse to volunteer services, but morally and ethically there was a clear-cut obligation to assist at the scene of the accident. What is a profession, after all, if not a public trust? And nursing is a profession whose express purpose is to serve the health needs of suffering humanity. Nurses who are unable to subordinate their personal feelings at a time when their professional services are so urgently needed not only bring criticism upon themselves but dishonor the fundamental ethical concepts upon which the nursing profession was founded.

Proceed to Frame 1-70.

1-70   Even though nurses may be under no *legal* obligation to provide emergency care to persons who are not within their normal work responsibilities, once they volunteer to give such emergency care they are legally obligated to do so in a reasonable manner. This simply means that they are expected to act as other reasonably prudent nurses would act under the same emergency circumstances.

If a nurse were to volunteer emergency care to someone to whom the nurse owed no special duty of care, which of the following would be true?

☐   The nurse would be expected to act no differently than any other citizen in giving such care.

☐   The nurse would be legally required to exercise no greater care than other nurses would exercise under similar circumstances.

☐   The nurse would be legally required to exercise the highest degree of care to assure the victim's well-being.

1-71

Two nurses licensed to practice in New Jersey are on a summer vacation in the Southwest, and while motoring through Arizona they come upon the scene of a serious railroad accident causing injury to many persons. Their discussion concerning whether or not to stop and give emergency care to the victims is as follows:

Nurse A: "I really think we should help out. I know we're not legally obligated to do so, but I believe we have a moral obligation to render help under these circumstances."

Nurse B: "Well, we may have no legal obligation to offer our help, but you know as well as I do that once we start caring for these people, we run the risk of being sued for malpractice if we don't act with 'reasonable care.'"

Which nurse (if either) is legally correct?

Nurse A   *Nurse B*   *Both nurses*   *Neither nurse*
☐   ☐   ☐   ☐

1-70   *The nurse would be legally required to exercise no greater care than other nurses would exercise under similar circumstances.*

We will discuss this concept in more detail shortly.

1-71   *Both nurses*

GOOD SAMARITAN STATUTES

Beginning in the late 1950s, as fears of medical malpractice suits began to permeate the medical profession, much attention was focused on the growing reluctance of physicians to give emergency assistance to victims of highway accidents and other similar medical emergencies. While fears of being sued by injured accident victims or their families undoubtedly were exaggerated—the risk of being sued for negligence occurring in daily practice has always been infinitely greater—surveys of doctors at the time clearly showed that they would not stop to treat injured persons at the scene of an accident because of the threat of litigation.

Thus came into being the rash of so-called Good Samaritan laws, passed by state and provincial legislatures in the hope that persons with the necessary knowledge and training would no longer be discouraged from going to the aid of accident victims out of fear of being sued. The first Good Samaritan law was enacted by California in 1959, and now all the states, as well as five of the ten Canadian provinces and one Canadian territory, have enacted Good Samaritan laws.

Originally, these laws expressly limited the liability of physicians only, but later encompassed other health-care professionals through legislative amendments. Nurses are frequently mentioned in the statutes, but some grant immunity only to registered nurses, while others include licensed practical or vocational nurses. Many of the laws extend immunity to ''any person,'' a term certainly broad enough to include doctors and nurses as well as persons without medical training.

There has never been any semblance of uniformity in state Good Samaritan laws. Some of them grant absolute immunity against liability to physicians and nurses who render emergency assistance; most extend immunity from liability only for ordinary but not gross negligence. A few statutes not only provide immunity from liability, but protect the doctor or nurse from even being sued. By far, the majority of the Good Samaritan laws confine immunity to care given to injured persons ''at the scene'' of an accident and in need of immediate medical attention or in imminent danger of loss of life or impairment of health. But this is not always the case. The Texas statute, for example, specifies that the ''scene'' may include a hospital, and California's law has also been construed to include certain emergencies in the hospital if the responding physician had no legal duty to render aid to the patient in question.

Because of the wide differences between jurisdictions in the scope, applicability, and coverage of these Good Samaritan laws, it is virtually impossible for a physician or nurse to know with reasonable certainty whether he or she really enjoys any legal advantage when rendering emergency care in a state that has such a law. For example, Nevada and Pennsylvania extend protection only to ''registered nurses,'' thus affording no immunity to licensed practical or vocational nurses who happen to be passing through those states. Because of problems like this, a number of legal commentators have concluded that the Good Samaritan laws as a whole are relatively useless and will never achieve their intended goals until there is greater uniformity among them.

Neither before nor since the enactment of the Good Samaritan laws have there been any reported cases against nurses who have been held liable for negligence in treating victims at the scene of an accident or other emergency. The few reported Good Samaritan cases against doctors have focused on the rendering of emergency care in the hospital setting. (These cases are cited in the Selected References at the end of Part 1.) In any event, all members of the nursing profession should recognize their ethical and moral obligation to render emergency medical assistance to persons in genuine need of such assistance, without regard to any possible legal protection afforded by state or provincial Good Samaritan laws. The responsible trained nurse has nothing to fear when acting competently and within the standard of care, taking into consideration the exigent circumstances. The giving of *reasonable care* should be all the protection needed. Still, the prudent nurse should not hesitate to procure and maintain adequate malpractice insurance coverage just in case someone decides to file suit in a Good Samaritan situation.

Recently, there has been some call for Good Samaritan legislation of the compulsory-assistance type. Vermont, Minnesota and the Province of Quebec have enacted compulsory-assistance statutes—laws requiring *all* persons to render aid to persons who are "exposed to grave physical harm," or containing similar language. The Vermont statute grants civil immunity to one who provides reasonable assistance "unless his acts constitute gross negligence or unless he will receive or expects to receive remuneration." The immunity given, therefore, is not absolute, and the question still remains as to when liability might attach to the careless acts of a well-intentioned samaritan. The Vermont statute, which is not limited to roadside accidents, provides for criminal penalties for failure to render assistance as required under the law. By contrast, the Quebec statute, which specifies that "every person must come to the aid of anyone whose life is in peril," provides no penalties for violation of its mandate. (Quebec Statutes 1975, chapter 6, section 2.) The Minnesota statute makes the failure to render "reasonable assistance at the scene of an emergency" a petty misdemeanor. Incidentally, most European countries have long had compulsory-assistance statutes, and studies made of their impact indicate that they have had a measurably positive effect on public attitudes toward giving assistance.

POINTS TO REMEMBER

1. The legal consequences of an act amounting to nursing malpractice cannot occur until a nurse-patient relationship exists between the parties.

2. The nurse-patient relationship is a legal status that arises whenever a nurse renders nursing care to another person.

3. How a nurse's services are engaged, by whom they are engaged, or whether they are technically engaged at all is of no significance insofar as the nurse-patient relationship is concerned. The act of providing nursing care is what creates the relationship.

4. Once a nurse-patient relationship comes into being, the law automatically imposes certain legal responsibilities upon the nurse with respect to the patient, and these are greater than the general legal responsibilities (i.e., the duty of care) the nurse owes to members of the general public.

5. Nurses are under no *legal* obligation to provide emergency care to those to whom they owe no special duty of care although they may have an *ethical* responsibility to provide such care. A special statute in Vermont is an exception to this widely recognized common law rule. A nurse (or other person) in that state has an affirmative obligation to render assistance to persons exposed to "grave physical harm."

6. In most jurisdictions Good Samaritan laws have been passed to encourage physicians and nurses to give emergency medical assistance to the victims of highway accidents, but because of the wide differences between the various state laws, nurses are not assured of any greater protection from malpractice suits than they already enjoy.

7. Nurses will not be held liable for malpractice in the giving of emergency medical care provided they do what other reasonable and prudent nurses would do under the same emergency circumstances.

NOTE: In the material that follows we will examine the legal principles at the heart of the nurse's liability for malpractice. You will learn about the nurse's legal duty of care, about legal standards of care, and how the law determines whether or not a nurse's conduct conforms to the particular standard of care applicable in a given situation.

The Nurse's Legal Standard of Care

1-72   You will recall that the law imposes an absolute duty on *every* person to act in a reasonable and prudent manner to avoid causing injury to others. When individuals do not act with reasonable care and cause harm to others, we say they are negligent, and they will be held legally liable to the injured persons.

This fundamental standard of conduct applies with equal force to the acts of nurses and other health-care professionals insofar as their *nonprofessional* activities are concerned. The standard is much higher, however, when it comes to the providing of *professional* services. Thus, because the nurse is regarded as a person possessing special skills and learning related to the art of nursing, the laws says that the reasonableness of the individual nurse's conduct must be measured against that of other reasonably prudent members of the nursing profession under the same or similar circumstances.

The duty to exercise reasonable care to avoid injury to others is an obligation the law imposes on

☐ laypersons only   ☐ professionals only   ☐ all persons   ☐ no one

---

1-73   In any given situation, the nature and degree of the reasonable care expected of someone may vary, depending on

☐   the individual's sense of social responsibility

☐   the individual's understanding of the law

☐   the individual's status as a professional

1-72 *all persons*	**1-73** *the individual's status as a professional*
	For a definition of the term "professional," see p. 66, Note A.

1-74   The higher standard of reasonable care expected of a professional person does not apply to all that person's actions but only to those that directly relate to professional functions and responsibilities.

Consider the following example:

A registered nurse and a plumber drive their automobiles to the local shopping center in order to do their grocery shopping. While they are there, their vehicles collide. There is evidence that both drivers were equally negligent.

In a court case arising out of this incident, the nurse would not be held to any higher standard of care for negligent conduct than the plumber because

☐ the nurse was not on the way to work at the time of the accident

☐ the nurse's conduct was not related to any professional nursing duties

☐ nurses and laypersons are presumed to be equally competent in driving automobiles

---

1-75   In the previous example, the negligent conduct occurred while the nurse was off duty. However, the negligence having occurred while the nurse was not officially on duty has no bearing on the applicable standard of care. The critical factor is whether or not the nurse's conduct involves the providing of professional nursing services to the person who suffers the harm.

If a passenger in the plumber's automobile was injured when the vehicles collided, and the nurse administered emergency first aid, the nurse   ☐ would   ☐ would not   be held to a high-standard of care than the plumber in so doing because

☐ a nurse has a legal responsibility to give first aid to injured persons

☐ the nurse would be carrying out a professional nursing function

☐ a layperson is not expected to know how to administer first aid

---

1-74 *the nurse's conduct was not related to any professional nursing duties*	**1-75** *would* ☐ If you checked the 1st box, ☑ reread Frames 1-66 through ☐ 1-71.

1-76   In each of the following fact situations, indicate whether the standard of care applicable to the nurse's conduct would be ordinary negligence or professional negligence (malpractice):

ordinary negligence	*professional negligence*	
☐	☐	Just before going off duty, a recovery room nurse is directed by the supervisor to raise the siderails on the bed of a patient still recovering from anesthesia. The nurse forgets and leaves without doing so. The patient later falls out of bed, fracturing his nose.
☐	☐	A pediatric nurse erroneously gives the wrong infant to the parents of a newborn when the mother is discharged from the hospital. Although the error is discovered by hospital personnel two days later, the parents bring suit for the mental anguish suffered.
☐	☐	In a hurry, a nurse on a coffee break accidentally collides with a gurney carrying a patient to the operating room for emergency surgery. The impact causes blood plasma being fed intravenously to shake loose and spill on the floor. The delay in getting replacement plasma hastens the patient's death.

1-76   *ordinary negligence*   *professional negligence*

☐	☑
☑	☐
☑	☐

If you are still uncertain about this distinction,
reread Frames 1-41 through 1-46.

1-77   For the most part, statutes that define and prescribe the areas of control of professional and practical nursing are drawn in broad, general terms and do not lay down legal guidelines for *specific* conduct. Statements of functions issued by nursing organizations likewise tend to lay down fairly general guidelines, although sometimes they can be quite specific.

By and large, however, it is the courts that have filled in most of the gaps by applying general legal principles to specific situations. The law of nursing malpractice has thus been developed principally by the courts as a part of the evolving common law.

The most common sources of the nurse's legal duty of care to patients are

☐   judicial pronouncements in court cases

☐   state and provincial nurse practice acts

☐   statements of functions by professional nursing organizations

---

1-78   The courts have generally expressed the nurse's legal duty of care in the following manner:

In the performance of professional nursing duties, a nurse is required to exercise the degree of care and skill which a reasonably prudent nurse with similar training and experience practicing in the same community would exercise under the same or similar circumstances.

A nurse's failure to exercise the required degree of care and skill is considered negligence, and the nurse will be held legally liable to the person who is harmed by the negligent conduct.

Which of the following situations would give rise to a charge of negligence on the part of a nurse?

☐   failure of the nurse to allay the patient's fears

☐   failure of the nurse to exercise reasonable care in treating the patient

☐   failure of the nurse to establish a good therapeutic relationship with the patient

---

1-77 *judicial pronouncements in court cases*

1-78 *failure of the nurse to exercise reasonable care in treating the patient*

1-79

An individual sues a general-duty hospital nurse for an act of alleged malpractice that occurred while the individual was a patient at the hospital.

If the patient is to win the suit, which of the following offers of proof would *best* establish the nurse's liability?

☐ proof that the nurse failed to carry out a standard nursing procedure prescribed by the hospital

☐ proof that the nurse failed to do what other nurses with similar skills and training would have done in the given situation

☐ proof that the nurse failed to follow a physician's standing order for the type of case in question

---

1-80   In determining whether a nurse acted with reasonable care in any given situation, the nurse's qualifications, experience, and training are major factors to be considered. The degree of care expected is a relative one; the conduct required of the nurse is only that required of other nurses with similar background and training under the particular circumstances presented.

A malpractice suit is filed against a licensed practical nurse for harm resulting from an alleged failure to properly execute the order of a registered nurse in carrying out a therapeutic procedure.

In determining the nurse's legal liability for malpractice, the court would take into consideration the following:

☐ only the nurse's specific conduct, not background or training

☐ the nurse's professional background and training as well as the specific conduct

☐ only the nurse's professional background and training

1-79 ☐ If you checked either the 1st
☑ or 3d box, see p. 66, Note B.
☐

1-80 *the nurse's professional background and training as well
as the specific conduct*

1-81   A registered nurse with 1 year of hospital experience normally would be expected to exercise a degree of care in carrying out professional nursing duties that

☐   equals

☐   is higher than

☐   is less than

that of a licensed practical nurse with 5 years' experience in the same hospital.

1-82   The single most crucial factor in determining whether a particular nurse acted with reasonable care in a given situation is

☐   how many years the nurse has had his or her license

☐   how the nurse's conduct compared with that of other nurses of similar background and experience

☐   how experienced the nurse is in a particular nursing specialty

---

1-83   *True   False*

☐   ☐   In determining an industrial nurse's liability for malpractice, a court probably would measure the nurse's conduct against that of a hospital surgical nurse.

☐   ☐   A nurse's previous experience in handling a certain type of case would be a pertinent factor in assessing his or her negligence in any similar case.

☐   ☐   A general-duty nurse employed by a nursing home would be held to the same standard of care as a general-duty nurse employed by a hospital when carrying out normal nursing functions.

1-81 *is higher than*	**1-82** *how the nurse's conduct compared with that of other nurses of similar background and experience*	**1-83** *False* *True* *True*

NOTE: Most states and provinces have recognized the expanded role of professional nurses by including in their nurse practice acts special provisions authorizing nurses with the requisite training to undertake many highly technical procedures previously considered beyond the scope of nursing practice. These changes reflect growing public trust in professional nursing and clear recognition that nurses with specialized training can undertake many independent nursing functions that once were deemed to be solely within the province of the physician.

While this increase in nursing specialization clearly has its rewarding aspects from a career standpoint, it has brought with it a decided increase in the nurse's legal accountability. Thus, as we shall see, the performance of the nurse-specialist is measured by a yardstick that is far more demanding than that of the nonspecialist.

Standard of Care of the Nurse-Specialist

1-84   When nurses have acquired the necessary education and training to engage in specialized fields of nursing such as pediatrics, anesthesiology, critical care, or surgical nursing, they are held to a higher standard of care than general-duty nurses in carrying out their duties, but only *while performing services in their specialty*. The standard of care expected of the nurse-specialist or nurse-practitioner (referred to in Canada as the nurse-clinician) is the degree of care and skill customarily exercised by other nurses who practice that specialty. Here again we see that the greater the nurse's educational background and training, the higher the standard of care generally expected by the law.

Nurse N is a certified registered nurse-anesthetist in a large hospital.

Under what circumstances would Nurse N be held to a higher standard of care than a general-duty nurse in the same hospital?

☐   when counting sponges used during an operation

☐   when monitoring circulatory and respiratory sufficiency during an operation

☐   when administering a preoperative sedative

1-85   Nurse N's conduct in the operating room would be measured against that expected of a reasonably prudent

☐   nurse-anesthetist   ☐   scrub nurse   ☐   anesthesiologist

---

1-84   *when monitoring circulatory and respiratory suffi-ciency . . .*

1-85   *nurse-anesthetist*

1-86

Nurse N, a duly certified nurse-practitioner under the state nurse practice act, is employed by a health maintenance organization (HMO). P, a 30-year-old male complaining of recent episodes of chest pain, is examined by Nurse N, who diagnoses muscle spasm and prescribes diazepam (Valium). The pain persists and P returns the following day, at which time he is seen by an emergency department physician who orders a chest x-ray and prescribes stronger medication for the "muscle spasms." P returns the following day because the pain now is constant, and a different physician orders an ECG. This reveals an acute myocardial infarction, and P is admitted immediately to the hospital for treatment. He later sues the HMO, Nurse N, and the first doctor for failure to diagnose his condition promptly.

Nurse N was not legally authorized to examine and diagnose P, especially since staff physicians were readily available.

True   *False*
☐   ☐

1-87   Nurse N's conduct in this case would be measured against that of

☐ other nurses employed by HMOs

☐ other nurse-practitioners in the same locality

☐ doctors specializing in cardiology

1-88   A finding by the jury that the first physician was negligent would automatically relieve Nurse N of any liability for negligence.

True   *False*
☐   ☐

1-86 *False*	**1-87** *other nurse-practitioners in the same locality*	**1-88** *False*

1-89

Nurse N is a pediatric nurse-specialist with 5 years' experience in that specialty. One day, a staff physician summons Nurse N, who is in the vicinity of the coronary intensive care unit, to assist in defibrillating a patient who has just gone into ventricular fibrillation.

In so assisting the physician, what legal standard of care would be applicable to Nurse N's conduct?

☐   the standard of care applicable to nurse-specialists in coronary care

☐   the standard of care applicable to general-duty nurses with similar experience in defibrillating patients

☐   the standard of care applicable to other nurse-specialists in pediatric nursing

Standard of Care of the Nursing Student

1-90   There is an important exception to the general rule regarding the standard of care to be applied to a nurse's conduct: When a nursing student performs duties customarily performed only by a registered nurse, the courts have held the nursing student to the higher standard of care of the registered nurse. This rule applies even though the duties may have been specifically assigned to the nursing student by the clinical instructor.

The reason for this exception is that a patient has a right to assume that all professional services furnished in the hospital, including nursing services, will be provided by persons with the requisite degree of professional training and skill.

Consider the following situation:

A nursing student is assigned by his clinical instructor to perform a complex nursing procedure normally performed only by registered nurses. The student's ineptness causes injury to the patient, who later sues him, claiming that the student's conduct did not meet the standard of care of other reasonably prudent *registered nurses*. In defense of his conduct the nursing student points out that:

A.   Nursing students ordinarily are not given assignments of the type in question and, accordingly, he should not be held liable.

B.   He should not be held liable because he was only following the orders of his clinical instructor.

C.   Since he is only a student, his conduct should be judged by the standard of care applicable to other nursing students under similar circumstances.

Which, if any, of these defenses would protect the student from liability?

A	*B*	*C*	*None of these*
☐	☐	☐	☐

1-89 *The standard of care applica-ble to general-duty nurses with similar experience . . .*	**1-90** *None of these*

1-91   The nursing student in the previous example could have avoided being held liable to the patient by proving that

☐ he performed the procedure in question at the specific direction of his clinical instructor

☐ he exercised the degree of care expected of reasonably prudent registered nurses in the same or similar circumstances

☐ he exercised the degree of care expected of other reasonably prudent nursing students in the same or similar circumstances

---

1-92   Where injury to a patient is caused by a nursing student in the course of clinical training, there is little doubt that the law's principal concern is with

☐ compensating the injured patient

☐ improving the quality of patient care

☐ punishing the student's negligent conduct

1-93

N is a nursing student who has been assigned to the medical ward of a local hospital to obtain clinical experience.

If N's conduct causes harm to a patient assigned to her care, she would be held liable for

☐ negligence

☐ malpractice

☐ neither of the above

1-91 ☐ ☑ ☐	**1-92** *compensating the injured patient*	**1-93** *malpractice*

1-94   Knowing one's own limitations of training and experience is a good rule for *every* nurse, but it is particularly important for nursing students to be aware of their limitations and to bring these to the attention of the clinical instructor whenever they are assigned tasks that call for skills they do not possess.

Acting with reasonable care may well require nursing students to decline to carry out tasks that they know they are not qualified to perform, *even at the risk of appearing insubordinate.*

Consider the following situation:

The charge nurse in a large hospital is suddenly diverted from her normal supervisory and administrative duties and is required to assist in a technical nursing procedure at a patient's bedside. She is somewhat irritated by this diversion, and when she notices a nursing student in the hallway, she directs the latter to take over for her. The student has never performed the nursing function in question but is too frightened to inform the charge nurse of this fact. His inexperience in carrying out the procedure results in harm to the patient.

Based on the foregoing fact situation, indicate whether the following statements are true or false.

True   False

☐   ☐   The student could not avoid personal liability for the harm done once he undertook to perform the procedure as ordered.

☐   ☐   The student could avoid personal liability for the harm done by pointing out that his fear of being regarded as insubordinate kept him from refusing the assignment.

☐   ☐   The student could avoid personal liability for the harm done by proving he was clearly untrained in the procedure in question.

1-95   In the described situation, what course of action should the nursing student have taken in order to avoid liability?

☐   He should have ignored the charge nurse's order, since he knew he could not give competent assistance to her.

☐   He should have protested his inexperience to the patient or a member of the patient's family.

☐   He should have informed the charge nurse of his inability to carry out the procedure and his consequent refusal to do so.

1-94   *True*
            False
            False

1-95   *He should have informed the charge nurse of his inability . . .*

1-96   Assume that the charge nurse in the previous example had directed a *registered* nurse to take over for her, instead of the nursing student. In what way (if any) would the situation differ?

☐   A registered nurse presumably would be more competent than a nursing student to carry out a technical nursing function.

☐   The situation would not differ in any respect from that involving the nursing student.

☐   The registered nurse would be held to a higher standard of responsibility than the nursing student and could not refuse to perform the assigned function.

1-97   The law's insistence that nurses not undertake to perform functions they are not qualified to perform is intended to

☐   bring about better and safer patient care

☐   protect the nurse and the hospital from liability suits

☐   assure a nurse's continued liability insurance coverage

NOTE: As we have shown, the mere fact that a nursing student is given a nursing assignment by the clinical instructor or by a unit or charge nurse does not absolve the student from personal liability for any harm caused. The nursing student who is directed to carry out an assignment that he or she is not qualified to perform and in which he or she is likely to harm the patient should immediately bring the matter to the attention of the clinical instructor or other responsible hospital staff member. In the final analysis, both patient and nursing student will benefit from the student's clear understanding of his or her legal responsibilities and forthright conduct in these difficult situations.

One final point: The fact that the nursing student may be held liable does not necessarily relieve the clinical instructor or charge nurse from liability for negligence in carrying out supervisory duties when a student is assigned a task clearly beyond his or her capabilities. This subject is covered in greater detail later in this course.

1-96 *A registered nurse presumably would be more competent than a nursing student to carry out a technical nursing function.*

1-97 *bring about better and safer patient care*

POINTS TO REMEMBER

1. Professional and lay persons alike are required to act with reasonable care, but the reasonableness of a professional person's conduct is measured not against the conduct of laypersons but against the conduct of other reasonably prudent members of the same profession.

2. The higher standard of care imposed on a professional person applies only to conduct that is related to that person's professional duties.

3. In the performance of professional duties, a nurse is required to exercise the degree of care and skill that a reasonably prudent nurse with similar training and experience would exercise under the same general circumstances.

4. When it is being determined whether or not a nurse acted with care in a given situation, the nurse's educational background and professional training are always taken into consideration.

5. The nurse who is a specialist is held to the higher standard of care that applies to other nurse-specialists who practice that specialty, but only while the nurse is performing services in that specialty.

6. Legally, every patient has the right to expect competent nursing care, even if provided by students as part of their clinical training. Thus, a nursing student will be held to the standard of care of the registered nurse when performing duties in a hospital that are customarily performed only by registered nurses.

7. When a nursing student does not possess the skills needed to carry out an assigned nursing function, acting with reasonable care requires that the student refuse to perform the function, even at the risk of appearing insubordinate.

Determining Negligent Conduct

1-98   It is sometimes said that professional negligence does not exist in a vacuum, which simply means that in determining what is negligent conduct, the "surrounding circumstances" must always be taken into account. The types of surrounding circumstances normally considered are (1) the nature and complexity of the nursing function involved, (2) the forseeability of harm if care is not exercised, (3) the nurse's known or presumed professional qualifications to perform that function, and (4) the urgency of the overall situation. All these play a vital part in every malpractice suit.

Which of the following statements *best* illustrates the point of the preceding paragraph?

- ☐ Negligent conduct usually involves a variety of surrounding circumstances.
- ☐ In the eyes of the law, all the surrounding circumstances must be considered in determining whether or not particular conduct is negligent.
- ☐ There are four major types of surrounding circumstances involved in every malpractice case.

1-99   Select from the following list *two* factors that would be legally significant surrounding circumstances in a malpractice suit against a general-duty nurse:

- ☐ the fact that the alleged malpractice involved nursing care customarily given by a nurse-specialist
- ☐ the fact the alleged malpractice occurred while carrying out a difficult and novel nursing procedure
- ☐ the fact that the nurse had been sued for malpractice on at least one prior occasion
- ☐ the fact that the nurse was generally antagonistic to the patients and was not well-liked

1-98 *In the eyes of the law, all the surrounding circumstances must be considered . . .*	**1-99** ☑ ☑ ☐ ☐

1-100   In view of the law's consideration of the surrounding circumstances in determining liability in a malpractice suit, how likely is it that two nurses sued for the same type of allegedly negligent conduct would fare *differently* in the outcome of their lawsuits?

- ☐   not likely
- ☐   quite possible
- ☐   impossible

1-101   As noted, one legally significant surrounding circumstance is the forseeability of harm to the patient if proper care is not exercised. Under the doctrine of forseeability, every person is held legally liable for all the reasonably forseeable consequences of negligent conduct, provided those consequences are naturally and proximately related to such conduct. Thus, an important aspect of determining whether a nurse has been negligent is the extent to which he or she is able to foresee that his or her actions (or inaction) will cause harm to the patient.

The doctrine of forseeability applies

- ☐   only to health care providers
- ☐   to everyone
- ☐   only to nurses

1-102   If most reasonably prudent nurses would anticipate harmful consequences to a patient from specific nursing conduct, whether acts or omissions, then proof of such conduct by a nurse would be a clear basis for holding the nurse liable for malpractice.

True   False
☐   ☐

1-100 *quite possible*	**1-101** *to everyone*	**1-102** *True*

1-103

Doctor D orders Nurse N to give an elderly female patient a particular medication, but the order fails to specify the route of administration.

What is the correct legal position of Nurse N?

☐ N can assume the doctor wished him to exercise his own judgment regarding the route of administration.

☐ N can assume the medication will not be harmful to the patient no matter how it is administered.

☐ N can assume that some harm is likely to result if the incomplete medication order is not clarified.

1-104

Pediatric Nurse N knows that a 6-year-old boy has experienced convulsions previously when his temperature rose above 102 degrees. Late one evening, Nurse N records a temperature of 102.5 degrees, but concludes this is a momentary spike. Shortly thereafter, the child has a violent seizure, goes into a coma, and dies two days later. The parents sue Nurse N for the child's wrongful death.

Which of the following most accurately characterizes Nurse N's legal position?

☐ N could not reasonably have forseen that her inaction might lead to the child's death.

☐ N could be held liable for all the consequences of her inaction, including liability for his death.

☐ N could be held liable, but only for the normal consequences of an episodic seizure.

1-103 ☐
        ☐
        ☑

1-104 *N could be held liable for all the consequences of her inaction . . .*

1-105   When a nurse's liability in a given situation is being determined, circumstances relating to the nurse's *personal* state of mind or physical condition are generally considered irrelevant. Since nurses are charged with responsibility for their patients' welfare, they are expected to maintain themselves in a physical and mental condition that will enable them to meet their normal professional responsibilities at all times.

> While on duty at the hospital, Nurse N receives a call from her husband who tells her he has been arrested for drunken driving. They argue vehemently and the conversation leaves Nurse N very distraught. Shortly thereafter, she forgets to disconnect a heat lamp, which causes severe burns to a patient.

Indicate which, if any, of the following would afford Nurse N a good defense in the patient's later lawsuit against her.

☐   N has no valid defense against the lawsuit.

☐   N can defend by showing that the heat lamp was set up by someone else before she came on duty.

☐   N can defend by showing that her failure to disconnect the lamp was due to her severe emotional state.

1-106   Under *ordinary* circumstances a nurse's claim of fatigue and inability to act with the customary degree of care and judgment would not be a relevant defense in a malpractice suit. Which of the following circumstances (if any) *might* be relevant in a malpractice action brought against a nurse?

☐   The nurse had been on duty continuously for 36 hours to help meet an acute shortage of nurses during a mass casualty situation at the hospital.

☐   The nurse had been up late the evening before as the result of getting stuck in a traffic jam on the way back from a holiday weekend.

☐   The nurse was exhausted from studying until 2 A.M. for a special nursing examination scheduled 2 days later.

1-105 *N has no valid defense against the lawsuit.*

1-106 ☑ If you checked either the 2d
☐ or 3d box, see p. 67, Note C.
☐

EXPLANATORY NOTES

Note A   (from Frame 1-73)

A word about terminology: The term "professional" is used in its primary dictionary sense, namely, "of, relating to, or characteristic of a profession." The intention is to distinguish professional activities (i.e., those which require special skills and learning) from those of a nonprofessional nature, which are performed by laypersons. Within this general context, the term professional is intended to apply to the acts of licensed practical nurses as well as registered professional nurses, at both the student and graduate level.

Proceed to Frame 1-74.

Note B   (from Frame 1-79)

The nurse's failure to comply with a standard hospital procedure or a physician's standing order would certainly appear to be evidence of a failure to exercise reasonable care, but this is not *necessarily* the case. Under some circumstances a nurse's rigid adherence to a particular standard procedure or a physician's standing order might actually be considered *unreasonable,* or even dangerous.

We must never forget that nurses are supposed to be aware of the total nursing needs of their patients, and if they carry out orders that they know are wrong and are likely to be harmful to their patients, they will be held legally liable for so doing. In the eyes of the law, the patient's welfare is paramount over any standard procedure or method of conduct.

Without knowing the particular circumstances, therefore, we cannot characterize the conduct as unreasonable or negligent merely because the nurse failed to follow the hospital's prescribed procedure or the physician's standing order.

Proceed to Frame 1-80.

Note C   (from Frame 1-106)

Both the second and third choices describe circumstances which are purely *personal* to the nurse, even though the third choice appears to have some relevance to the nurse's professional activities. Nevertheless, a nurse who is too fatigued to carry out the normal patient care responsibilities because of a decision to stay up late to study for an examination has acted neither with reasonable care nor in the patients' best interests.

The test of reasonableness in this situation is what other reasonably prudent nurses would have done under the circumstances. And here the answer becomes clear: The prudent nurse either would have *avoided* becoming fatigued by getting the proper amount of sleep or (alternatively) would have informed the nursing supervisor of his or her fatigued condition and consequent inability to work on the assigned shift.

In contrast with the latter two situations, the first one describes unusual emergency circumstances which were *not of the nurse's own making,* and these would be sufficient to alter the usual rule regarding the irrelevance of the nurse's personal physical condition.

Proceed to Frame 1-107.

1-107   A nurse who is suddenly and unexpectedly confronted with an emergency situation presenting imminent (perhaps life-threatening) danger to a patient is not expected to use the same degree of prudence and judgment that he or she would use under normal circumstances. In an emergency a nurse's duty is merely to exercise the degree of care and skill that an ordinarily prudent nurse of similar training and experience would exercise under similar circumstances.

> Five hospital nurses are sued in separate malpractice actions involving different types of negligent conduct. At the trials of these malpractice suits, all the nurses *admit* they deviated from the normal standard of care but each raises a particular circumstance in defense.

Which of the five nurses (if any) has raised an issue that might alter the standard of care normally expected?

- ☐ Nurse A, who claims that the patient in question was someone she had never attended before

- ☐ Nurse B, who claims that he was actually off duty at the time the nursing care in question was given

- ☐ Nurse C, who claims that she was directed by the head nurse to assist in an emergency procedure with respect to which she had no prior experience

- ☐ Nurse D, who claims that vitally needed resuscitation equipment which he ordered was not brought to the patient's room because of a sudden strike of paramedical personnel at the hospital

- ☐ Nurse E, who claims that she gave the patient an injection with an unsterile needle because his condition was rapidly deteriorating and time did not permit her to obtain a sterile needle

---

1-108   In emergency circumstances, a nurse is not legally required to exercise reasonable care in treating a patient.

                                True   *False*
                                   ☐   ☐

1-107   ☐   At this point you may wish to
            ☐   review the material in Frames
            ☑   1-64 through 1-71 dealing with
            ☑   the nurse's responsibility to
            ☑   give emergency care to some-
                one.

1-108   *False*

1-109   The fact that a nurse is legally considered a minor (under the pertinent state law) will not in and of itself exempt him from liability for negligence in carrying out his nursing duties. This fact emphasizes the need for all nurses to be fully aware of their legal responsibilities in caring for patients. Age and relative inexperience will not shield them from liability for negligent conduct if they are sued.

Which *two* of the following would be considered *legally significant* in assessing a nurse's liability for an act of malpractice?

- ☐ the fact that the nurse graduated with honors from a highly rated nursing school
- ☐ actual experience as a nurse
- ☐ the particular conduct complained of
- ☐ prior status as a licensed practical nurse
- ☐ the fact that the nurse is legally a minor

1-110   When a nursing student is treating hospitalized patients as a part of nursing training, the student's exposure to liability (i.e., risk of being sued for malpractice) is   ☐ greater than   ☐ the same as   ☐ less than   a registered nurse's exposure to liability.

1-111   The fact that a nurse who is sued for malpractice is a minor

- ☐ is of no legal significance in determining the outcome of the case
- ☐ will usually resolve the case in the nurse's favor
- ☐ is a clear indication that the nurse probably was negligent

1-109 *actual experience as a nurse* *the particular conduct complained of*	**1-110** *the same as* The importance of this conclusion can not be overemphasized. If in doubt, reread Frames 1-90 through 1-97.	**1-111** *is of no legal significance in determining the outcome of the case*

Violation of Statutes

1-112   Earlier it was pointed out that statutes *generally* do not lay down legal guidelines for specific types of nursing functions, but this is not *always* the case. Sometimes the applicable standard of care is expressly set forth in a statute that prohibits a particular type of nursing activity or function, and in this situation deviation from the standard of care is shown by proof of the statutory violation.

A provincial statute states that nurses shall not perform nursing duties during any period in which they are suffering contagious or communicable diseases. Nurse N applies for work at a small hospital in the province, knowing that she has TB at the time. After three patients at the hospital contract TB, it is discovered that Nurse N was the infecting carrier.

What would be necessary to hold Nurse N liable for the resulting harm to the three patients?

- ☐ proof of her negligence in treating one or more of the patients
- ☐ proof of her knowing violation of the provincial statute
- ☐ proof of her violation of the standard of care normally applicable when a nurse has a contagious disease

---

1-113   The nurse practice act of State X expressly prohibits a nurse from prescribing medication for a patient except upon the specific order of a licensed physician. Nurse N, certified as an OB/GYN nurse-practitioner by the Nurses Association of the American College of Obstetrics and Gynecology, and employed in a family planning clinic in State X, prescribes birth control pills to a patient, acting entirely on her own.

The fact that Nurse N is appropriately certified as an OB/GYN nurse-practitioner   ☐ will   ☐ will not   protect her against a claim that she violated the nurse practice act of State X.

1-114   The language of the nurse practice act in the previous frame is an example of

- ☐ a statutory impediment
- ☐ a standard of care
- ☐ a suggested guideline

1-112 *proof of her knowing violation of the provincial statute*	**1-113** *will not*	**1-114** *a standard of care*

1-115

The nurse practice act of State Y provides that only a licensed professional nurse may administer inoculations. Nurse N, who is licensed as a practical nurse in State Y, is employed by Doctor D as her office assistant. One day, concerned over the large number of patients waiting to see the doctor, N takes it upon herself to administer a polio booster shot to a two-year-old child. The needle breaks in the child's buttock, and cannot be removed without surgery. The parents sue both Doctor D and Nurse N for the resulting damages.

In a lawsuit of this type, proof of N's violation of the state's nurse practice act would be

☐ sufficient legally to hold N liable for the child's injuries

☐ taken into consideration, but would not be legally significant on the issue of N's liability

☐ of little legal importance on the issue of N's liability

1-116   Apart from N's violation of the statute in the previous frame, the standard of care by which her conduct would be measured in this case would be

☐ that of a licensed practical nurse

☐ that of a licensed professional nurse

☐ that of a reasonably prudent office nurse

NOTE: A nurse's proven violation of a statute will not automatically hold him or her liable unless there is a clear cause-and-effect relationship between his or her violation of the statute and the harm or injury which the patient suffered. We refer to this as the rule of proximate causation and will discuss it in more detail in a later part of this course.

1-115   *sufficient legally to hold N liable for the child's injuries*

1-116   *that of a licensed professional nurse*

1-117   When the major issue in a malpractice case is the nurse's failure to conform to a standard of care outlined in a statute, in what manner is negligence (if any) proved?

- ☐ by the testimony of other nurses as to what they would have done under the circumstances

- ☐ by the testimony of experts in the field of nursing as to what should have been done under the circumstances

- ☐ by proof of the nurse's violation of the statute that prescribed the standard of care

---

OTHER APPLICABLE STANDARDS OF CARE

In addition to the general standards applicable to nursing practice laid down in state and provincial statutes, some very specific standards have been promulgated by the Joint Commission on Accreditation of Hospitals, by national, provincial, and state nursing associations, and by various nursing specialty groups. In actual practice, however, the most significant regulation of the nurse's professional conduct comes from the state or provincial nurse practice act and the rules and regulations issued thereunder by the respective boards of nursing.

The state and provincial boards of nursing are customarily delegated broad authority, including the authority (1) to prescribe regulations setting forth educational requirements and admission standards for licensure of nurses and, in some states and Canadian provinces, nurse-practitioners; (2) to delineate the tasks nurses and nurse-practitioners are permitted to carry out either independently or in collaboration with physicians; and (3) to establish criteria and administrative mechanisms for disciplining nurses who violate the rules, including authority to impose appropriate penalties.

Professional nursing is continually expanding its statutory basis for practice, with increasing numbers of states and Canadian provinces amending their nurse practice and medical practice acts so as to make more explicit those nursing functions that are deemed independent and do not require specific physicians' orders. The overlapping nature of many medical and nursing functions—such as those relating to the making of diagnoses and the establishment of treatment plans or regimens—has made it difficult at times to determine who is primarily responsible and should be held legally liable when a diagnosis proves to be wrong or a particular treatment regimen results in injury to the patient. These scope of practice issues are discussed at greater length in Part 5.

1-117   *by proof of the nurse's violation of the statute that prescribed the standard of care*

POINTS TO REMEMBER

1. Whether or not an act constitutes negligent conduct depends not only on the act itself but on all the surrounding circumstances.

2. Four surrounding circumstances deemed to be of prime concern are (1) the nature of the nursing function involved, (2) the nurse's qualifications to perform that function, (3) the forseeability of harm if care is not exercised, and (4) the urgency of the overall situation.

3. Under ordinary circumstances, a nurse's personal state of mind or physical condition is not considered relevant as a defense to a malpractice claim.

4. In an emergency a nurse is not held to the same standard of care expected under normal circumstances.

5. Being a minor does not, in and of itself, exempt a nurse from liability for acts of malpractice.

6. When a statute lays down a standard of nursing conduct, liability normally will result upon clear proof of violation of the statute and harm flowing therefrom.

SELECTED REFERENCES—PART 1

Common Law and Statutory Law Distinguished

In re Davis' Estate, 35 A. 2d 880 (N.J. 1944)

Tort Law Defined

74 *Am Jur 2d,* TORTS § 1
Freeman v. Busch Jewelry Co., 98 F. Supp. 963 (Ga. 1951)

Tort Law and Contract Law Distinguished

W. Prosser, *Handbook of the Law of Torts,* 4th ed., West Publishing, St. Paul, 1971, § 92,
    pp. 613–622
74 *Am Jur 2d,* TORTS § 23
Bankers Fidelity Life Ins. Co. v. Harrison, 123 S.E. 2d 438 (Ga. 1961)

Concept of Legal Liability

Continental Insurance Co. v. Echols, 243 S.E. 2d 88 (Ga. 1978)
Stuyvesant Insurance Co. v. Bournazian, 342 So. 2d 471 (Fla. 1977)

Negligence Defined

W. Prosser, *Handbook of the Law of Torts,* 4th ed., West Publishing, St. Paul, 1971,
    §§ 35–36, pp. 149–163
Annotation, 59 ALR 1263
Palsgraf v. Long Island R. Co., 162 N.E. 99 (N.Y. 1928)

Malpractice Defined

Matthews v. Walker, 296 N.E. 2d 569 (Ohio 1973)
Kosberg v. Washington Hospital Center, Inc., 394 F. 2d 947 (D.C. 1968)
Valentin v. La Société Francaise, 172 P. 2d 359 (Cal. 1956)

Negligence and Malpractice Distinguished

Ratliff v. Employer's Liability Assurance Corp., Ltd., 515 S.W. 2d 225 (Ky. 1974)
Kambas v. St. Joseph's Mercy Hospital of Detroit, 205 N.W. 2d 431 (Mich. 1973)
Duling v. Bluefield Sanitorium, 142 S.E. 2d 754 (W. Va. 1965)

Creation of the Nurse-Patient Relationship

C. Murphy, "Models of the Nurse-Patient Relationship," in *Ethical Problems in the Nurse-Patient Relationship*, C. Murphy and H. Hunter (eds.), Allyn and Bacon, New York, 1982, pp. 8–25

Osborne v. Frazor, 425 S.W. 2d 768 (Tenn. 1968)

Burrows v. Hawaiian Trust Company, 417 P. 2d 816 (Haw. 1966)

Noland v. Brown, 129 S.E. 2d 477 (N.C. 1963)

Harvey v. Silber, 2 N.W. 2d 483 (Mich. 1942)

Standard of Care Applicable to Nurses Generally

D. Guariello, "The Legal Boobytraps in Nursing Standards," *RN*, 47(6):19 (June 1984)

D. A. Forgey, "Hospital Liability: Taking a Turn for the Nurse," *For the Defense*, 23:9 (July 1981).

W. Morris, "The Negligent Nurse, the Physician, and the Hospital," *Baylor L. Rev* 33:109 (1981).

W. T. Eccard, "A Revolution in White—New Approaches in Treating Nurses as Professionals," *Vanderbilt L. Rev.* 30:839 (1977).

Standards of Practice, American Nurses Association, 1973

Annotations, 51 ALR 2d 970; 99 ALR 2d 599

Hammond v. Grissom, 470 So. 2d 1049 (Miss. 1985)

Daniel v. St. Francis Cabrini Hospital of Alexandria, 415 So. 2d 586 (La. 1982)

Wood v. Rowland, 592 P. 2d 1332 (Col. 1979)

Fraijo v. Hartland Hospital, 99 Cal. App. 3d 331 (Cal. 1979)

Stone v. Sisters of Charity of House of Providence, 469 P. 2d 229 (Wash. 1970)

Standard of Care of Nurse-Specialists

61 *Am Jur 2d*, PHYSICIANS & SURGEONS § 26

W. Prosser, *Handbook of The Law of Torts*, 4th ed., West Publishing, St. Paul, 1971, § 32, pp. 161–166

Restatement (Second) TORTS § 299A, Comment d

W. Regan, "Nurse Specialists: Authority and Accountability," *Regan Report on Nursing Law*, 24(5):1 (Oct. 1983)

M. Cushing, "When Medical Standards Apply to Nurse Practitioners," *Amer. J. Nurs.*, 82:1274 (Aug. 1982)

Parks v. Perry, 314 S.E. 2d 287 (N.C. 1984)

Czubinsky v. Doctors Hospital, 188 Cal. Rptr. 684 (Cal. 1983)

Tice v. Hall, 303 S.E. 2d 832 (N.C. 1983)

Warren v. Canal et al., 300 S.E. 2d 557 (N.C. 1983)

Whitney v. Day, 300 N.W. 2d 380 (Mich. 1981)

Gugino v. Harvard Community Health Plan, 403 N.E. 2d 1166 (Mass. 1980)

Sesselman v. Muhlenberg Hospital, 306 A. 2d 474 (1973)

Standard of Care of Nursing Students

H. Creighton, *Law Every Nurse Should Know,* 4th ed., W. B. Saunders, Philadelphia,
    1981, pp. 137–141
N. Hershey, "Student, Instructor, and Liability," *Am. J. Nurs.* 65:122–3, (Mar. 1965)
Carter v. Anderson Memorial Hospital, 325 S.E. 2d 78 (S.C. 1985)
Habuda v. Trustees of Rex Hospital, 164 S.E. 2d 17 (N.C. 1968)
Honeywell v. Rogers, 251 F. Supp. 841 (1966)
Payne v. Garvey, 142 S.E. 2d 158 (N.C. 1965)
O'Neil v. Glens Falls Indemnity Co., 310 F. 2d 165 (Neb. 1962)
Miller v. Mohr et al, 89 P. 2d 807 (Wash. 1939)
Nickley v. Eisenberg, 239 N.W. 426 (Wis. 1931)

Standard of Care in an Emergency

D. Louisell and H. Williams, *Medical Malpractice,* Matthew Bender & Co., New York,
    1983, § 9.05
M. Mancini and A. Gale, *Emergency Care and the Law,* Aspen Systems, Rockville, Md.,
    1981
W. Prosser, *Handbook of The Law of Torts,* 4th ed., West Publishing, St. Paul, 1971, § 33,
    pp. 169–170
Anthony v. Hospital Service District No. 1, 477 So. 2d 1180 (La. 1985)
Bartimus v. Paxton Community Hospital, 458 N.E. 2d 1072 (Ill. 1983)
Lunsford v. Board of Nurse Examiners, 648 S.W. 2d 391 (Texas 1983)
Murphy v. Rowland, 609 S.W. 2d 292 (Texas 1981)
Ulma v. Yonkers General Hospital, 384 N.Y.S. 2d 201 (N.Y. 1981)
Piehl v. The Dallas General Hospital, 571 P. 2d 149 (Ore. 1977)
Christian v. Wilmington General Hospital Association, 135 A. 2d 727 (Del. 1957)
Landsberg v. Kolodny, 302 P. 2d 86 (Cal. 1956)
Robinson v. Wirts, 127 A. 2d 706 (Pa. 1956)
Huffman v. Lundquist, 234 P. 2d 34 (Cal. 1951)
Wallstedt v. Swedish Hospital, 19 N.W. 2d 426 (Minn. 1945)

Good Samaritan Laws and Their Effect

R. Tuttle, "Hospital Emergency Rooms—Application of Good Samaritan Laws," *Med.
    Tr. Tech. Q.,* 31:141 (Fall 1984)
J. Horsley, "You Can't Escape the Good Samaritan Role—Or Its Risks," *RN,* 44(5):87
    (May 1981)
F. J. Helminski, "Good Samaritan Statutes: Time for Uniformity," *Wayne L. Rev.* 27:217
    (1980)
M. Lipman, "Can You Afford to be a Good Samaritan? Yes!" *RN* 37:90 (September 1974)
Annotation, 39 ALR 3d 222
Colby v. Schwartz, 78 Cal. App. 3d 885 (Cal. 1979)
McKenna v. Cedars of Lebanon Hospital, 93 Cal. App. 3d 282 (Cal. 1979)

Hamburger v. Henry Ford Hospital, 284 N.W. 2d 155 (Mich. 1979)
Gragg v. Neurological Associates, 263 S.E. 2d 496 (Ga. 1979)
Wallace v. Hall, 244 S.E. 2d 129 (Ga. 1978)

Compulsory Assistance Statutes

Note, "Creation of a Duty Absent a Special Relationship—Legal Duty Based on a Moral Obligation," *Whittier L. Rev.* 6:605 (1984).
Restatement (Second) TORTS § 314, comment c. Vermont Statutes Annotated, Title 12, § 519 (Supp. 1973). Minnesota Statutes, § 604.05, (Sub. 1) (1984).
Quebec Statutes 1975, chapter 6, section 2.
Soldano v. *O'Daniels,* 141 Cal App. 3d 443, 190 Cal. Rptr. 310 (1983)

Determining Negligence—Surrounding Circumstances

D. Louisell and H. Williams, *Medical Malpractice,* Matthew Bender & Co., New York, 1983, § 9.05
57 *Am Jur 2d,* NEGLIGENCE § 1
Restatement (Second) TORTS § 11
Chapman v. Carlson, 240 So. 2d 263 (Miss. 1970)
Long v. Sledge, 209 So. 2d 814 (Miss. 1968)
Lince v. Monson, 108 N.W. 2d 845 (Mich. 1961)
Fowler v. State, 78 N.Y.S. 2d 860 (N.Y. 1948)

Concept of Forseeability of Harm

Harper & James, *The Law of Torts,* vol. 2, Little, Brown & Co., Boston, 1956, § 16.5, p. 907
W. Prosser, *Handbook of The Law of Torts,* 4th ed., West Publishing, St. Paul, 1971, § 43, pp. 250–270
Mercy Hospital v. Larkins, 174 So. 2d 408 (Fla. 1965)

Standard of Care—Violation of Statutes

W. Prosser, *Handbook of the Law of Torts,* 4th ed., West Publishing, St. Paul, 1971, § 36, p. 190
Restatement (Second) TORTS, § 285
Central Anesthesia Associates v. Worthy, 325 S.E. 2d 819 (Ga. 1985)
McCarl v. State Board, 396 A. 2d 866 (Pa. 1978)
Barber v. Reinking, 411 P. 2d 861 (Wash. 1966)
Richardson v. Gregory, 281 F. 2d 626 (D.C. 1960)

Part Two
Special Rules of Liability

Part 2

INTRODUCTORY NOTE

Is the nurse who has committed an act of malpractice held liable even though the nurse is employed by a physician or a hospital? Is it possible that the physician or hospital can be held liable and the nurse escape liability? To what extent is the nurse's employment status a factor in liability for malpractice? Are the school nurse and industrial nurse *more* likely or *less* likely to be sued for malpractice than their general-duty colleagues? These are some of the problems treated in Part 2 of this course, in which we will examine in greater depth the nature and extent of the nurse's liability.

The various legal doctrines explained in this part will give you insight into the ways in which the law fixes liability for acts of malpractice and will show how you may be subjected to a greater exposure to liability based upon such factors as your state of employment or the unique legal status of your employer. The fundamental doctrines to be covered in Part 2 are the rule of personal liability, the liability of the nurse for the acts of others, the doctrine of *respondeat superior,* the doctrines of charitable immunity and governmental immunity, and the special liability of occupational health nurses.

Rule of Personal Liability

2-1   If there is one rule that all nurses should know and clearly understand, it is the fundamental rule of law that *every person is liable for his or her own tortious conduct.* (Remember: A tort is a private legal wrong.) This is called the rule of personal liability.

While the rule of personal liability is simple enough, it is often misunderstood. Stating the rule in a different way may help clarify its meaning: The law does not permit a wrongdoer (in the tort-liability sense) to avoid legal liability for his or her own wrongdoing even though someone else also may be sued and held legally liable for the wrongful conduct in question under another rule of law.

The rule of personal liability is a rule that

☐   protects nurses against lawsuits for malpractice

☐   holds everyone personally liable for his or her own tortious conduct

☐   makes some persons liable for the tortious conduct of others

---

2-2   The rule of personal liability applies to the conduct of

☐   nurses only

☐   doctors and nurses only

☐   professional persons only

☐   everyone

2-3

A private physician tells his office nurse to execute a medical order that both know to be improper. The physician assures the nurse that he will take full responsibility for any harmful consequences. The patient is harmed and sues the nurse for the conduct in question.

The physician's verbal assurance to his nurse will adequately protect the nurse from legal liability to the patient.

True   *False*
☐   ☐

2-1 *holds everyone personally lia-ble for his or her own tortious conduct*	2-2 *everyone*	2-3 *False* If you checked the wrong an-swer, turn to p. 91, Note A.

2-4

While employed as a general-duty nurse in a hospital, Nurse N negligently injures a patient.

Assuming that under the applicable law the hospital can be held liable for the negligent acts of its employees, which of the following conclusions (if any) would apply?

- ☐ If the injured person sues and collects damages from the hospital, Nurse N cannot be held personally liable.

- ☐ Nurse N cannot be held liable under any circumstances since N's hospital employer has agreed to assume liability for its nurses' negligent conduct.

- ☐ Both Nurse N and N's hospital employer can be held liable for N's negligent conduct.

2-5   The law will absolve nurses from personal liability for their negligent conduct

- ☐ if they are employed by hospitals that are insured against malpractice claims
- ☐ if they can show they were carrying out the specific orders of a physician
- ☐ in both of the above instances
- ☐ in neither of the above instances

2-4 *Both Nurse N and N's hospital employer can be held liable for N's negligent conduct.*

2-5 *in neither of the above instances*

2-6   The rule of personal liability becomes particularly pertinent when applied to the acts of nurses who are supervised by other nurses. In every instance the fundamental rule is the same: *The nurse who is negligent is always personally liable even though someone else also may be sued and held liable.*

Nurse N (a registered nurse) directs Nurse P (a practical nurse) to perform a nursing function which the latter is not qualified to carry out. P follows N's orders without question, however, and harm results to the patient, who thereupon sues both N and P.

	Yes	No
If P is found to be negligent, can N also be held liable if N too is found to be negligent?	☐	☐
If N is found to be negligent, would P thereby be relieved of liability?	☐	☐

Supervisor's Liability for the Acts of Subordinates

2-7   While all professional persons are held liable for their own negligent conduct (malpractice), there are certain circumstances under which a person who supervises others may be held liable for the negligent acts of those he or she supervises. Thus, a nursing supervisor is expected to know whether the one to whom he or she has assigned specific nursing duties is competent to perform them with or without supervision. The supervisor's inability to properly evaluate the patient's nursing needs and the nurse's capabilities will be sufficient to hold the supervisor liable for any harm that results to the patient.

A nursing supervisor may safely assume that

☐ a registered nurse is competent to carry out any assigned nursing function

☐ some patients' needs cannot be delegated to a nurse even though he or she is a registered nurse and experienced in many phases of nursing

☐ a practical nurse can never carry out a nursing function as well as a registered nurse

---

2-6   *Yes*

No

At this point you may wish to review Frames 1-90 through 1-97.

2-7   *some patients' needs cannot be delegated to a nurse . . .*

2-8 A nursing supervisor gives Nurse N a routine nursing assignment which, as a registered nurse, N should be able to perform without difficulty. Nevertheless, N's negligence causes the patient to be seriously burned.

Under these facts, which of the following would be true?

☐ The supervisor can be held liable because he made the nursing assignment in question.

☐ The supervisor can be held liable for failing to ascertain Nurse N's competence to perform the assignment.

☐ Nurse N alone can be held liable for her negligence in carrying out an assignment clearly within her capabilities.

2-9 An operating-room supervisor directs a nursing student to assist at major abdominal surgery even though the supervisor knows the student has assisted during minor surgical procedures on only two prior occasions. As a result of the student's negligence, a laparotomy sponge is left in the patient, with serious consequences.

On what basis could the nursing student be held liable?

☐ for failure to discuss his or her limitations with the supervisor prior to assisting at the surgery

☐ for lack of care in counting the sponges

☐ for both of the above

☐ for neither of the above

2-10   On what basis could the operating-room supervisor be held liable?

☐ for the assignment of the nursing student despite the knowledge of the latter's limited qualifications to assist at major surgery

☐ for failure to supervise the nursing student more closely during the operation

☐ for both of the above

☐ for neither of the above

2-8 ☐ ☐ ☑	2-9 *for both of the above*	2-10 *for both of the above*

ASSIGNMENT PROBLEMS FACED BY SUPERVISORY NURSES

Supervisory nurses have responsibilities that necessarily put them at greater risk of personal liability, so a little further discussion of their legal position is in order. To begin with, the basic rule is clear: every nurse, whether subordinate or supervisor, is expected to provide the same degree of care that a reasonably prudent nurse with the same level of expertise and training would give under comparable circumstances. Since it is a supervisor's job to supervise, he or she is held to the standard of care of other reasonably prudent supervisors in the same or similar circumstances. What does the law expect of such persons?

Whether the title is head nurse, charge nurse, operating room supervisor, cardiac care unit supervisor, recovery room supervisor, emergency room supervisor, or simply the unit manager, nurses in charge are directly responsible for the quality of care rendered by everyone working under their overall area of responsibility. The list may include nurses, licensed practical nurses, nursing students, medical and surgical technicians, special duty nurses, nurses' aides, orderlies, and other persons who have direct patient care functions.

A major part of the supervisor's responsibility is the making of careful nursing assignments, sometimes in the face of drastic staffing shortages. Even though the standards of the Joint Commission on Accreditation of Hospitals (JCAH) require hospitals to maintain a sufficient number of duly licensed registered nurses on duty ''at all times'' to plan, supervise, and evaluate nursing care, as well as to give patients the professional nursing care they require, supervisors often find themselves forced to ''float'' nurses from their normally assigned units to others that may call for nursing skills they simply do not possess. The legal risks of so doing are apparent (for supervisor and float nurse alike), but this does not always solve the *practical* problems supervisory nurses have to face when dealing with staffing crises not of their own making.

Supervisors who believe their units are inadequately staffed must make their views known to hospital administration promptly and emphatically, *preferably in writing*. They should carefully document incidents in which patients have been endangered through lack of proper staffing, pointing out how substandard assignments expose patients to physical harm and the hospital as well as themselves to consequent malpractice suits. The failure to take vigorous action of this type will inevitably lead to the emotional trauma of litigation and an unnecessary challenge to a supervisor's professional competence.

POINTS TO REMEMBER

1. It is a fundamental rule of law that every person is legally responsible for his or her own tortious conduct. This is called the rule of personal liability.

2. Under the rule of personal liability a wrongdoer cannot avoid legal liability for his or her own wrongful conduct, even though someone else may share that liability under some other rule of law.

3. Physicians cannot alter the rule of personal liability by their agreement to assume responsibility for the negligent acts of their nurses. In the final analysis, nurses will always be held liable for their own negligent conduct.

4. Supervisors ordinarily will not be held liable for the negligent acts of those whom they supervise since all professional persons are held liable for their own negligent conduct.

5. A supervisor *may* be held liable for the acts of someone he or she supervises if the supervisor is either negligent in making an assignment clearly beyond the latter's capabilities or does not provide adequate supervision of a nurse or nursing student who, because of inexperience, requires close supervision in carrying out a specific function.

6. A nursing supervisor who believes that crisis-staffing with float nurses will jeopardize patient safety and precipitate litigation should document his or her position and promptly inform the hospital administration.

Doctrine of *Respondeat Superior*

2-11   The preceding frames explained the rule of personal liability. Now we turn to a related legal doctrine that has a significant effect upon the nurse's legal liability: the doctrine of *respondeat superior* ("let the master respond").

The doctrine of *respondeat superior* is a legal doctrine that holds an employer liable for the negligent acts of his or her employees which occur while they are carrying out his or her orders or are otherwise serving the employer's interests. Since most nurses are employed by others, this doctrine assume a position of great importance and accordingly should be clearly understood.

What is the legal effect of the doctrine of *respondeat superior?*

☐   It establishes the legal relationship of employer-employee.

☐   It absolves an employee of personal liability for his or her negligent acts.

☐   It creates liability on the part of an employer for the negligent acts of his or her employees.

2-12   In what way does the doctrine of *respondeat superior* affect the nurse's personal liability for a negligent act?

☐   It shifts the nurse's liability for negligence to the employer and thereby relieves the nurse of all personal liability.

☐   It subjects the nurse's employer to liability for the nurse's negligence but does not relieve the nurse of personal liability for the conduct in question.

☐   It has no effect on the nurse's liability for negligence in that he or she is held solely responsible.

2-11   *It creates liability on the part of an employer for the negligent acts of his or her employees.*

2-12   *It subjects the nurse's employer to liability for the nurse's negligence . . .*

2-13   The doctrine of *respondeat superior* applies (1) only when there is an employer-employee relationship and (2) only with respect to negligent acts committed within the scope of the employment. The theory behind the doctrine is that one who is an employer should be held legally responsible for the conduct of those persons (employees) whose actions he or she has a right to direct or control.

> Supervisory Nurse S and general-duty Nurse N are employed by Hospital H. In the course of treating a patient, S (negligently) directs N to give the patient the wrong medication, and in the process of administering the drug, N (negligently) injures the patient.

Who can be held liable to the patient for the resulting harm?

☐ only Nurse S

☐ only Nurse N

☐ only Hospital H

☐ both nurses, but not the hospital

☐ all three parties

2-14   Why would Nurse S *not* be held liable under *respondeat superior* for Nurse N's negligence?

☐ because S was not N's employer

☐ because both nurses were negligent

☐ because *respondeat superior* does not apply in a case where two employees are equally negligent

---

2-13 *all three parties*

2-14 *because S was not N's employer*
The liability of nursing supervisors is discussed on p. 91, Note B.

2-15   Bear in mind that *respondeat superior* holds the employer liable only for negligent conduct that occurs within the scope of the employment relationship.

> Nurse N is employed by a hospital in a large city. While on a summer vacation in an adjoining state N has occasion to give emergency care to a victim of a highway accident. N's negligence causes further injury and the victim later sues for malpractice.

Why would the doctrine of *respondeat superior* not apply in this case?

- ☐ because the care that was given took place in a state in which the nurse was not employed

- ☐ because the negligent conduct did not occur within the scope of the nurse's employment

- ☐ because the negligent conduct arose out of emergency care

---

2-16   If the nurse had not been on vacation, would the doctrine of *respondeat superior* apply to N's conduct in giving the emergency care?

Yes   *No*

☐   ☐

2-17   Under *respondeat superior,* an employer might be held liable for a patient's injury even if the nurse-employee who rendered the care is found not to be negligent.

True   *False*

☐   ☐

2-15 *because the negligent conduct did not occur within the scope of the nurse's employment*	2-16 *No* If you checked Yes, see p. 91, Note C.	2-17 *False*

If you checked Yes, see p. 91, Note C.

EXPLANATORY NOTES

Note A   (from Frame 2-3)

Although many nurses undoubtedly share your view, this is not correct. As persons with professional training, nurses must always do what their education, training, and experience indicate is best for their patients, and if they knowingly perform acts that do not meet the required standards of care, they will be held personally liable. In other words, they cannot avoid legal responsibility for the consequences of their own negligent conduct, regardless of any assurances given to them by well-intentioned (but legally mistaken) physicians.

In the given example, the physician also will be held liable to the injured patient, and it is more than likely that the physician's malpractice insurance policy is broad enough to cover the neglect of his office nurse under the described circumstances. The fact remains, however, that *the rule of personal liability cannot be bypassed merely on the verbal assurances of a physician,* and the nurse would be well advised to exercise his or her own professional judgment notwithstanding such assurances.

Proceed to Frame 2-4.

Note B   (from Frame 2-14)

It is important to note that a nurse with supervisory responsibility is not held liable merely because a nurse to whom he or she has assigned nursing duties negligently injures a patient. The supervisor is liable only for his or her own negligence in carrying out his or her supervisory duties. Note also that the supervisor's liability is based upon his or her own conduct, while the hospital's liability under *respondeat superior* arises by virtue of its employer status. The nurse with supervisory responsibilities is not the employer of the nursing personnel who work under his or her direction.

As a general rule, a nursing supervisor can assume that a subordinate nurse's registration, license, or other form of certification qualifies the individual to carry out the usual responsibilities assigned to persons with such evidence of nursing skills. However, the supervisor can be held liable for making an assignment to a nurse who he or she has reason to believe may carry out the task negligently.

Proceed to Frame 2-15.

Note C   (from Frame 2-16)

It is remotely possible (but not likely) that the nurse, as an employee of the hospital in question, would be expected to give emergency care to highway-accident victims within his or her own city, but this theoretical obligation would certainly not extend to highway-accident victims in an adjoining state. (See, however, the exceptions noted on page 47.)

You must not forget that the *respondeat superior* doctrine applies only to an employee's acts of negligence that occur in the course of his or her employment, and the giving of emergency care to highway-accident victims is not normally a part of a nurse's employment duties. As pointed out in Part 1, while there is no *legal* obligation that nurses render such care outside their normal employment settings, the ethics of the profession encourage such humanitarian assistance.

Proceed to Frame 2-17.

2-18   Since most nurses are not self-employed but work for others, the doctrine of *respondeat superior* significantly affects their legal liability for acts of negligence. In the absence of both an employment relationship and negligent conduct, however, the doctrine will not apply.

Consider the following situation:

Nurse N is employed by Doctor D, and Nurse F, a friend of Nurse N, is employed by Doctor Z. Both doctors have their offices in the same building. One day, as the nurses are leaving for lunch together, they notice an elderly lady in obvious respiratory distress in the lobby of the building. Nurse N recognizes the lady as a patient of Doctor D, and immediately runs back to summon Doctor D to the lobby. Meanwhile, Nurse F goes to the victim's aid, but injures her in the attempt.

The patient later dies and her estate sues both Doctor D and Doctor Z, claiming negligence on the part of Nurse F.

Assuming Nurse F was in fact negligent, against whom would the doctrine of *respondeat superior* apply in this case?

☐ against Doctor D only

☐ against Doctor Z only

☐ against both doctors

☐ against neither doctor

2-19   Indicate which of the following legal doctrines are directly relevant in the given fact situation:

☐ emergency care rule

☐ establishment of a nurse-patient relationship

☐ rule of personal liability

☐ none of the above

2-18 ☐ ☐ ☐ ☑	If you did not select the correct answer, turn to p. 94, Note A.	**2-19** ☑ ☑ ☑ ☐	

2-20 The doctrine of *respondeat superior* is primarily concerned with the following three elements:

- ☐ nurse-patient-physician
- ☐ employer-employee-negligent conduct
- ☐ hospital-nurse-physician

2-21 The rule of *respondeat superior* ordinarily does not apply when the nurse offers his or her services as a private-duty nurse since the relationship thus established is not one of employer-employee. The private-duty nurse is considered an independent contractor who is held legally responsible for his or her own conduct. This does not apply, however, when the private-duty nurse works under the direction, supervision, and control of a hospital, nursing home, home health agency or private physician.

The doctrine of *respondeat superior* does not apply to the negligent conduct of a nurse when he or she is employed (select two)

- ☐ by someone who is uninsured against malpractice claims
- ☐ by a particular person as a private-duty nurse
- ☐ by an employer who legally cannot be sued for the negligence of his or her employees

---

2-22 Assume negligent conduct in the course of his or her duties on the part of each of the following nurses. With respect to which of them would the doctrine of *respondeat superior* apply?

Would apply	*Would not apply*	
☐	☐	A registered nurse employed by a hospital
☐	☐	A private-duty nurse employed by a hospitalized patient
☐	☐	A practical nurse employed by a convalescent individual at home
☐	☐	A private-duty nurse employed by a hospital
☐	☐	A practical nurse employed by a physician

2-20	2-21	2-22 *Would apply*	*Would not apply*	
☐	☐	☑	☐	If you checked two or more wrong boxes, turn to p. 94, Note B.
☑	☑	☐	☑	
☐	☑	☐	☑	
		☑	☐	
		☑	☐	

EXPLANATORY NOTES

Note A   (from Frame 2-18)

This was a fairly complex problem, but a little careful analysis should help clarify the matter. Doctor D could not be held liable because *respondeat superior* applies only to the act of an employee, and the negligent act in this case was committed by Doctor Z's nurse.

Theoretically, Doctor Z could be held liable since the negligent nurse was Z's employee; however, this would not be sufficient to hold Doctor Z liable under *respondeat superior* because you will recall that Nurse F was on lunch hour and was not acting within the scope of the employment by Doctor Z at the time of the incident.

The correct response, therefore, is that *neither* doctor could be held liable. Just by way of review, *respondeat superior* holds an *employer* liable for the negligent act of an *employee* which arises out of and in the course of the *employment*. All three elements must be present or else the employer cannot be held liable. In the given example, neither doctor would be held liable because Doctor D's nurse committed no negligent act, and Doctor Z's nurse (who *did* commit a negligent act) was not acting within the scope of her employment at the time.

Proceed to Frame 2-19.

Note B   (from Frame 2-22)

Respondeat superior generally applies to the acts of a nurse employed by a hospital, home health-care agency, or private physician. Thus, you should have had little difficulty in deciding that the rule applies to the first and last nurses listed—the registered nurse employed by the hospital and the practical nurse employed by the physician. Private-duty nurses are *usually* (but not always) employed by private persons, and when they *are* so employed, they are solely responsible for their own conduct. The second and third examples illustrated this type of employment status—the private-duty nurse employed by the hospitalized patient and the practical nurse employed by the convalescent individual at home.

The fourth example was perhaps more troublesome since the private-duty nurse was employed by a hospital rather than by a private person. Nevertheless, the legal responsibility in such a situation is the same as if the nurse were a full-time staff nurse at the hospital. Remember: The doctrine of *respondeat superior* is strictly tied to the nurse's *employment status at the time of the alleged malpractice*, not the employment status he or she usually enjoys.

Proceed to Frame 2-23.

2-23   Even though the doctrine of *respondeat superior* provides the injured patient with another party to sue, it does *not* relieve negligent nurses of their own liability. Thus, if the employer is otherwise blameless for the negligent conduct of a nurse-employee but is obligated under *respondeat superior* to pay damages to the injured patient, the employer has the legal right to recover in a separate action against the nurse-employee the amount the employer has thus been required to pay.

> Nurse N, employed by a large midwestern hospital, commits an act of malpractice in the course of nursing duties which results in serious injury to Patient P.

> Under these facts, which of the following statements would be true?

> ☐   P can sue either Nurse N or the hospital for N's negligent conduct, but not both.

> ☐   If P is successful in a suit against N's employer and the latter pays the judgment rendered in the case, N can be held liable to the hospital for the judgment paid.

> ☐   If P is successful in a suit against Nurse N and N pays the judgment, N is legally entitled to recover from the hospital the amount thus paid.

NOTE: It bears repeating that while the doctrine of *respondeat superior* gives the patient someone else to sue, it does not relieve the negligent nurse of his or her ultimate liability to the patient. Moreover, an employer who is required to pay a judgment because of the negligence of a nurse-employee is less likely to seek reimbursement from the nurse than to terminate his or her employment. Thus, while *respondeat superior* affords the nurse a certain degree of protection against being sued personally, it is *not* (and should not be thought of as) a shield against liability for acts of malpractice.

2-24   Who benefits the *most* from the doctrine of *respondeat superior:* the nurse, the nurse's employer, or the injured person?

> ☐   the nurse, because he or she can avoid liability for negligent conduct

> ☐   the employer, who can always recover any damages paid from the negligent nurse-employee

> ☐   the injured person, who is given an additional party to sue for damages who is generally in a better financial position to make payment

---

2-23   ☐
          ☑
          ☐

2-24   *the injured person, who is given an additional party to sue for damages . . .*

POINTS TO REMEMBER

1. The doctrine of *respondeat superior* holds an employer legally liable for the negligent acts of his or her employees that arise out of and in the course of the employment. The legal basis of *respondeat superior* is an employer-employee relationship, with the employer being held responsible for the acts of those whom he or she has a right to supervise or control.

2. Even though *respondeat superior* may apply in a particular case, the negligent employee is always liable for his or her own negligent conduct and may be sued alone or jointly with the employer.

3. Ordinarily (but not always) the doctrine of *respondeat superior* applies to the acts of nurses when they are employed by a hospital, nursing home, or a private physician.

4. Ordinarily (but not always) the doctrine of *respondeat superior* does not apply when nurses offer their services as private-duty nurses. However, when private-duty nurses come under the direct supervision and control of a physician, nursing home, or hospital, the doctrine *will* be applicable to their conduct.

5. Employers who are required (under *respondeat superior*) to pay damages to injured persons because of the negligence of their employees have the legal right to recover from such negligent employees the amounts thus paid.

2-25   In what way is the doctrine of *respondeat superior* related to the rule of personal liability?

- ☐ It completely nullifies the rule of personal liability.

- ☐ While it creates an additional liability, it does not hold negligent employees free from liability for their own conduct.

- ☐ It forces the injured person to sue someone who is blameless for the negligent acts of his employee.

Hospital Liability under *Respondeat Superior*

2-26   With a few exceptions, which we will discuss shortly, a hospital generally is held liable (under *respondeat superior*) for the negligent acts of *all* its employees—including, of course, its nurses. Many of the lawsuits brought against hospitals involve claims arising out of nursing malpractice, and when liability is proved such claims generally are paid by the hospital's liability insurance carrier.

A hospital's liability under *respondeat superior* applies to

- ☐ the acts of physicians and nurses only

- ☐ the acts of professionals only

- ☐ the acts of nonprofessionals only

- ☐ the acts of all the hospital's employees

2-27   The underlying reason for holding a hospital liable under *respondeat superior* is that

- ☐ the hospital unquestionably is in a better financial position to pay malpractice claims than is its negligent employee

- ☐ the hospital has the legal right and authority to exercise direction and control over its employee's actions

- ☐ the rule of personal liability does not apply to the acts of a hospital employee

2-25 *While it creates an additional liability, it does not hold negligent employees free from liability for their own conduct.*	**2-26** *the acts of all the hospital's employees*	**2-27** ☐ ☑ ☐

NOTE: Thus far in this discussion of *respondeat superior* we have concerned ourselves solely with acts of negligence committed by a nurse when performing nursing functions in a professional capacity, but the doctrine applies with equal force to negligent conduct of a nonprofessional nature. For example, if a nurse employed by a nursing home were to take a patient's blood sample to an outside laboratory by automobile and while en route were to injure a pedestrian, the nurse's negligence in driving the automobile (clearly not a professional nursing act) would nevertheless make the nursing home-employer liable to the pedestrian under the doctrine of *respondeat superior*.

2-28   Before one could determine whether or not the doctrine of *respondeat superior* would apply to the conduct of a nurse in a given situation, one would have to know

- ☐ who employed the nurse and paid for his or her services
- ☐ whether the negligent act arose out of the nurse's professional (i.e., nursing) or nonprofessional activities
- ☐ who had the legal right to direct and control the nurse's activities at the time the negligent act was committed

2-29   If a hospital were to engage the services of a private-duty nurse for general-duty nursing over a weekend, would the hospital be liable under *respondeat superior* for the nurse's negligent acts?

Yes   *No*
☐   ☐

2-30   *Any* negligent act or omission on the part of an employed nurse, whether in a professional capacity or not, will give rise to liability on the part of the nurse's employer so long as the act or omission occurred within the scope of the employment, i.e., while on duty during working hours.

True   *False*
☐   ☐

2-28 *who had the legal right to direct and control the nurse's activities at the time the negligent act was committed.*	**2-29** *Yes*	**2-30** *True*

NOTE: We come now to a special application of the doctrine of *respondeat superior* that has particular relevance for nurses engaged in operating room activities. This special application of the rule arises from the fact that an employee (the nurse) may serve two employers (the doctor and the hospital) simultaneously . . . even if only for brief periods of time.

The "Borrowed Servant" Doctrine

2-31   Ordinarily, a staff physician is not liable for the failure of a hospital nurse to carry out reasonable orders in treating a patient. The mere fact that a physician gives instructions— whether verbally, on the chart, or in some other manner—does not create an employer-employee relationship between the physician and the nurse. Indeed, in many, if not most, instances the physician does not know *which* nurse will actually be assigned to execute the instructions. The nurse is still under the direction and control of the hospital, and the hospital *only* will be held liable for any negligence on the nurse's part in carrying out those instructions.

Indicate whether the following statements are true or false.

True   *False*

☐   ☐   A hospital is liable under *respondeat superior* for the acts of all nurses in its employ, but not when they are carrying out the orders of attending physicians.

☐   ☐   General-duty nurses, but not their hospital-employers, will be held liable if they deviate from the orders of an attending physician and the patient suffers injury.

☐   ☐   The attending physician, but not the hospital, will be held liable for the negligence of a hospital nurse when executing the physician's medically sound order.

☐   ☐   Generally, a hospital-employed nurse is considered to be under the direction and control of the hospital, regardless of whose orders the nurse is carrying out.

2-31   *True*   *False*
☐   ☑
☐   ☑
☐   ☑
☑   ☐

2-32

Doctor D performs a thoracotomy and gives written orders for the postoperative care of the patient. One order calls for giving the patient intramuscular injections of an antibiotic at stated intervals. In administering the injection ordered, Nurse N strikes the patient's sciatic nerve, resulting in nerve damage and a "foot drop" condition.

Assuming Nurse N's negligence in giving the injection, who is the party most likely to be held liable to the patient under the rule of *respondeat superior*?

☐   Nurse N

☐   the hospital

☐   Doctor D

☐   both Doctor D and the hospital

2-33   There are special circumstances in which the courts have imposed legal liability upon an attending physician or surgeon for a hospital nurse's negligence, while absolving the hospital of its normal liability as the nurse's employer. This exception to the rule of *respondeat superior* usually arises when a hospital nurse, although not in the regular employ of an operating surgeon, technically becomes the surgeon's temporary employee ("borrowed servant") while working under the direct supervision and control of the surgeon during an operation. This special application of the *respondeat superior* rule is thus aptly called the "borrowed servant" doctrine.

The "borrowed servant" doctrine applies to an OR nurse's conduct

☐   whenever a hospital assigns him or her to operating room duty

☐   whenever the OR nurse's activities require special skills and he or she is subject to the direct control of the surgeon

☐   whenever the operating room nurse and the surgeon jointly agree that it should apply

---

2-32   ☐   If you did not choose the cor-
           ☑   rect answer, turn to p. 119,
           ☐   Note A.
           ☐

2-33   *whenever the OR nurse's ac-
           tivities require special skills
           and he or she is subject . . .*

2-34   The key to the borrowed servant doctrine is the matter of control. Before the physician or surgeon can be held liable, it must be shown that he or she had the right to control the assisting nurse in details relating to the *specific act* that produced the injury for which liability is sought to be imposed. Unless such control can be shown, either the hospital (or some other physician present) will be held liable for the nurse's negligent conduct under *respondeat superior*.

In the following fact situations, who (apart from the nurse) would be held liable for the nurse's conduct?

Hospital	Doctor	
☐	☐	A scrub nurse negligently prepares the operating room for surgery.
☐	☐	An OR nurse improperly counts the sponges used during an operation.
☐	☐	A nurse-anesthetist improperly administers anesthesia at a rate prescribed by the surgeon.
☐	☐	An OR nurse improperly positions an electrosurgical machine, causing burns to the patient.

2-35   During abdominal surgery, an anesthesiologist directs a nurse in the operating room to intubate a patient. The nurse does so improperly, causing injury to the patient's mouth and teeth.

Indicate whether the following are true or false.

True	False	
☐	☐	The anesthesiologist, but not the surgeon, could be held liable for the nurse's negligence under the "borrowed servant" theory.
☐	☐	The surgeon, but not the anesthesiologist, could be held liable for the nurse's negligence under the "borrowed servant" theory.
☐	☐	The hospital, but neither the surgeon nor the anesthesiologist, could be held liable for the nurse's negligence under the *respondeat superior* theory.
☐	☐	The nurse, but no one else, could be held liable for the harm caused by the nurse's negligence.

2-34 Hospital	Doctor		2-35 True	False
☑	☐		☑	☐
☑	☐		☐	☑
☐	☑		☐	☑
☑	☐		☐	☑

2-36   While the "borrowed servant" rule most often applies to operating room situations, it is equally applicable in theory to other situations in the hospital context. The critical factor in each case is whether the physician in fact becomes the nurse's temporary employer by exercising direct control over the nurse's acts.

A physician can avoid liability under the "borrowed servant" rule by proving

☐ the nurse was assigned by the hospital

☐ the nurse was carrying out a routine nursing function

☐ the nurse was not in the operating room at the time of the incident

---

2-37   In a non-operating room situation, and in the absence of any special circumstances, an attending physician will not be held liable for a nurse's negligence in carrying out treatment prescribed by the physician.

True   *False*
☐   ☐

2-38   As a general rule, a nurse   ☐ will   ☐ will not   be considered the "borrowed servant" of a physician or surgeon whenever the nurse is directed by the physician to perform a specific nursing procedure at a patient's bedside.

2-36 *the nurse was carrying out a routine nursing function*	**2-37** *True*	**2-38** *will not*

THE "CAPTAIN OF THE SHIP" DOCTRINE

An offshoot of the "borrowed servant" doctrine is the "captain of the ship" doctrine, which imposes liability on the surgeon in charge of an operation for the negligence of any of his or her nonphysician assistants during the time an operation is in progress, even though they remain employees of the hospital. This rather harsh legal doctrine has not gained universal acceptance, and even in those few jurisdictions where it is followed its use is restricted to acts of negligence that occur in the operating room, in the presence of the surgeon, and under his or her immediate direction.

Even in the operating room, many courts make a distinction between nursing acts that are "medical" in nature and those considered to be essentially routine administrative or clerical tasks. In this sense, the "captain of the ship" doctrine has been held totally inapplicable to preoperative preparations and postoperative care. Thus, it does not apply to the negligent acts of nurses during preliminary cleaning and preparation of the operating room, sterilization of the instruments to be used, making ready the sterile drapes, placing the patient on the operating table, or any of the myriad acts carried out by nurses in the recovery room after surgery has been completed.

Those jurisdictions that do not adhere to the "captain of the ship" doctrine take the position that a surgeon's mere presence in the operating room is not enough to make the surgeon liable for the negligence of nurses who have been assigned by the hospital to assist during surgery. This is especially true where the nurse is a trained and certified anesthetist or other operating room specialist. Clearly, there is a trend away from the "captain of the ship" doctrine and toward the recognition of the independent professional nature of nursing, both in and out of the operating room.

The "borrowed servant" and "captain of the ship" doctrines, as you have seen, are simply special applications of the *respondeat superior* doctrine. They are of far greater importance to the hospital and physician than to the nurse because they fix liability upon those parties for acts they did not directly supervise or carry out. The legal phrase characterizing this form of substituted liability is *vicarious liability*.

NOTE: In recent years the courts, with increasing frequency, have held hospitals liable for all manner of acts performed within the hospital. The doctrine of hospital corporate negligence (an independent basis of hospital liability) was first enunciated in the landmark case of *Darling v. Charleston Community Hospital,* 211 N.E. 2d 53 (Ill. 1965), where the court found the hospital failed to comply with various standards designed to insure patient safety, including the JCAH standards, the rules and regulations of the state health department, and the hospital's own bylaws and regulations. Subsequent court decisions in other states have reinforced that independent theory of liability. Nevertheless, *respondeat superior* continues to play an important role in determining who ultimately is liable for the nurse's negligent acts or omissions. The doctrine has several notable exceptions, however, which we will now examine.

Doctrine of Charitable Immunity

2-39   The first important exception to the *respondeat superior* doctrine can have far-reaching financial consequences for nurses who practice in a few American states. In these states the doctrine of *charitable immunity* applies, which holds that a charitable (i.e., nonprofit) hospital cannot be held liable in tort by a person who has been injured due to the negligence of a hospital employee. The practical effect of this rule is to force the injured person to sue the negligent hospital employee personally.

     In a state that recognizes the charitable immunity doctrine, which of the following classes of nurses would be affected the most?

☐   school nurses

☐   occupational health nurses

☐   nonprofit hospital nurses

☐   public health nurses

2-40   In a state that adheres to the charitable immunity doctrine, would a proprietary (profit-making) hospital be liable for the negligent acts of its nurses under *respondeat superior*?

            Yes   *No*
             ☐   ☐

2-39   *nonprofit hospital nurses*   2-40   *Yes*

                                                              If you checked the wrong an-
                                                              swer, turn to p. 119, Note B.

2-41   What is the significant legal consequence when the charitable immunity rule applies to hospital care in a particular jurisdiction?

☐   An injured patient cannot prevail in a suit against a charitable hospital whose negligent employee caused the injury.

☐   A negligent charitable hospital employee is protected against being held personally liable by the injured patient.

☐   The law in that jurisdiction permits the injured patient to hold both the hospital and its negligent employee liable.

NOTE: At one time, many jurisdictions adhered to the charitable immunity rule. Today the vast majority of jurisdictions have abolished the rule either directly by statute or indirectly by judicial decision. Approximately 35 jurisdictions have rejected the rule in its entirety, while several others have retained the rule in varying degrees by limiting the amount of damages recoverable (e.g., New Jersey permits recovery only up to $10,000), by limiting the amount recoverable only to the extent of existing liability insurance (as in Maine and Rhode Island), or limiting recovery only to paying patients (as in Georgia).

Two states—Arkansas and Colorado—have categorically declined to abandon the charitable immunity rule. Thus, nurses who practice in charitable (nonprofit) hospitals in those states run a greater risk of being sued and being held personally liable for their acts of negligence in treating patients. And, of course, nurses also run the risk of being sued and being held personally liable for negligently caused patient injuries in those states mentioned above that have placed limits on the amount of damages a patient can recover from a charitable hospital.

In Canada the doctrine of charitable immunity has not been adopted. Accordingly, a charitable hospital in Canada can be held liable for the negligence of its employees under the usual rule of *respondeat superior*.

2-41 *An injured patient cannot prevail in a suit against a charitable hospital. . . .*

Doctrine of Governmental Immunity

2-42   Another exception to the *respondeat superior* doctrine comes into play when the nurse's employer is a state or provincial government. The common-law rule of *governmental immunity* provides that state and provincial governments cannot be held liable for the negligent acts of their employees while carrying out governmental activities. However, some states and provinces have changed this rule by statute, and in these particular jurisdictions the doctrine of *respondeat superior* continues to apply to the acts of nurses employed by the state or provincial government. Consider the following situation:

> Public Nurse N is employed by State X in one of its mental health clinics. While performing encephalography on a patient, N negligently injures his scalp.

Under these facts can the patient sue State X for his injury?

Yes   *No*   *Can't be sure*
☐   ☐   ☐

2-43   If State X has *not* passed any special legislation with respect to liability for acts of its employees, against whom can suit be brought by the patient for his injury?

☐   only Nurse N

☐   only State X

☐   both Nurse N and State X

☐   none of the above

2-44   If State X *has* enacted a statute waiving (relinquishing) its governmental immunity, against whom can suit be brought by the patient for his injury?

☐   only Nurse N

☐   only State X

☐   both Nurse N and State X

☐   none of the above

2-42 *Can't be sure* No information has been given about the state's position on immunity; hence, we really don't know enough to make a proper choice.	**2-43** *only Nurse N*	**2-44** *both Nurse N and State X*

GOVERNMENTAL IMMUNITY FROM TORT SUITS

The law relating to charitable and governmental immunity has undergone significant change over the past decade, with the states having almost completely eliminated charitable immunity as a basis for denying recovery of damages by a patient injured through negligence in a nonprofit hospital. In general, the states have been slower to reject immunity of government-operated hospitals, although there is clearly a trend in that direction.

In those states that still adhere to the doctrine of governmental immunity, the courts have stuck to their basic legal position that a state, in its discharge of purely governmental functions, should not (and therefore cannot) be held liable in tort. Some have cited the dire economic consequences to the state if it were forced to pay for the tortious conduct of its agents and employees. On the other hand, many states, either by legislation or judicial decision, have substantially rejected immunity, either completely or by allowing damage claims up to a specified dollar amount, or the amount of the state's existing liability insurance coverage.

The following states are the few that still adhere to the doctrine of governmental immunity and will not allow a claimant to sue the state to recover damages for the negligence of its employees: Alabama, Delaware, Maine, Maryland, North Dakota, South Dakota, Virginia, Wisconsin, and Wyoming. It bears repeating that nurses who practice in state-operated hospitals or other medical facilities in these states are more likely to be sued personally, a fact that makes the purchase of professional liability insurance protection a virtual necessity. This issue is discussed more fully in Part 8.

Liability of the School Nurse

2-45   In the United States the rules relating to governmental immunity affect not only nurses employed directly by state governments but also nurses employed by school districts. This is because education is a state function in the United States and a school district is therefore legally considered a subdivision of the state government. Accordingly, a nurse employed by a school district will be subject to the same legal liabilities for tortious conduct as other government employees are subject to in that jurisdiction.

The school nurse employed in a state that is immune from tort liability is exposed to a   ☐ greater   ☐ lesser   risk of personal liability than a school nurse in a state that has waived its immunity to tort liability.

2-46

Nurse N is a school nurse in State X, which has waived its immunity to tort liability.

If Nurse N commits a negligent act while in the employ of a school district in State X, which of the following would apply?

☐ The rule of *respondeat superior* would apply to N's conduct, making the school district liable.

☐ The rule of *respondeat superior* would not apply to N's conduct, making the nurse the only party against whom suit could be brought.

2-47   If State X in the above example had not waived its immunity to tort liability, which of the following would apply?

☐ Nurse N could expect to be sued and held liable personally for the negligent conduct.

☐ The state would most likely bring suit against Nurse N to recover the damages paid out because of the negligence.

☐ The person injured as a result of Nurse N's negligence would have no legal basis for suing Nurse N or State X.

2-45 *greater*	**2-46** *The rule of* respondeat superior *would apply to N's conduct, making the school district liable.*	**2-47** *Nurse N could expect to be sued and held liable personally. . . .*

2-48 The school nurse is held to the same standard of care applicable to other professional nurses with comparable backgrounds and training and working in similar circumstances, unless that standard is modified by statute.

School Nurse N administers an anticonvulsant drug to a 7-year-old child during school hours, pursuant to parental consent and a physician's order. Hurried, Nurse N negligently administers too large a dose, however, causing the child to suffer a severe reaction and consequent injury requiring hospitalization.

In a lawsuit brought by the child's parents, Nurse N's conduct would be measured against

- ☐ that of reasonably prudent general-duty hospital nurses
- ☐ that of reasonably prudent special-duty nurses
- ☐ that of reasonably prudent school nurses
- ☐ all of the above

2-49 In the previous example, assume that the state law specifically provides that a school nurse who administers medications to a child pursuant to parental consent and a physician's written order cannot be held liable for ordinary negligence in so doing, and that gross or willful negligence is the only basis for holding a nurse liable.

This statute would

- ☐ have no effect on the outcome of this case
- ☐ absolve the nurse of liability in this case
- ☐ establish the standard of care governing this case

> NOTE: In point of fact, nearly a dozen states now have laws regulating the administration of medications by school nurses and other school personnel. The Connecticut statute is one that provides immunity to nurses for ordinary negligence, as in the example just given.

2-48 *that of reasonably prudent school nurses*	**2-49** *establish the standard of care governing this case*

2-50   School nurses usually are not under the direct supervision of physicians, which makes their position legally more perilous than that of nurses who work under the direct supervision of physicians. For this reason, school nurses should be especially alert to their legal responsibilities and exercise the utmost in good judgment in all that they do.

Nurse N is the school nurse for a large school in a jurisdiction which has *not* waived its immunity to tort liability. One morning a 16-year-old girl reports to the nurse, complaining of moderately severe abdominal cramps. The nurse decides that the girl is experiencing simple menstrual cramps and applies a hot water bottle to the affected area. Her condition worsens and the child eventually is removed to the hospital, where her condition is diagnosed as acute appendicitis. The child dies in surgery because of the delay in treatment attributable to the nurse's conduct.

In a malpractice suit alleging the foregoing facts, who could be held liable for the child's death?

☐   the nurse alone

☐   the school district alone

☐   both the nurse and the school district

2-51   Because they work in a nonmedical environment, school nurses must exercise considerable independent judgment and must be able to recognize and treat most of the ailments and injuries that schoolchildren experience. One of their chief tasks, of course, is knowing how to identify those conditions that require immediate medical attention, and making the necessary arrangements therefor.

What would be the *most significant* professional qualification of a nurse hired by a school district as a school nurse?

☐   the nurse's ability to work closely with school officials in assessing the health status of students

☐   the nurse's ability to exercise independent nursing judgment in critical emergency situations

☐   the nurse's ability to properly counsel students on their medical and dental health problems

2-50 *the nurse alone*	**2-51** *the nurse's ability to exercise independent nursing judgment. . . .*

NOTE: In Canada there is no statutory rule of immunity that precludes the bringing of a suit directly against a local school board for the negligence of one of its nurses. The usual practice is for the injured person (or his or her legal representative) to join in one suit both the school board and the nurse in question.

2-52   As a brief review, match the letter of each of the legal doctrines below with its appropriate description.

A. *Respondeat superior*

A nonprofit hospital cannot be held liable for the negligence of its employees. ☐

B. Rule of personal liability

An employer is liable for the negligent acts of his or her employees committed in the scope of their employment. ☐

C. Charitable immunity rule

A governmental body cannot be sued for the negligent acts of its employees. ☐

D. Governmental immunity rule

Every person is held liable for his or her own negligent conduct. ☐

2-52   [C]
       [A]
       [D]
       [B]

POINTS TO REMEMBER

1. As a general rule, hospitals are liable under *respondeat superior* for the negligent acts of *all* their employees.

2. The key element in deciding whether or not *respondeat superior* will apply in a given case is whether another party had the right to direct and control the nurse's activities with respect to the incident in question.

3. The "borrowed servant" doctrine is a special application of the *respondeat superior* doctrine. It provides that a temporary employer (usually the operating surgeon) is held liable for the negligent acts of nurses in the operating room or elsewhere done under his or her direction and control. Routine nursing functions are not held to be within the purview of the operating surgeon's "borrowed servant" liability.

4. In a few states of the United States, the doctrine of *respondeat superior* does not apply to employees of certain types of hospitals. In these states the doctrine of charitable immunity still applies. Under this doctrine a nonprofit hospital is legally immune from suit for the negligent acts of its employees. The doctrine of charitable immunity does not apply in Canada.

5. In some jurisdictions the common law doctrine of sovereign (governmental) immunity applies, which provides that no claim can be brought against the state or province for the negligent acts of its employees.

6. In American states that adhere to the governmental immunity rule, the local school board (which is considered a branch of the state government) cannot be held liable for the negligence of one of its employees.

7. In Canada a local school board *can* be sued for the negligence of one of its employees, there being no special rule of immunity applicable to school boards in Canada.

8. Whenever a special exception to the doctrine of *respondeat superior* applies, the nurse is exposed to a greater risk of personal liability for his or her negligent conduct.

> NOTE: Since many nurses are employed by the United States and Canadian govern-
> ments, a brief discussion of their liability is in order. We will not be discussing the liability
> of nurses who work for state or provincial governments—only those employed by the
> federal government in both the United States and Canada.

Liability of Federal Government Nurses

2-53   Prior to 1946, the United States government could not be sued for the torts of its
employees. In that year the Congress enacted the Federal Tort Claims Act (FTCA), permitting
such suits to be brought by nongovernment individuals who have suffered injury or loss of
property due to the negligent acts of Federal employees. Acts of medical negligence (malpractice) are included.

In view of the enactment of the Federal Tort Claims Act (FTCA), the United States
government is   ☐ immune from suit   ☐ subject to suit   for the negligent acts of its
employees.

2-54   Which of the following (if any) is (are) correct?

The FTCA permits

☐ injured Federal government employees to sue the government for injuries they
incur at work

☐ the Federal government to sue one of its negligent employees for injury caused a
nongovernment person

☐ someone not employed by the Federal government to sue the latter for the
negligent conduct of one of its employees

☐ none of the foregoing

2-53   *subject to suit*

2-54   *someone not employed by the
Federal government to sue
the latter for the negligent
conduct of one of its employees*

2-55   By assuming liability for the negligent acts of its employees under the FTCA, the

United States government   ☐ is subject to   ☐ is not subject to   the rule of *respondeat*

superior.

NOTE: Since 1966, nurses employed by the Veterans Administration have been accorded statutory immunity from suit for their negligent acts performed in the course of their employment. 38 U.S.C. 4116.

Since 1970, nurses employed by the United States Public Health Service have been accorded similar immunity. 42 U.S.C. 233.

This does not mean that the United States cannot be held liable for the negligent conduct of nurses who work for the Veterans Administration or the Public Health Service. It *does* mean that the nurses themselves cannot be held *personally liable,* a rather significant advantage over the nurse who is not employed by the United States government.

The Canadian government also has enacted legislation that makes it possible for an injured patient to sue the government for the negligence of its medical employees. By virtue of the Crown Liability Act, the rule of *respondeat superior* applies to the conduct of all nurses employed by the Dominion of Canada.

2-55   *is subject to*

Liability of the Occupational Health Nurse

2-56   The occupational health nurse faces a risk of personal liability that in some cases exceeds and in some cases is less than the liability of other classes of nurses. This is because of the unique interplay between the doctrine of *respondeat superior* and state workers' compensation laws.

All state and provincial workers' compensation laws mandate the compensation of employees who are injured while at work in accordance with specific compensation schedules. These same laws make this remedy the injured employee's *sole remedy against the employer,* and thus deny the employee the legal right to sue the employer for damages even if the employer's negligence was the prime cause of his injury.

Indicate which of the following, if any, is a legal consequence of a state or provincial workers' compensation law:

☐   It affords a statutory compensation remedy to an injured employee that makes it unnecessary to sue his or her employer for damages.

☐   It effectively deprives an injured employee of the right to sue the employer for damages incurred in an on-the-job injury.

☐   Both of the above

☐   Neither of the above

2-57   In eight or nine states, an employee injured on the job can sue any person (other than his or her employer) whose negligence caused the injury, including a coworker. In most states, however, the immunity from suit granted the employer is also extended to coworkers of the injured employee. Thus, a nurse employed by a company in a state with such a law, and whose negligence causes harm to a fellow employee, would be protected from civil liability for his or her actions.

Based on the foregoing, in a state that accords immunity from suit against the employer and coworkers of an injured employee, a negligent nurse is in a more protected legal position than is a general-duty nurse employed by a hospital.

True   *False*

☐   ☐

2-56 *Both of the above*	**2-57** *True*

2-58   If the nurse (1) is engaged by the employer as an independent contractor, or (2) works for an employer in a state whose workers' compensation law provides immunity from suit only to the employer, the nurse can be held personally liable for his or her negligent conduct that causes injury to an employee.

> Nurse N is an occupational health nurse employed by a manufacturer in a state that has not granted immunity from suit to coworkers of an employee injured while on the job. Doctor D is the plant physician, and in D's absence Nurse N's activities are guided by special medical directives which cover both routine and emergency situations.

> During Doctor D's absence one day, Nurse N negligently evaluates an employee's signs of illness. The employee suffers a permanent disability as the direct result of N's negligence.

Which of the following would most likely be held liable to the disabled employee in this case?

☐   the manufacturing concern

☐   Doctor D

☐   Nurse N

2-59   If Doctor D's standing order to Nurse N was: "In every case do whatever you think is in the patient's best interests," which of the following would be true?

☐   Doctor D automatically would be held liable for all Nurse N's negligent acts under the doctrine of *respondeat superior*.

☐   The lack of specific guidelines for N to carry out nursing functions would expose N to greater liability for negligent conduct.

☐   Nurse N could avoid liability for any negligent conduct by pointing to the broad authority granted by Doctor D.

2-58   *Nurse N*   **2-59**   ☐   If you selected the wrong an-
                                         ☑   swer, turn to p. 119, Note C.
                                         ☐

SPECIAL PROBLEMS ARISING OUT OF HOME HEALTH CARE

The extremely rapid growth of home health care over the past several years has brought into focus some potential legal liability issues based on care provided in the home setting. When the Medicare program introduced the concept of diagnostic-related groups (DRGs), the trend toward early discharge of patients from hospitals accelerated dramatically. Today, home-care agencies of many varieties—including extensions of hospital services, visiting nurse and community health nurse services, and a vast number of home-health agencies offering a combination of professional nursing and nonprofessional services—are vying with each other to capture a share of the lucrative home-care market.

While there is little doubt that home care is less costly and more humane for the elderly than long-term institutionalization, it brings with it its own set of problems, especially those attributable to more complex therapies and the use of highly technical equipment. Patients who used to be treated only in the hospital are now being treated at home with IV therapy, parenteral nutrition, enterostomal care, diabetes care, postoperative cardiology care, pulmonary care, etc.—in many cases calling for oxygen tanks, tubes, indwelling catheters, and a variety of complex monitoring devices. In these circumstances, the danger of injury to the patient through some form of negligence is ever present. The opportunities for equipment failure, in particular, increase enormously where the equipment is not under the day-to-day control of trained technicians as in the hospital setting.

The legal problems most likely to arise out of home health-care services are (1) determining who has primary legal responsibility for establishment of the fundamental home-care plan, as well as continuing legal responsibility once the plan is initiated, (2) the normal standard-of-care problems associated with the provision of nursing services, and (3) fixing legal responsibility for the reliable performance and safety of the equipment used. Since there have been no reported legal decisions as yet dealing with home care per se, one can only speculate as to how many of these problems ultimately will be resolved. But one would predict that when a malpractice suit is brought, everyone associated with the patient's care at home—the hospital, the home-care agency, the prescribing or treating physician, the equipment manufacturer, and the individual home-care nurse will be joined as defendants in the litigation until it can be decided exactly who is responsible for what.

In any event, the legal doctrines discussed earlier, such as the rule of personal liability and the doctrine of *respondeat superior,* will continue to be the basic guidelines for deciding most fact situations. What must still be determined by the courts, however, are the specific standards of care to be applied to home health care. Clearly, there is a fundamental legal obligation on the part of the home-care agency to (1) exercise care in the selection of competent and experienced nursing personnel, (2) carefully train such personnel in the use of specialized equipment and medical technologies, (3) develop operational guidelines and protocols for the provision of home care designed to assure close communication between all the involved parties (especially the handling of potential emergencies), and (4) assure the safety and reliability of all medical equipment used.

Although there is, as yet, no national certification body for home-care nursing, clinical nurse-specialists are likely to play an increasingly greater role in home care, particularly since they will be readily able to provide the specialized services called for, such as IV antibiotic therapy, respiratory therapy, and parenteral nutrition. The absence of immediate medical backup may prove to be a problem in some cases, but by and large well-trained nurses will be able to function capably in the home environment where they should find their nursing skills utilized to the fullest. The unique scope-of-practice problems faced by nurse-specialists are dealt with at length in Part 4.

EXPLANATORY NOTES

Note A   (from Frame 2-32)

Certainly, Nurse N would not be held liable in this case under the doctrine of *respondeat superior,* even though N would still be held liable for personal negligence. Do not forget: *respondeat superior* is a substituted liability doctrine.

Since the administration of an intramuscular injection is a common nursing function, Doctor D would not be held liable for the nurse's negligence merely for having ordered the injection.

Under the given facts, only the hospital would be held liable under *respondeat superior*.

Proceed to Frame 2-33.

Note B   (from Frame 2-40)

It should be noted that the charitable immunity rule is an exception to the basic doctrine of *respondeat superior*. Accordingly, unless it specifically applies in a given case, the usual rule of *respondeat superior* will continue to apply. The concept of charitable immunity is a dwindling legal doctrine that has all but vanished from American law. When applicable at all, it applies only to so-called charitable (nonprofit) hospitals. For this reason, negligent conduct that occurs in a profit-making hospital would be subject to the doctrine of *respondeat superior*.

Proceed to Frame 2-41.

Note C   (from Frame 2-59)

There is little doubt that the lack of clear working guidelines for carrying out nursing functions would expose Nurse N to greater liability for negligent conduct. As a matter of fact, following such an open-ended standing order would not only expose a nurse to greater liability for malpractice but might also be the grounds for a criminal charge of practicing medicine without a license. In the final analysis, the rule of personal liability will always hold nurses personally responsible for their negligent conduct, and all the more so where they have no clear guidelines from the company physician.

The intelligent occupational health nurse must not rely on a "do-whatever-you-think-is-proper" standing order as authority for his or her functions, and he or she should ignore or challenge any such order for the reasons mentioned above. Incidentally, most courts also would hold the company physician liable for negligence in supervision in a case of this type, but our primary concern here is with the nurse's conduct.

Proceed to Part 3.

POINTS TO REMEMBER

1. Under the Federal Tort Claims Act (FTCA), the United States government has consented to be sued for the negligent acts of its employees. The doctrine of *respondeat superior* applies, therefore, to the United States government.

2. In all essential respects the principles of malpractice law apply in the same manner to nurses who are in private or government practice.

3. By virtue of special statutory enactments, nurses employed by the United States Public Health Service and by the Veterans Administration have complete immunity from personal liability for acts of negligence in the course of their government nursing duties. These statutes do not affect the rights of aggrieved patients from suing the government for the injuries they have sustained, however.

4. The Canadian government likewise has waived its immunity against suit and can be held liable for the negligent acts of any of its employees so long as they are committed in the scope of the employment.

5. Because of the joint effect of the doctrine of *respondeat superior* and workers' compensation laws, occupational health nurses are sometimes exposed to a greater risk of being sued for negligent conduct than all other classes of nurses.

6. Since workers' compensation laws generally prevent an employee from suing an employer for an injury incurred in the course of the employment, in many states the employee whose injury is aggravated by the malpractice of the company nurse can sue only the nurse, and not the employer.

SELECTED REFERENCES—PART 2

Rule of Personal Liability

W. Prosser, *Handbook of the Law of Torts*, 4th ed., West Publishing, St. Paul, 1971, § §
   46–51, pp. 291–313
74 *Am Jur 2d*, TORTS, § 10, p. 628
Annotations, 51 ALR 2d 970, 60 ALR 475
Dessauer v. Memorial General Hospital, 628 P. 2d 337 (N. Mex. 1981)
Hiatt v. Groce, 523 P. 2d 320 (Kan. 1974)
Brady v. Roosevelt Steamship Co., 317 U.S. 575 (1943)

Supervisor's Liability for Acts of Subordinates

Bowers v. Olch, 260 P. 2d 997 (Cal. 1953)
Valentin v. La Société Francaise de Bienfaisance, 172 P. 2d 359 (Cal. 1946)

Doctrine of *Respondeat Superior*

W. Prosser, *Handbook of the Law of Torts*, 4th ed., West Publishing, St. Paul, 1971, § 458
53 *Am Jur 2d* § 417

Hospital Liability Under *Respondeat Superior*

D. Louisell and H. Williams, *Medical Malpractice*, Matthew Bender & Co., New York,
   1983, § 16.08
Variety Children's Hospital v. Perkins, 382 So. 2d 331 (Fla. 1982)
Su v. Perkins, 211 S.E. 2d 421 (Ga. 1974)
Sesselman v. Muhlenberg Hospital, 306 A. 2d 474 (N.J. 1973)
Darling v. Charleston Memorial Hospital, 211 N.E. 2d 253 (Ill. 1965)

Borrowed Servant Doctrine

Restatement (Second) Agency § § 226–227
Baird v. Sickler, 433 N.E. 2d 593 (Ohio 1982)
Truhitte v. French Hospital, 180 Cal. Rptr. 152 (Cal. 1982)
City of Somerset v. Hart, 549 S.W. 2d 814 (Ky. 1977)
Hudmon v. Martin, 315 So. 2d 516 (Fla. 1976)
Martin v. Perth Amboy General Hospital, 250 A. 2d 40 (N.J. 1968)
Buzan v. Mercy Hospital, 203 So. 2d 11 (Fla. 1967)

Captain of the Ship Doctrine

D. Louisell and H. Williams, *Medical Malpractice*, Matthew Bender & Co., New York, 1983, § 16.07

J. Greenlaw, "Liability for Nursing Negligence in the Operating Room," *Law, Medicine, and Health Care* 10(10):222 (Oct. 1982)

B. McVey and R. Walsh, "Medical Malpractice—Who is the captain of the ship?" *Federat Ins L Couns Q* 27:331 (Summer 1977)

Annotation, 29 ALR 3d 1065

Kitto v. Gilbert, 570 P. 2d 544 (Col. 1977)

Sparger v. Worley Hospital, 547 S.W. 2d 582 (Tex. 1977)

Thomas v. Hutchinson, 275 A. 2d 23 (Pa. 1971)

Mazur v. Lipschutz, 327 F. 2d 42 (3d Cir. 1964)

McConnell v. Williams, 65 A. 2d 246 (Pa. 1949)

Ybarra v. Spangard, 154 P. 2d 687 (Cal. 1944)

Doctrine of Charitable Immunity

D. Louisell and H. Williams, *Medical Malpractice*, Matthew Bender & Co., New York, 1983, § 17.04

A. Bottari, "The Charitable Immunity Act," *Seton Hall L. J.*, 5:61 (Fall 1980)

Williams v. Jefferson Hospital Association, 442 S.W. 2d 243 (Ark. 1969)

Rhoda v. Aroostock General Hospital, 226 A. 2d 530 (Me. 1967)

Hemenway v. Presbyterian Hospital Association of Colorado, 419 P. 2d 312 (Col. 1966)

Doctrine of Governmental Immunity

Gallegos v. Southern Nevada Memorial Hospital, 577 F. Supp. 824 (Nev. 1983)

Williamson v. Jones, 336 N.W. 2d 489 (Mich. 1983)

Hall v. Roberts, 548 F. Supp. 498 (Va. 1982)

Neal v. Donahue, 611 P. 2d 1125 (Okla. 1980)

Gregory v. Martyak, Kapish, et al, 408 A. 2d 188 (Pa. 1979)

Perry v. Kalamazoo State Hospital, 273 N.W. 2d 421 (Mich. 1978)

Ramsay v. Prince Georges County, 308 A. 2d 217 (Md. 1973)

Maine Revised Statutes Annotated, Title 14, § 1803

Liability of the School Nurse

S. Cohn, "Legal Issues in School Nursing Practice," *Law, Medicine & Health Care* 12:219 (Oct. 1984)

M. Kinne, "Accidents," *J. School Health*, 52 (9):564–5 (Nov. 1982)

H. Creighton, "School Nurses: Legal Aspects of their Work," *Nurs. Clin. N. Amer.* 9:467 (Sept. 1974)

Standards for School Nurse Services, National Education Association, Washington, D.C. (1970)

Liability of Federal Government Nurses

Immunity of V.A. nurses - 38 U.S.C. § 4116
Immunity of U.S.P.H.S. nurses - 42 U.S.C. § 233
Mendez v. Belton, 739 F. 2d 15 (1st Cir. 1984)
Apple v. Jewish Hospital & Medical Center, 570 F. Supp. 1320 (N.Y. 1983)
Lojuk v. Quandt, 706 F. 2d 1456 (7th Cir. 1983)
Baker v. Barber, 673 F. 2d 147 (6th Cir. 1982)

Liability of the Occupational Health Nurse

E. A. Bowyer, "The Liability of the Occupational Health Nurse," *Law, Medicine and Health Care* 11(5):224 (Oct. 1983)

M. L. Brown, *Occupational Health Nursing: Principles and Practices,* Springer Publishing, New York, 1981

M. Cushing, "An Occupational Nurse's Liability," *Amer. J. Nurs.,* 81(12):2207 (Dec. 1981)

M. Mancini, "The Law and the Occupational Health Nurse," *Amer. J. Nurs.,* 79(9):1608 (Sept. 1979)

Cooper v. National Motor Bearing Co., 288 P. 2d 581 (Cal. 1955)

Home Health Nursing

P. G. Stitt, "Home Health Care Innovations in Health Care Delivery," *Hawaii Med. J.,* 44:166 (May 1985)

J. Powers and C. Burger, "Home Health Care vs. Nursing Home Care for the Elderly," *J. Tenn. Med. Assoc.,* 78(4):227 (April 1985)

"Home Care Today," Interview with Elsie Griffith, R.N., *Amer. J. Nurs.,* 84(3):341 (March 1984)

J. Arbeiter, "The Big Shift to Home Health Nursing," *RN,* 47(11):38 (Nov. 1984)

S. Weinstein, "Specialty Teams in Health Care," *Amer. J. Nurs.,* 84(3):342 (March 1984)

I. Trail, "The Legal Implications of Community Nursing Care," *Nurs. Clin. N. Amer.,* 9:463 (Sept. 1974)

Caring Magazine, National Association for Home Care, Washington, D.C. (All issues)

Matter of David Gentile Nursing Service, 483 N.Y.S. 2d 796 (N.Y. 1985)

Homemakers v. Gonzalez, 400 So. 2d 965 (Fla. 1981)

Part Three
Specific Types of Negligent Conduct

Part 3

INTRODUCTORY NOTE

In Part 1 we discussed the general legal principles that apply to nurses in carrying out their customary duties, and in Part 2 we discussed some of the special rules of liability. Now we shall see examples of how these concepts are applied in specific fact situations. Many nursing functions and responsibilities have been the subject of court cases, thereby providing authoritative guidelines to proper conduct in future similar cases.

It should be noted that the profession of nursing has undergone dynamic changes within the past decade or so. The nurse has evolved from being the handmaiden of the physician to a recognized professional assistant in carrying out many patient care functions.

Earlier views of the nurse as the physician's aide in carrying out numerous dependent functions have been superseded by changes in nursing curricula and educational standards qualifying the nurse to perform many independent functions without the necessity of medical orders or direct medical supervision. Notwithstanding these changes in the activities carried out by nurses, the case law does not reveal any undue exposure to liability *solely* because of this expanded role in providing patient care services. Following the general rules outlined earlier in this course, liability is always predicated on failure to exercise the degree of care and skill expected of the nurse—or the nurse-specialist—under similar circumstances.

It would be impossible to cover the entire gamut of factual situations that have been before the courts, but the cases which are included herein are considered representative of the more common problems encountered in nursing malpractice suits during recent years.

Patient Safety Errors

3-1   A nurse is required to exercise ordinary or reasonable care to safeguard and protect his or her patient from any known or reasonably foreseeable harm. The courts have held this to be as much the nurse's responsibility as that of the physician. Many of the nurse's routine patient care activities relate to the safety and security of the patient, and the nurse is expected to perform these acts without any special medical order or supervision.

Under what circumstances will a nurse be held legally responsible for seeing that no harm comes to his or her patient?

☐ only when the nurse is engaged to care for the patient as a private-duty nurse

☐ only when the nurse has been specifically directed to protect the patient against harm

☐ whenever the nurse is assigned to caring for the patient

3-2 which   A nurse's responsibility to safeguard and protect his or her patient from harm is one

☐ requires either a written or verbal order from a physician or nurse-supervisor

☐ the nurse must exercise independently of any special medical order or supervisory directive

☐ the nurse must exercise only when employed by a hospital, nursing home, or other health care institution

---

3-3   The nurse's responsibility to protect his or her patient from harm includes harm that might result from carrying out a physician's specific order.

True   *False*

☐   ☐

| **3-1** *whenever the nurse is assigned to caring for the patient* | **3-2** *the nurse must exercise independently of any special medical order or supervisory directive* | **3-3** *True* |

3-4

P, a 76-year-old female hospitalized for treatment of congestive heart failure was known to lapse into a semicomatose state from time to time. When lucid, she constantly complained of being cold and asked for hot water bottles around her legs. No specific doctor's orders were given for these complaints, but Nurse N was given general instructions by supervisory Nurse S to "keep the patient warm."

Nurse N, irritated by P's constant complaints, placed several excessively hot heating pads around P's legs while P was semicomatose, disregarding the patient's immediate objection to the intensity of the heat. Upon checking the patient an hour later, it was noted that she had sustained serious burns on her legs, requiring extensive remedial measures, P later sued Nurse N, Nurse S, her treating physician, and the hospital for the injuries sustained.

What was the *legal* duty owed by Nurse N with respect to the safety of patient P?

☐   the duty to respond immediately to all requests for nursing care made by P

☐   the duty to safeguard and protect P from any known or reasonably foreseeable harm

☐   the duty to do whatever the doctor ordered

3-5   What was the principal foreseeable danger to guard against in this case?

☐   the danger that P might sustain burns while in a semiconscious state

☐   the danger that P's general condition might worsen

☐   the danger that P might attempt to move the heating pads to another area of her body

---

3-4 ☐ If you checked the 1st or 3d
          ☑ box, turn to p. 139, Note A.
          ☐

3-5 *the danger that P might sus-
         tain burns while in a semi-
         conscious state*

3-6   The kind and degree of nursing care necessary to protect a patient from harm will always depend upon the particular circumstances of the case. The prime determinant of the type of care necessary is the patient's physical and mental capacity to contribute to his or her own safety and security.

What *legal* significance would be attached to the fact that P was an elderly patient in a weakened condition who occasionally lapsed into a comatose state?

□ P would be expected to be more aware of the possible harm she might sustain while in a comatose condition.

□ The foreseeability of harm to P would be greater, and the degree of care to protect against such harm also would be greater.

□ No particular legal significance would be attached since the degree of care expected of the nursing staff would not differ merely because of these factors.

3-7   Which of the following actions would have afforded *better*, and nevertheless *reasonable*, protection against the type of occurrence that eventually led to P's injuries?

□ Nurse S could have assigned staff nurses other than Nurse N to check on P's condition every ten minutes

□ The hospital could have issued standing orders never to apply heating pads to semicomatose patients.

□ Nurse N could have double-checked the temperature of the heating pads after P complained about the intensity of their heat.

3-6 □	3-7 □
☑	□
□	☑

3-8   Supervisory Nurse S gave Nurse N specific instructions to keep Patient P warm. If a jury was to decide that Nurse N was negligent in fulfilling his or her legal responsibilities to P, what likely effect would this have on Nurse S's liability?

☐   No liability would result since the instructions in question were well within the capabilities of a trained nurse.

☐   Nurse S would be held liable for failing to check on P's condition personally.

☐   Nurse S would be held liable for giving only general instructions to Nurse N about keeping Patient P warm.

NOTE: You will recall that a nursing supervisor can be held liable if he or she assigns a task to an individual who is not competent to perform that particular task. A general instruction to "keep the patient warm" is not the type of nursing task that calls for particularized nursing skills, and it is highly unlikely that a nursing supervisor would be held liable for harm resulting from giving such a simple and routine order.

The important thing to note is that a nurse never should rely blindly on someone else's orders and use them as a shield for his or her own negligent conduct. The test is always the same: How would other reasonably prudent nurses have acted in a similar situation?

3-9   Assuming Nurse N's negligence in this case, who else would probably be held liable for N's conduct?

☐   the doctor and the hospital

☐   the hospital

☐   no one else

3-8   *No liability would result since the instructions were well within the capabilities of a trained nurse.*

3-9   *the hospital*

3-10   All nurses should be especially alert to the hazards of smoking by patients who may not be mentally aware of the dangers involved or physically able to protect themselves from causing fires and being burned. Under no circumstances should a nurse accommodate a patient's plea to smoke, regardless how persistent, when the forseeability of harm to the patient or others clearly dictates that he or she should not be permitted to smoke.

P, a 42-year-old male of below-average intelligence, was hospitalized with paralysis of his arms and his vocal cords. Nurse N, assigned to care for P, knew him to be a lifelong pipe smoker and frequently lit P's pipe for him and permitted him to smoke. N's only orders from Nurse S, her supervisor, were not to leave him alone when smoking, and N followed these orders faithfully. One day P's bed caught fire and he suffered burns that resulted in his death. His pipe (which was lit) and some matches were found on the floor near his bed.

P's estate sues Nurses N and S for malpractice in failing to protect P from harm. At the trial, Nurse N testifies she was not in the room at the time the fire began and has no way of knowing how P's pipe might have been lit. Nurse S testifies that he had given Nurse N strict orders not to leave P alone while he was smoking and that N is a competent and diligent nurse in all respects.

What was the *legal* duty owed by Nurse N with respect to the safety of Patient P?

☐   the duty to light his pipe for him and see that it was out when she left the room

☐   the duty to safeguard and protect him from any known or reasonably foreseeable danger

☐   the duty not to leave him unattended while he was smoking his pipe

---

3-11   What was the principal foreseeable danger to guard against in this case?

☐   the danger that P might fall asleep while smoking

☐   the danger that P might burn himself while attempting to light his pipe

☐   the danger that P might attempt to smoke his pipe while unattended

---

3-10 ☐
          ☑
          ☐

3-11   *the danger that P might at-
           tempt to smoke his pipe while
           unattended*

3-12   What *legal* significance would be attached to the fact that P was of below-average intelligence and could neither move his arms nor speak?

- ☐ P would be expected to know the greater risk presented by his smoking (in view of his condition) and would be expected to assume full responsibility for any consequent harm.

- ☐ The foreseeability of harm from his smoking would be greater, and the degree of care to protect P against such harm would be proportionately greater.

- ☐ No particular legal significance would be attached since the degree of care expected of the nursing staff would not differ merely because of these factors.

3-13   Which of the following actions would have afforded *better*, and nevertheless *reasonable*, protection against the type of occurrence that eventually led to P's death?

- ☐ Nurse S could have assigned staff nurses to check on P's smoking every 10 minutes.

- ☐ Nurse N could have removed P's pipe and matches from his room and forbidden his smoking while in the hospital.

- ☐ Nurse N could have posted a sign near the entrance to P's room forbidding all persons to light P's pipe without first consulting her or Nurse S.

3-12	☐
	☑
	☐

3-13	☐
	☐
	☑

3-14   Under the given facts, what is the only *positive* conclusion that can be drawn with respect to the incident in question?

- ☐ that a passerby probably lit P's pipe for him

- ☐ that P was not adequately protected against a reasonably foreseeable type of harm

- ☐ that P probably attempted (unsuccessfully) to light his pipe by himself since no nurse was around to light it for him

---

3-15   Not all malpractice claims and suits against nurses are related to errors in carrying out technical nursing procedures. In point of fact, one of the most common causes of such claims and suits is falls from beds, examining tables, or x-ray tables. The prudent nurse always should be alert to the possibility of falling by a patient who is elderly, is under sedation, has suffered a head injury, complains of blacking out, or has not fully recovered from the effects of an anesthetic. Failure to anticipate serious injury to a patient with any of these symptoms is pure and simple negligence.

P, an elderly woman who had just undergone an ECG, was removed by Nurse N to an unattended holding room on a stretcher that had no siderails. After being left alone for an hour, P tried unsuccessfully to attract Nurse N's attention. Finally, P got off the stretcher and while trying to reach the bathroom fell and broke her hip.

Was P's fall and broken hip a reasonably foreseeable consequence of leaving her on the stretcher in the manner indicated?

Yes	*No*
☐	☐

3-14   *that P was not adequately protected against a reasonably foreseeable type of harm*

3-15   *Yes*

3-16   Assuming that the hospital had no policy on the use of bedrails for patients undergoing ECGs, which of the following conclusions would be most accurate?

- ☐ In the absence of any hospital policy on the matter, Nurse N could not be held liable for P's injuries.

- ☐ Even without any hospital policy on the matter, Nurse N had a legal duty to protect P from injury, including a possible fall.

- ☐ In the absence of any hospital policy on the matter, the hospital could not be held responsible for P's injuries.

3-17   From the standpoint of the degree of care required in this case, what would probably be the single most important fact a jury would consider in a suit brought by P against Nurse N?

- ☐ the fact that P was left unattended for over an hour

- ☐ the fact that P was impatient and careless

- ☐ the fact that the hospital had no policy on siderails

NOTE: As pointed out in the preceding example, injuries resulting from falls are a common cause of claims against nurses—based on the nurse's simple negligence in failing to safeguard his or her patient from reasonably foreseeable harm. Although the problem of falls concerns all categories of patients, the one category that deserves particular mention is the elderly patient. The nursing student should become sensitive to the mobility problems of older patients.

Clearly, hospital policy in most instances will dictate the necessity for side rails and other forms of restraint to prevent or reduce the hazard of falls. But often the problem boils down to the simple matter of leaving the patient unattended when he or she should not be left alone. How long, and under what circumstances, a patient may be left alone depends on the facts of each case; but the exercise of reasonable care demands that the nurse be alert to the possibility of a serious fall whenever the patient is elderly, has had a sedative, is recovering from the effects of anesthesia, is semiconscious, or is known to suffer dizzy spells.

3-16   *Even without any hospital policy on the matter, Nurse N had a legal duty to protect. . . .*

3-17   *the fact that P was left unattended for over an hour*

Following Physicians' Orders

3-18   Nurses are authorized to perform many acts which, under other circumstances, would constitute the unauthorized practice of medicine. This is particulary true in emergency situations. In addition, a nurse is legally required to carry out any nursing or medical procedure directed by a duly licensed physician *unless* the nurse has reason to believe that harm will come to the patient from the execution of the order.

Under what circumstances can a nurse legally carry out a purely medical procedure?

☐   under no circumstances, since this would constitute the unauthorized practice of medicine

☐   only when ordered to do so by a licensed physician or in an emergency

☐   whenever the patient's condition so requires and no physician is available to order the procedure

---

3-19   Which of the following most accurately states the nurse's legal duty with respect to carrying out a physician's order to perform some medical procedure?

☐   Unless the nurse believes the patient will be harmed, he or she must carry out any procedure ordered by the physician.

☐   The nurse must exercise independent judgment on whether or not a particular medical procedure will prove effective before carrying it out.

☐   The nurse has the duty to follow the physician's orders without question, at the risk of losing his or her license.

NOTE: Under no circumstances should nurses carry out physicians' orders directing them to commit acts they know, or should know, to be *unlawful*. If they do, they will subject themselves to criminal liability, whether or not a patient suffers injury, and they cannot avoid such liability by claiming they were merely following the doctor's orders. As mentioned earlier, however, we will not dwell upon the criminal aspects of nursing law in this course.

3-18   *only when ordered to do so by a licensed physician or in an emergency*

3-19   *Unless the nurse believes the patient will be harmed, he or she must carry out any procedure ordered by the physician.*

3-20   In order to meet his or her legal responsibility to the patient, the nurse who is directed to carry out a medical act must understand both *how* to execute the medical procedure in question and the *effect* of the procedure on the patient.

> Nurse N, a first-year nursing student, is directed by a staff physician to administer a local anesthetic to a patient at a bedside operative procedure. Under the particular state nursing practice act the administration of anesthetics is described as a medical function.

> Under the described circumstances, would Nurse N be acting illegally by carrying out the physician's order?

                              Yes   *No*
                               ☐   ☐

3-21   In order to avoid legal liability in this situation, what would be expected of Nurse N?

☐   Nurse N should get the prior approval of the supervising nurse.

☐   Nurse N should verify the fact that the physician is duly licensed.

☐   Nurse N should know how to administer the anesthetic and be knowledgeable of its effect on the patient.

3-22

Nurse N is given an order by a physician to perform a medical procedure that N has reason to believe will result in harm to the patient.

Which of the following accurately states the legal consequences of carrying out or refusing to carry out the procedure?

☐   By carrying out the procedure with due care, Nurse N cannot be held legally liable for any harm to the patient.

☐   By refusing to carry out the procedure, Nurse N may lose his or her license to practice as a nurse.

☐   By carrying out the procedure without question, Nurse N can be held legally liable for any harm that results to the patient.

3-20 *No*	**3-21** *Nurse N should know how to administer the anesthetic . . .* *For amplification of this response, turn to p. 139, Note B.*	**3-22** *By carrying out the procedure without question, Nurse N can be held legally liable . . .*

3-23   Where harm to the patient is a distinct possibility, reasonable care calls for the nurse to question the physician concerning his or her recommended treatment, thereby alerting the physician to the potential harm that may result. If the nurse does not question the physician's order and harm *does* result to the patient, the nurse is clearly negligent and can be held liable to the patient for his or her own negligent conduct.

How can a nurse avoid legal liability for potential harm to a patient resulting from a procedure carried out under a physician's direct order?

- ☐ by questioning the physician and then proceeding only if the physician agrees to assume full responsibility
- ☐ by noting his or her objections to the ordered treatment on the patient's chart
- ☐ by not carrying out the procedure

3-24   What is the *fundamental* reason why a nurse should *not* follow a physician's order when the nurse has reason to believe some harm will result to the patient?

- ☐ A reasonably prudent nurse should never carry out an act calculated to be dangerous or harmful to the patient.
- ☐ A nurse may lose his or her license to practice by blindly following orders that prove harmful to patients.
- ☐ A nurse is likely to have his or her malpractice insurance canceled if he or she is involved in too many malpractice suits.

3-25

A physician writes the following order: "Patient to be walked 5 minutes every day *without fail*." Nurse N, about to get the patient up the following day, is told by her: "I'm terribly sick. My head is swimming, and I feel faint." Nurse N, referring to the doctor's order, insists that the patient walk, but the patient falls and is injured in the process.

Who is *likely* to be held liable for the harm caused?

- ☐ the doctor only
- ☐ the nurse and the doctor
- ☐ the nurse only

3-23   ☐ For information concern-
          ☐ ing the correct procedure
          ☑ to follow, turn to p. 139,
             Note C.

3-24   ☑
          ☐
          ☐

3-25   ☐ If you are uncertain about
          ☐ the correct answer, turn to
          ☑ p. 139, Note D.

EXPLANATORY NOTES

Note A   (from Frame 3-4)

Both the first and third items are directly related to the patient's safety, but neither represents a legal duty of care with respect to the patient's safety. The courts always express legal duties in general terms, thereby permitting the pertinent legal rules (or standards) to be applied in a variety of fact situations. The second item expresses a rule in this manner.

Proceed to Frame 3-5.

Note B   (from Frame 3-21)

It is highly unlikely that a first-year nursing student would know, or would be expected to know, how to administer an anesthetic for a bedside surgical procedure. The given example was chosen expressly to illustrate that apart from the *legality* of carrying out a physician's order, there is the separate issue of the nurse's potential *liability* for attempting to carry it out if the nurse (1) does not know how to perform the procedure, and (2) is not aware of the effect of the procedure on the patient.

Proceed to Frame 3-22.

Note C   (from Frame 3-23)

The nurse who is directed to carry out a medical order that he or she is not qualified to perform or which the nurse believes will result in harm to the patient should immediately bring the matter to the attention of the nursing supervisor or a responsible hospital official in the event the supervisor is unavailable. If the nurse is a student, he or she should bring the matter to the attention of the nursing instructor or a responsible hospital official in the event the instructor is unavailable. As mentioned in an earlier note, both patient and nurse will benefit from a clear understanding by the nurse of his or her legal responsibilities and forthright conduct in these difficult situations.

Proceed to Frame 3-24.

Note D   (from Frame 3-25)

In retrospect, the doctor's order may have been too inflexible, but since walking a patient is a rather routine medical order, there is no basis for finding the doctor negligent on that basis alone. The nurse, however, is supposed to exercise independent professional judgment in a situation such as this, and the nurse's inflexibility is legally unpardonable. While it is possible that both the doctor and the nurse would be held liable for the harm caused the patient, most courts would fix the blame on the nurse, whose (unsuccessful) defense would be that she was "just following the doctor's orders."

Proceed to Frame 3-26.

3-26   A nurse's intervention may take the form of requesting the physician to clarify an order or objecting to carrying out the order when the nurse *knows* it to be harmful or erroneous. This responsibility to protect the patient from harm applies to all types of nursing activities, from the most simple to the most complex.

> Nurse N, a certified registered nurse-anesthetist, is directed by the operating surgeon to administer a general halogenated anesthetic to the patient. Knowing the anesthetic agent in question to be contraindicated because of the patient's past history of hepatitis, Nurse N suggests to the surgeon a more appropriate substitute. The surgeon dismisses the nurse's suggestion and repeats the order to administer the original anesthetic drug.

Why should, or should not, Nurse N follow the surgeon's direct order in this instance?

☐ Nurse N should not follow the order, since it is N's primary responsibility to determine the appropriate anesthetic agent.

☐ Nurse N should not follow the order, since N has a primary legal responsibility to protect the patient from harm.

☐ Nurse N should follow the order, since N gave the surgeon a second opportunity to consider the order and change it as suggested.

3-27   Indicate which of the following classes of nurses is authorized to challenge a physician's order:

☐ private-duty nurses   ☐ occupational health nurses   ☐ nurse-specialists

☐ general-duty nurses   ☐ licensed practical nurses   ☐ all nurses

---

3-26 *Nurse N should not follow the order, since N has a primary responsibility to protect the patient from harm.*

3-27 *all nurses*

PHYSICIANS' ASSISTANTS AND NURSES

What is the nurse's legal duty with respect to following or challenging the order(s) of a legally certified physician's assistant? This brings into focus the entire issue of the relationship between physicians' assistants and the hospitals, nursing homes, and other facilities in which they work. Since the mid-1970s, many state legislatures have enacted statutes defining physicians' assistants and delineating the scope of the services they may provide and the degree of medical supervision they require. There is still a considerable amount of confusion concerning these matters, and nursing organizations have raised many objections about the broad authority granted physicians' assistants under many of these laws.

The Joint Commission on Accreditation of Hospitals has recognized physicians' assistants as being part of the hospital's medical staff, and the few court cases discussing the point have supported this position. In 1979, the Washington State Nurses Association challenged a regulation promulgated by the State Board of Medical Examiners (pursuant to statutory authority) authorizing physicians' assistants to issue prescriptions for medications and to write medical orders for patient care. The Nurses Association took the position that the State Board of Medical Examiners had exceeded its statutory authority in granting such broad delegated medical authority, and that this would, in effect, require nurses to execute prescriptions issued by physicians' assistants as well as by physicians.

The court ruled in favor of the Board of Medical Examiners, stating in part, "Two provisions in the statutes authorizing physicians' assistants to practice medicine indicate a legislative intent to create an agency relationship. . . . These provisions for control and responsibility indicate that the actions of the assistant are to be considered as actions of the supervising physician." *Washington State Nurses Association v. Board of Medical Examiners*, 605 P. 2d 1269 (Wash. 1980).

On the matter of carrying out a physician's assistant's orders, the Iowa Attorney General has ruled that "if the physician's assistant can carry out the intent of the physician under whose supervision he acts and performs his duties . . . only by giving certain orders to a nurse, then he has a legal right to give those orders and the nurse is under a legal obligation to obey them." Iowa Attorney General Opinion No. 78-12-41, Dec. 30, 1978. By the same token, to the extent the nurse has a legal duty to challenge a physician's order, the nurse has the same duty to challenge orders transmitted by a physician's assistant.

3-28   The nurse must be tactful and courteous in questioning a physician's order, and must be prepared to justify his or her position. Challenging a physician's apparently harmful order calls for a keen awareness of the physician's professional and psychological position, but the responsible nurse must *never* permit a fear of rebuke by the physician to override a fundamental concern for the welfare and safety of the patient.

Consider the following case:

A hospital staff physician writes an order for an unusually large dose of a drug for a patient, and three staff nurses have serious doubts concerning the quantity of the drug ordered. Each broaches the subject to the physician in a different manner:

Which of these nurses has sufficiently alerted the physician to the possible danger involved in carrying out the order?

☐ Nurse A: "Doctor, I simply will *not* give Mrs. P such a massive dose of _____. I'm sure it will harm her. Are you sure you know what you are doing?"

☐ Nurse B: "Doctor, I see you have ordered an injection of 30 mL _____ for Mrs. P. That is a much larger dose than we usually give, and since it might be harmful in that dosage, I thought I'd better check with you. Did you really intend it to be 30 mL?"

☐ Nurse C: "Doctor, will you please explain to me why you have ordered such a large dose of _____ for Mrs. P? All the nurses I've spoken to say that you must have made an error and I'm afraid to risk giving the injection unless you can give me a good explanation."

3-29   Which nurse has brought the matter to the physician's attention in the manner *most likely* to bring about the desired result?

Nurse A   *Nurse B*   *Nurse C*
☐   ☐   ☐

3-28   ☑
            ☑
            ☑

3-29   *Nurse B*

For information about a related problem, turn to Note A, p. 148.

3-30

P, a female patient of Doctor D, was noted to be anemic in her thirty-fifth week of pregnancy, and the doctor immediately ordered a blood transfusion in the emergency room of the local hospital. Doctor D set the amount of blood to be administered at 1000 mL and injected the needle and started administering saline solution prior to the actual transfusion of blood. Doctor D then set the stopcock on the saline solution at the desired rate and left, giving Nurse N instructions only to continue with the procedure.

After the saline solution had been administered, Nurse N connected the container of blood and set the stopcock at the same rate of flow that earlier had been set by Doctor D. The latter returned while the blood was still being transfused and commented that all was in order. When P had received the full 1000 mL of blood, she was permitted to leave the emergency room but was brought back shortly thereafter, suffering from pulmonary edema. She died, despite all efforts to save her and her child.

P's estate sues Nurse N for alleged malpractice in failing to slow down the rate of flow of the blood being transfused. At the trial all the testifying physicians agree that the attack of pulmonary edema was principally due to the transfusion of such a large quantity of blood into a patient in the last stages of pregnancy and that the *rapid rate of flow* was a contributing factor that probably hastened the patient's death.

The facts as stated indicate that Nurse N   ☐ did have   ☐ did not have

the necessary qualifications to carry out the transfusion.

3-31   Establishment of the rate of flow of blood in this case would be

☐ a matter for Nurse N's personal judgment

☐ a matter of medical judgment for the physician

☐ a matter of hospital policy

3-30   *did have*

3-31   *a matter of medical judgment for the physician*

3-32   What was Nurse N's legal duty with respect to carrying out the transfusion that was begun by Doctor D?

☐ Nurse N was required to challenge Doctor D's decision to transfuse such a large quantity of blood at such a rapid rate.

☐ Nurse N was required to follow Doctor D's orders unless there was some reason to suspect harm would result to the patient.

☐ Nurse N should have slowed the rate of flow of the blood in the exercise of independent professional judgment.

3-33   If Nurse N, *acting on his or her own,* had slowed the rate of flow of the transfusion but P nevertheless died of pulmonary edema, what legal consequence would this have?

☐ Doctor D could sue Nurse N for malpractice.

☐ Nurse N could be charged with practicing medicine without a license.

☐ Nurse N would avoid liability by having acted in the patient's best interests.

3-34   Accepting as true the proposition that the quantity and rapid rate of flow of the blood transfused into the patient was the probable cause of death, who most likely would be held liable for P's death in this case?

☐ Doctor D

☐ Nurse N

☐ the hospital

3-32 ☐ ☑ ☐	**3-33** *Nurse N could be charged with practicing medicine without a license.* The scope of nursing practice issues are discussed more fully in Part 4.	**3-34** *Doctor D*

POINTS TO REMEMBER

1. The nurse is legally required to exercise reasonable care to safeguard his or her patient from any known or reasonably foreseeable harm.

2. The safety and security of the patient is a paramount responsibility of the nurse although the physician shares this legal responsibility.

3. A nurse is legally authorized and required to carry out any nursing or medical procedure he or she is directed to carry out by a duly licensed physician unless the nurse has reason to believe harm will result to the patient from doing so.

4. Where there is no medical reason to question a physician's order, failure to carry out such an order will subject the nurse to liability for any consequent harm to the patient.

5. To meet his or her legal responsibility in carrying out a physician's order, the nurse must know *how* to execute the procedure in question as well as the *effect* of the procedure on the patient.

6. When a nurse has reason to question a physician's order, he or she should do so tactfully, but directly, keeping in mind the fundamental rule that the patient's safety is always of paramount concern.

7. If there are reasonable grounds for believing some harm will come to the patient if he or she carries out a physician's order, the nurse has a legal duty *not* to follow the order. The nurse should bring the matter immediately to the attention of the supervisor (or instructor, in the case of a nursing student). If the supervisor or instructor is not available at the moment, the matter should be brought to the attention of a responsible hospital official.

8. The above legal rules with respect to following or challenging orders given by a physician apply with equal force to orders given to the nurse by a physician's assistant acting on behalf of the physician employer.

Observation and Diagnosis Errors

3-35   Except in an emergency situation where a physician is not available, or where specifically authorized by statute, it is unlawful for a nurse to *medically* diagnose a patient's condition for the purpose of instituting positive treatment or therapeutic measures. This is clearly the province and function of the physician. However, the professional nurse is always authorized to make a *nursing diagnosis,* in order to evaluate those factors (physical, mental, sociological, and economic) that may have an influence on the patient's recovery. The nurse may then take appropriate steps based on such diagnosis to prevent complications or anything that might worsen the patient's condition.

Under what circumstances may a nurse make a diagnosis?

☐   whenever the nurse believes he or she has sufficient experience to be able to do so

☐   whenever the nurse is required to evaluate the patient's condition to determine the specific needs for nursing care

☐   under no circumstances, since this is the physician's sole responsibility

---

3-36   What type of diagnosis is a nurse *prohibited* from making?

☐   one that involves evaluating the patient's state of mind or reaction to a particular course of treatment

☐   one that involves evaluating external influences affecting the patient's condition, such as family relationships or financial problems

☐   one that involves medical judgments concerning the patient's condition for the purpose of instituting specific treatment

---

3-37   In an emergency a nurse legally may make a medical diagnosis and undertake whatever medical treatment is necessary before a physician can be summoned and arrives.

True   *False*
  ☐   ☐

3-35 ☐	3-36 ☐	3-37 *True*
☑	☐	If you checked the wrong an-
☐	☑	swer, turn to p. 148, Note B.

3-38   One of the fundamental legal responsibilities of the nurse is the duty to keep accurate records of the patient's physical and mental condition (e.g., temperature, pulse, and other overt physical signs, as well as emotional behavior). This responsibility is one that is shared by practical and registered professional nurses alike, but the registered nurse, because of special training, has the additional responsibility of *interpreting* and *evaluating* the patient's symptoms and reactions to any nursing or medical regimen and reporting them to the physician so he or she may make appropriate adjustments in the prescribed treatment.

Recording and reporting the patient's physical signs and general emotional behavior is the responsibility of

☐   all nurses

☐   registered nurses only

☐   practical nurses only

3-39   Why is the registered nurse held to a higher standard of care than the practical nurse with respect to reporting the patient's reactions and symptoms?

☐   because the registered nurse is more directly involved in patient care

☐   because the registered nurse has been trained to evaluate and interpret reactions and symptoms and to make judgments thereon concerning essential action necessary

☐   because practical nurses are not expected to concern themselves with reactions and symptoms of their patients

---

3-38 *all nurses*	**3-39** ☐ The respective roles of the ☑ R.N. and L.P.N. are dis- ☐ cussed on p. 149, Note C.

EXPLANATORY NOTES

Note A   (from Frame 3-29)

What happens if the nurse discreetly challenges the physician's order but the physician nevertheless chooses to proceed with the treatment? Should the nurse simply remain silent? Not if the nurse really cares about the patients and at the same time wants to protect both himself or herself and the hospital from possible liability. There is a growing trend for the courts to hold hospitals liable for a nurse's failure to report obvious negligence to another physician in a position to correct the situation before the patient is harmed. The reasonably prudent nurse, therefore, will not simply challenge the physician but will follow through with a prompt report of the matter to the appropriate hospital authority. In short, "going through the motions" will not protect the nurse or hospital employer from legal liability when a physician's course of conduct is clearly calculated to harm a patient.

Proceed to Frame 3-30.

Note B   (from Frame 3-37)

It is well established that in an emergency situation a nurse may perform any medical act deemed necessary to preserve life or limb. The reasonableness of the nurse's conduct in such a situation is always gauged by the surrounding circumstances, and the nurse is not held to the standard of nursing care expected under more normal circumstances. In all cases involving emergency care it is expected that the nurse will summon medical assistance as soon as possible, and the legal privilege of making medical judgments and undertaking medical acts in an emergency is limited to those immediate, at-the-scene measures deemed absolutely necessary to save life or limb.

Proceed to Frame 3-38.

Note C   (from Frame 3-39)

Both the R.N. and L.P.N. share the common objective of rendering skillful nursing care to the ill, injured, or infirm, but the L.P.N.'s legal status, as determined by state and provincial licensure laws, is considerably more restricted due to the more limited educational background of the L.P.N. Both the R.N. and the L.P.N. are required to have the same basic concepts of nursing care (including the necessary manual skills), but the R.N. has a much greater responsibility for (1) assessing the nursing needs of patients, (2) evaluating the incapacities of patients, (3) judging how much the patient can do for himself or herself and how much assistance he or she needs, and (4) understanding and observing the effects of the treatments and medications administered. The R.N., by training, has been prepared to structure a comprehensive nursing care plan to fit the needs of the individual patient.

The L.P.N., by contrast, is authorized to perform *selected* nursing acts, and then only under the direction of a physician, dentist, or R.N. In the institutional setting the L.P.N. generally works in a close relationship with the R.N. and under the R.N.'s direct supervision. The L.P.N.'s concern for proper patient care is every bit as great as that of the R.N., and in some areas continuing shortages of R.N.'s have imposed many additional responsibilities on L.P.N.'s. It is clear, however, that the L.P.N. is not authorized to supervise, manage a nursing unit, or teach. While the L.P.N. may perform many of the same nursing functions performed by R.N.'s, he or she must always be aware of his or her legal limitations in areas where the professional judgment expected of an R.N. is called for.

Proceed to Frame 3-40.

3-40

Prior to delivery of Patient P's child, Doctor D made a small incision to relieve the constrictive muscle surrounding the cervix. D left the incision unsutured, but pelvic packs were inserted to control bleeding. Nurse N informed Doctor D while D was still at the hospital that she believed the patient was bleeding too much, but each time D insisted her condition was normal.

Doctor D then instructed Nurse N in how to measure the rate of flow of the bleeding and gave orders to call if the postpartum flow was greater than normal. One hour later Nurse N noted excessive bleeding but did not take the patient's blood pressure, temperature, pulse, or respiration, nor did she call Doctor D because, in her opinion, D would not have come back to the hospital anyhow. A relief nurse who came on duty 30 minutes later could not locate the patient's pulse and immediately called Doctor D, but by the time D arrived the patient had died from the hemorrhage.

P's estate sues Doctor D and Nurse N for their alleged malpractice in treatment.

What legal duty did Nurse N have with respect to keeping track of P's vital signs?

☐ the duty to record vital signs as soon as the patient's condition began to deteriorate

☐ the duty to record vital signs at regular intervals and to report significant changes to the physician

☐ the duty to use her best professional judgment concerning the desirability of or need for recording vital signs

---

3-41   Would Nurse N's failure to note the patient's blood pressure, pulse, respiration, and temperature represent a departure from the standard of care expected in such a situation?

Yes   *No*
☐   ☐

3-40 *the duty to record vital signs at regular intervals and to report significant changes . . .*

3-41 *Yes*

3-42   What *significant* error in judgment did Nurse N make in this case?

☐   Nurse N misjudged the seriousness of the patient's condition until it was too late.

☐   Nurse N assumed that Doctor D would not be responsive to any emergency call on her part.

☐   Nurse N assumed that the patient's condition would improve rather than worsen.

3-43   What would a reasonably prudent nurse have done under the circumstances of this case?

☐   He or she would have taken the patient's vital signs regularly and would have called Doctor D as soon as he or she determined the patient's bleeding was excessive.

☐   He or she would have waited until the patient's bleeding was serious enough to ensure that Doctor D would respond to an emergency call.

☐   He or she would have informed the patient's family of the situation so that they might prevail upon Doctor D to take appropriate remedial action.

3-44   If Doctor D is held liable for malpractice in failing to suture the incision immediately after the baby was delivered, will Nurse N thereby be relieved of liability for her conduct?

Yes   *No*
☐   ☐

3-42 ☐ ☑ ☐	**3-43** ☑ ☐ ☐	**3-44** *No* If you checked the wrong answer, turn to p. 162, Note A.

Failure to Communicate

3-45 Nurses must continually evaluate a mass of information and findings, and as soon as they become aware of significant medical data, dangerous circumstances, or a dramatic worsening of the patient's condition, they are required to communicate this to the treating physician at once. Their failure to communicate these observations can have disastrous consequences and will certainly increase the chances for malpractice litigation.

A mother brought her two young boys to the hospital's emergency department for treatment of rashes and fever. She specifically mentions to Nurse N that she had taken several ticks from the body of one of the children, but Nurse N fails to communicate this information to Doctor D, the emergency department physician. As a result, Doctor D diagnoses measles rather than Rocky Mountain spotted fever, and the condition of both children deteriorates rapidly, with one child dying several days later. Doctor D eventually makes the correct diagnosis and is able to treat the second child successfully.

In a lawsuit brought by the parents of the deceased child against the hospital, Doctor D, and Nurse N, whom would a jury most likely find *primarily* liable for the child's wrongful death?

☐ Nurse N, because the nurse failed to communicate the vital information that could have saved the child's life

☐ Doctor D, because it was the physician's responsibility to make an accurate diagnosis and prescribe accordingly

☐ the hospital, because it guarantees the quality of care provided to all patients seeking care in its emergency department

---

3-46 If Nurse N is held liable, is it likely that the hospital employer will also be held liable?

Yes No
☐ ☐

3-45 *Nurse N, because the nurse failed to communicate the vital information that could have saved the child's life*

3-46 *Yes*

3-47   With respect to the matter of communication, indicate whether the conclusions set forth below are true or false.

True	False	
☐	☐	It is the nurse's legal duty to observe and report to the treating physician all significant changes in the patient's condition.
☐	☐	It is the nurse's legal duty to communicate abnormal data about a patient to the physician only when the nurse believes the physician will take appropriate action based thereon.
☐	☐	In deciding whether or not to communicate significant data to the treating physician, it is the nurse's responsibility to determine what is significant and what is not.
☐	☐	A nurse cannot be held liable for failing to contact a physician about a patient's worsening condition when the nurse knows from past experience the physician would not respond to the call.
☐	☐	When a nurse cannot locate the patient's physician to report vital information about his or her worsening condition, the nurse should communicate the information to a supervisor.

3-48   The fundamental reason why a nurse should communicate essential facts and information about a patient's worsening condition to the treating physician is

☐ to comply with hospital regulations

☐ to comply with specific medical orders

☐ to reduce the risk of harm to the patient

3-47	True	False	**3-48**	*to reduce the risk of harm to the patient*
	☑	☐		
	☐	☑		
	☑	☐		
	☐	☑		
	☑	☐		

Improper Supervision

3-49   Negligence in supervision is a growing cause of malpractice claims against registered professional nurses. The registered nurse who is a supervisor, unlike other categories of nurses, is legally and professionally responsible for directing and supervising the activities of practical nurses, nurse's aides, and other nurses involved in direct patient care. Ordinarily, supervisors are held liable only for their *own* negligence in caring for a patient, but they can also be held liable, under certain circumstances, for the negligence of someone they are supervising.

Which of the following classes of nurses can be held liable for negligence in supervision?

☐   practical nurses

☐   registered nurses

☐   nursing students

3-50   Why would a practical nurse not be held liable for negligence in supervision?

☐   because practical nurses are generally prudent and careful

☐   because practical nurses are not competent to supervise others

☐   because practical nurses are not legally or professionally responsible for supervising others

---

3-51   In general, a nursing supervisor's potential liability is   ☐ greater than   ☐ the same as   ☐ less than   that of other hospital-based nurses.

3-49 *registered nurses*	**3-50** ☐ ☐ ☑	**3-51** *greater than*

3-52   A nursing supervisor, as a specialist, is held to the standard of care of the reasonably prudent nursing supervisor in carrying out professional and administrative responsibilities. This includes not only the making of staff assignments, but his or her conduct in other supervisory situations.

> Supervisory Nurse S was informed by staff Nurse N that one of his patients who was recovering from major surgery showed clear signs of advancing tetanus. Supervisor S chose not to call the patient's physician because he knew the physician was out of town at a medical conference, nor did S summon any other physician for a period of three days. By that time, the patient's condition had so deteriorated that all efforts to save him were futile.

Nurse S's liability, if any, in this case would be based on

☐ her negligence in supervising Nurse N

☐ the doctrine of *respondeat superior*

☐ the rule of personal liability

3-53   The supervisor who assigns duties to an otherwise competent nurse cannot be held liable for the latter's negligence in carrying out those duties *simply because he or she is the nurse's supervisor*. Under the rule of personal liability, every person is legally responsible for his or her own negligent conduct.

> Nurse S is a supervisory nurse in a general hospital and Nurse N is S's subordinate. Both are registered nurses with several years of experience in all phases of nursing. Nurse S assigns Nurse N to a pediatric unit, and while there, Nurse N negligently administers an overdose of a medication to an infant.

Will Nurse S be held liable for Nurse N's negligent conduct under these circumstances?

Yes   No
☐   ☐

3-52   *the rule of personal liability*   **3-53**   *No*

3-54   Liability for negligence in supervision is generally based upon (1) failure of the supervisor to determine which of the patient's needs he or she can safely assign to a subordinate nurse or (2) failure of the supervisor to give closer personal supervision to a subordinate who requires such supervision.

A malpractice suit is filed against Supervisory Nurse S for injuries resulting from a nursing student's negligence in catheterizing a patient. At the trial it is shown that Nurse S was aware of the student's limited experience with catheterization procedures at the time she made the assignment. The jury finds Nurse S negligent and holds her liable for the injuries to the patient.

Which one or more of the following actions on Nurse S's part might have shielded her from liability in this situation?

☐   She could have performed the procedure herself in a safe manner.

☐   She could have directed the nursing student in the performance of the procedure, to ensure it was done safely in her presence.

☐   She could have assigned the procedure to a nurse she knew to be capable of carrying it out safely.

3-55   On what grounds (if any) might the nursing student in the previous frame also be held liable?

☐   He could be held liable for failing to meet the standard of care expected of his supervisor.

☐   He could be held liable for attempting to carry out a procedure clearly beyond his capabilities.

☐   He could not be held liable since he was only a nursing student.

3-54   ☑
          ☑
          ☑

3-55   *He could be held liable for attempting to carry out a procedure clearly beyond his capabilities.*

3-56   What is the general rule regarding the legal liability of a supervisory nurse?

- ☐ The supervisory nurse cannot be held liable for acts of negligence on the part of registered nurses he or she supervises, but can be held liable for acts of negligence on the part of practical nurses or nurse's aides whom he or she supervises.

- ☐ The supervisory nurse is not automatically liable for all acts of negligence on the part of those whom he or she supervises, but may be held liable where he or she is negligent in supervising others.

- ☐ The supervisory nurse cannot be held liable for acts of negligence on the part of nurses whom he or she supervises since each nurse is liable for his or her own negligent conduct.

3-57   It should be noted that even though a supervisory nurse may be held liable for the negligence of subordinates, this liability is not based on the doctrine of *respondeat superior,* since this doctrine is applicable only to persons or legal entities who are in a master-servant or principal-agent relationship. Supervisory nurses are not the employers (masters) of the nurses who work under their supervision, even though they exercise their authority on behalf of their hospital or nursing home employer.

Patient P, injured while being treated in Hospital H, files suit against Supervisory Nurse S for the negligent acts of Nurse N, who had been assigned by Nurse S to care for him.

If P is to prevail in his suit against Nurse S, he will have to prove

- ☐ that Nurse S stood in the same legal position as Nurse N's employer because of the authority to supervise granted to Nurse S

- ☐ that Nurse S was negligent in his own right and not because of any secondary or derivative liability imposed on him

- ☐ that Nurse S is liable because a supervisor is always responsible for the acts of subordinates

---

3-56 ☐
          ☑
          ☐

3-57 *that Nurse S was negligent in his own right. . . .*

SUPERVISORS AND THE MAKING OF FLOAT ASSIGNMENTS

Whatever the title—head nurse, charge nurse, patient care supervisor, or other comparable designation—the nursing supervisor is the person legally in charge. This means he or she is not only directly responsible for supervising the work of floor-duty nurses, but the services of Special Duty nurses, nursing students, nurses' aides, orderlies, and technicians as well. In short, the nursing supervisor is responsible for seeing to it that all medical orders on his or her unit are executed promptly and skillfully, and that all appropriate measures are taken to insure patient safety.

The supervisor is usually less concerned about his or her legal liability for the acts of nursing personnel in routine nursing settings than when circumstances are not routine and the supervisor has to make "float" assignments. Floating nurses to understaffed hospital units presents legal problems for all parties involved, but they can be especially troublesome to the nursing supervisor, who often has to make on-the-spot decisions that can have a significant impact on patient safety. The legal rules are those outlined in the preceding frames, and are easy enough to understand; it is their application to specific float situations that is often difficult.

The supervisor who is forced to float a nurse to a specialty unit (pediatrics, intensive care, coronary care, emergency department) with full knowledge of the nurse's limitations in that nursing specialty, will be held legally liable for any consequent injury to patients who suffer harm because of the nurse's negligence. The conscientious nursing supervisor who must make staffing assignments with inadequate numbers of trained nurses should not permit the situation to get out of hand. The supervisor should make hospital administration fully aware of the potential harm to patients as well as his or her greatly increased personal legal liability for acts of negligence committed by improperly trained staff nurses. Documenting his or her concerns and maintaining records of all communications to the appropriate hospital authorities will aid considerably if the supervisor is later forced to defend the making of such assignments in court.

POINTS TO REMEMBER

1. Except in an emergency, or when authorized by statute, a nurse may not lawfully make a *medical* diagnosis of a patient's condition for the purpose of instituting treatment.

2. A professional nurse is legally authorized to make a *nursing* diagnosis to determine appropriate steps necessary to prevent complications or a worsening of the patient's condition.

3. A nursing diagnosis is one that involves the evaluation of all physical, mental, sociological, and economic factors that have an influence on the patient's recovery.

4. In a life-threatening emergency a nurse may make a medical diagnosis and undertake whatever treatment is necessary before a physician can be summoned and arrives.

5. A fundamental legal responsibility of the nurse is to keep accurate records of the patient's physical and mental condition.

6. Because of additional training, the professional nurse is held to a higher standard of care than the practical nurse in *evaluating* the patient's reactions and symptoms.

7. Although supervisory nurses ordinarily are held liable only for their own negligent acts, under certain circumstances they can also be held liable for negligence in supervising others.

8. Negligence arising out of supervision applies only to professional nurses since a practical nurse has neither the legal authority nor the responsibility to exercise professional supervision over subordinates.

9. Supervisory negligence may result from assigning a task to a subordinate that is clearly beyond the latter's capabilities and from failing to give closer supervision to someone who requires such supervision.

10. Even though a supervisor may be held liable for supervisory negligence, the negligent subordinate nevertheless is not thereby relieved of liability for his or her own negligent conduct.

Medication Errors

3-58   Mistakes in administering medications are among the most common causes of malpractice suits against nurses. Liability of the nurse may result from administering the wrong dose to the wrong patient or at the wrong time, or failing to administer the proper medication at the right time or in the properly prescribed manner. A frequent cause of medication errors by nurses is misreading a doctor's order or failing to check with the doctor when the order is questionable.

> In a hurry, a physician writes an incomplete and partially illegible medication order. Nurse N, in an effort to be efficient and in order not to bother the physician with questions, decides which drug was intended, the dosage form, and the route of administration of the drug. Nurse N's judgment proves wrong, and the patient suffers serious harm.

On what basis could Nurse N be held liable for failing to have exercised reasonable care?

☐   for failing to question the physician concerning the incomplete and partially illegible medication order

☐   for showing more concern for the doctor than for the patient

☐   for prescribing a drug without proper legal authority

3-59

> Patient P goes to Doctor D's office for treatment of a dislocated thumb, and Doctor D asks the office nurse, Nurse N, to secure Novocain for local anesthesia. Nurse N orders a medical technician (also employed by Doctor D) to get the drug, but the latter, by mistake, hands Nurse N a bottle labeled Adrenalin. Nurse N does not check the label and prepares the hypodermic for Doctor D. Thirty minutes after receiving the injection, Patient P dies from a systemic reaction to the Adrenalin.

What conduct on the part of Nurse N would legally constitute unreasonable care in this case?

☐   requesting a technician to get the drug

☐   failing to check the label on the drug

☐   preparing the hypodermic before showing the drug to the doctor

---

3-58 ☑ Amplification of the nurse's ☐ responsibilities in drug ad- ☐ ministration can be found on p. 162, Note B.	**3-59** *failing to check the label on the drug*

3-60   Would Doctor D have a right to assume that the hypodermic prepared by Nurse N contained the proper drug in the proper dosage?

Yes   *No*

☐   ☐

3-61   Who could be held liable to P's estate in this case?

☐ only Nurse N

☐ only Doctor D

☐ only the technician

☐ both Nurse N and Doctor D

☐ Nurse N, Doctor D, and the technician

3-62   Many medication errors involve faulty technique in giving injections, usually resulting in nerve injury to the patient. Certainly, not every nerve injury following an injection is attributable to faulty technique on the part of the nurse, but where the onset of nerve injury is immediate and not otherwise explainable, the nurse generally is held liable for negligence in giving the injection.

Practical Nurse N gives a 5-year-old patient an intramuscular injection in his left buttock. Immediately thereafter the child experiences a painful, burning reaction at the site of the injection. A hematoma, ecchymosis, and sloughing soon develop at the site of the injection, necessitating additional medical care and surgery.

The facts as stated prove that Nurse N was negligent in giving the injection.

True   *False*

☐   ☐

3-60 *Yes*	**3-61** ☐	**3-62** *False*
As a general rule the answer is "yes." The facts in a specific case might prove otherwise, however.	☐ ☐ ☐ ☑	If you checked True, turn to p. 163, Note C.

EXPLANATORY NOTES

Note A   (from Frame 3-44)

Throughout this course it has been stressed repeatedly that every professional person is liable for his or her own negligent conduct (malpractice), and this frame illustrates this principle once again. The fact that the physician is held liable for personal negligent conduct does not mean that the nurse is free from liability for his or her negligent conduct. As a matter of fact, many of the more recent malpractice cases have involved both the physician and the nurse, and in a number of these cases both parties have been held liable for their concurrent acts of negligence. Remember: The rule of personal liability is always operative, and it should serve as a constant warning to nurses that they must act with reasonable care at all times.

Proceed to Frame 3-45.

Note B   (from Frame 3-58)

Perhaps no aspect of nursing care is fraught with more risk than that relating to the administration of drugs. It has been reliably estimated that nearly one out of every seven medication orders in hospitals is erroneously carried out, emphasizing the extreme caution that must be exercised by all nurses who handle drugs. In no other area of nursing practice is there a greater need for independent and intelligent judgment, and the wise nurse will *always* question an ambiguous or incomplete medication order. The courts are not as lenient and forgiving as they once were, and more and more nurses are being held liable for medication errors as the number and potency of new drugs continue to increase.

Many physicians permit their office nurses to authorize prescription refills by telephone without direct orders from the physician. While this practice is permissible, since the nurse is merely acting as a conduit for information, it should be clearly noted that a nurse is not permitted to *prescribe* and will be held personally liable for the untoward consequences of advising a patient what medication to take, *even though the drug may be purchased without a physician's prescription*. This type of activity is to be deplored since it involves the area of medical diagnosis, and the office nurse would be well advised to refrain from giving gratuitous advice concerning medications over the telephone.

Proceed to Frame 3-59.

Note C   (from Frame 3-62)

There have been cases in which the very fact of nerve injury following an injection has been submitted as proof of negligence, but most courts do not accept this proposition and require *some* proof of negligence on the part of the nurse. Most medical practitioners would agree that unforeseen and undesirable reactions from an injection can result from causes other than negligence, including the emotions and allergies of the patient, non-traumatic arthritis associated with the injection (but not due to negligence), and the internal condition of the patient before or after an operation. Nurses administering injections are not held liable where the resulting injury is not directly related to improper technique in administering the injection. For this reason, the correct response to this frame is a negative answer.

Proceed to Frame 3-63.

Negligence in Caring for Mentally Ill Patients

3-63   Earlier it was pointed out that the nature and quality of nursing care legally required to protect patients from harm are based on the patients' physical conditions and on their ability to contribute to their own safety and security. This rule assumes particular importance when the patients are suffering some form of mental illness that prevents them from appreciating the risk of harm to which they may be exposed.

      Which of the following factors is legally significant in determining the degree of care required to protect a patient from harm?

☐   the status of the attending nurse as a general-duty nurse or as a specialist

☐   the type of hospital the patient is in (TB, general, mental)

☐   the patient's physical and mental condition

3-64   Why is the nurse held to a higher standard of care in safeguarding a mentally ill patient?

☐   because this type of patient is the one who most frequently brings lawsuits

☐   because a mentally ill person frequently does not appreciate his or her exposure to potential harm

☐   because state and provincial statutes generally impose a higher standard of care with respect to the treatment of mentally ill persons

---

3-65   Rank the following patients in order of the quality and degree of nursing care necessary to protect each of them from any foreseeable harm (use 1, 2, and 3, placing a 1 in the box before the patient requiring the most care):

☐   a 41-year-old woman about to undergo a hysterectomy

☐   a 72-year-old alcoholic with a schizophrenic syndrome

☐   a 10-year-old girl convalescing with a fractured leg

3-62 *the patient's physical and mental condition*	**3-64** ☐
	         ☑
	         ☐
		3-65 ③
		         ①
		         ②

3-66   When there is neither any prior history nor any present indication that the patient is dangerous to others or to himself or herself, the degree of care and watchfulness expected of the nurse is less. Correspondingly, the degree of alertness must be heightened where suicide has been repeatedly threatened or the patient has known assaultive tendencies.

Indicate whether the nurse would be expected to exercise normal care or special care in supervising each of the following patients, basing your answer solely on the characteristics noted.

Normal care	*Special care*	
☐	☐	The patient has a violent temperament.
☐	☐	The patient is scheduled for surgery.
☐	☐	The patient is mentally retarded.
☐	☐	The patient is a paranoid schizophrenic.

3-67

Patient P is convalescing from leg surgery and is permitted to move about in a wheelchair. He has been unruly on several occasions and on one occasion four attendants were required to hold him down in bed. Nurse N, the head nurse on P's floor, issues no special orders with respect to P's supervision.

Yes	*No*	
☐	☐	Is P's described conduct such that it is reasonably foreseeable he may cause injury to someone?
☐	☐	Would Nurse N be justified in taking special precautions in supervising P's care?
☐	☐	If P causes injury to someone, can Nurse N be held liable for failing to order closer supervision of him?

3-66 *Normal care*	*Special care*		**3-67** *Yes*	*No*
☐	☑		☑	☐
☑	☐		☑	☐
☐	☑		☑	☐
☐	☑			

3-68   The prudent nurse must learn how to assess the suicidal potential of a patient before the act is committed. The nurse should know that the older patient is much more likely to commit suicide than the younger or middle-aged patient; that although women make more suicide attempts than men, men successfully commit suicide at a rate twice that of women; and that almost all successful suicides have a history of at least one prior attempt.

Patient P, a 39-year-old woman, was suffering from cancer, and had undergone a left mastectomy, followed shortly by a right pleural effusion and oophorectomy. After being informed that the cancer had metastasized, P became severely depressed and, while at her daughter's home, attempted suicide by strangling herself with a towel. She was admitted to the psychiatric ward of Hospital H, where she openly expressed the desire to commit suicide and even asked members of the nursing staff to assist in this process.

Although P was ordered to be placed under "constant supervision" by the staff physician, one week after being admitted, and while under the direct care of Nurse N, she was permitted to prepare her own bath. Forty minutes elapsed before Nurse N checked on her again, at which time she found the bathroom door locked. When it was finally opened, P was found fully clothed submerged in the water-filled bathtub. The medical examiner ruled drowning as the cause of P's death.

P's estate sues Nurse N for malpractice, claiming negligence in N's supervision of P.

What was Nurse N's legal duty in this case?

☐   to exercise sufficiently close supervision over P to protect her from harming herself or others

☐   to comply with all reasonable medical orders regarding P's treatment

☐   to stay with P every minute of the day

3-69   Would the fact that P had attempted suicide on one prior occasion indicate a sufficiently self-destructive intent to mandate extra care on the part of the nurses assigned to care for her?

Yes	No
☐	☐

3-68 *the duty to exercise sufficiently close supervision over P to protect her from harming herself. . . .*	**3-69** *Yes*

3-70   What significant legal difference (if any) would there be in this case had P never previously attempted suicide?

☐   N could not be held liable at all.

☐   N would be held liable only if it could be shown that N did not exercise reasonable care in allowing P to draw her own bath.

☐   There would be no significant legal difference.

3-71   Which of the following would have afforded Nurse N a *reasonable* legal defense in the lawsuit?

☐   the testimony of experts that not all persons who threaten suicide actually carry out their threat(s)

☐   proof that N monitored P several times while P was taking her bath

☐   proof that hospital policy did not require nurses to check on patients while they were bathing

---

3-70   ☐
☑
☐

3-71   *proof that N monitored P several times while P was taking her bath*

3-72   Reasonable care in treating suicidal patients requires prompt recognition of the frequently overlooked warning clues to suicide—whether verbal, behavioral, or otherwise. One of the most widespread myths about suicide is: "People who talk about it won't actually do it." In fact, almost all suicidal patients give verbal clues to those around them. Evidence of depression, disorientation, and deeply emotional dependency patterns are particularly associated with suicidal tendencies, and reasonable care requires the nurse to recognize and cope with these symptoms *promptly,* to forestall the possibility of suicide before the idea gets too firmly rooted in the patient's mind.

Which of the following remarks made to a nurse by a patient would be indicative of a suicidal intent?

☐   "I give up. I can't take this pain much longer."

☐   "If I can't walk again, what's the point of going on like this?"

☐   "I won't be a problem much longer. Anyway, I'm worth more dead than alive."

3-73   Which of the following statements is the *most accurate*?

☐   Suicidally inclined persons almost always exhibit some overt signs of their suicidal tendencies.

☐   Suicidally inclined persons generally give clues to their suicidal tendencies which, if recognized by the nurse in time, may permit the nurse to prevent the suicide from occurring.

☐   Suicidally inclined persons are easily identified by the fact that they are depressed, disoriented, and emotionally dependent.

NOTE: Nearly all suicidal patients have ambivalent feelings, so they cry out for help before they attempt to kill themselves. Seizing upon this ambivalence, the concerned nurse will reinforce the part of the patient that wants to live, by emphasizing the patient's importance to family and friends; by discussing the effects of suicide on any surviving dependents; and by discussing other hard times in the past, and how the patient coped with them. The wise nurse also will involve the patient's family, friends, coworkers, and clergyman in the process of support through this crisis period. In the final analysis, sensitivity, warmth, concern, and consistency are probably the most meaningful help a nurse can give a suicidal patient.

3-72   ☑
           ☑
           ☑

3-73   *Suicidally inclined persons generally give clues to their suicidal tendencies which, if recognized by the nurse in time. . . .*

POINTS TO REMEMBER

1. Medication errors are a common cause of malpractice claims against nurses and usually involve misreading of a medication order or failing to check with the physician when the order is ambiguous or incomplete.

2. Another major cause of malpractice claims is faulty technique in giving injections.

3. While not all nerve injuries due to injections are due to negligence, where the onset of pain, ecchymosis, and sloughing is immediate, the likelihood of malpractice is great.

4. A nurse is not authorized to *prescribe* medications and may be held personally liable for the untoward consequences of advising a patient what medications to take.

5. When there is no prior history nor any present indication that the patient is dangerous to himself or others, only the normal degree of care is expected of the nurse to safeguard the patient.

6. When patients are suffering some form of mental illness, their ability to contribute to their own safety and security is considerably diminished. This situation calls for the exercise of a higher degree of care with respect to the safety of mentally ill persons.

7. Most patients with suicidal tendencies give verbal or behavioral clues to their destructive intent, and the careful nurse will always be alert to these clues to prevent suicide from occurring.

SELECTED REFERENCES—PART 3

Patient Safety Errors

M. Knight, "Our Safety Net Keeps Patients From Falling," *RN*, 48(12):9 (Dec. 1985)
J. Greenlaw, "Failure to Use Siderails: When Is It Negligent?" *Law, Medicine & Health Care*, 10(6):125 (June 1982)
Annotation, 51 ALR 2d 970, § 2
Wooten v. United States, 574 F. Supp. 200 (Tenn. 1983)
Thomas v. St. Joseph's Hospital, 618 S.W. 2d 791 (Tex. 1981)
Beaches Hospital v. Lee, 384 So. 2d 234 (Fla. 1980)
University Community Hospital v. Martin, 328 So. 2d 858 (Fla. 1976)
McDowell Hospital v. Minks, 529 So. 2d 360 (Ky. 1975)
Cavanaugh v. South Broward Hospital District, 247 So. 2d 769 (Fla. 1971)
Smith v. West Calcasieu-Cameron Hospital, 251 So. 2d 810 (La. 1971)
Clark v. Piedmont Hospital, 162 S.E. 2d 418 (Ga. 1968)
Hospital Authority of St. Mary's v. Eason, 148 S.E. 2d 499 (Ga. 1966)
Shay v. St. Raphael Hospital, 210 A. 2d 664 (Conn. 1965)
D'Antoni v. Sara Mayo Hospital, 144 So. 2d 643 (La. 1962)
Oldis v. La Société de Bienfaisance Mutuelle, 279 P. 2d 184 (Cal. 1955)

Duty to Follow or Not Follow Physicians' Orders

70 *Corpus Juris Secundum*, PHYSICIANS & SURGEONS § 54, p. 976
W. Regan, "When Nurses Fail to Follow Doctors' Orders: Disaster," *Regan Report on Nursing Law*, 26(7):1 (Dec. 1985)
A. Tamiello and D. Gill, "When Following Orders Can Cost You Your License," *RN*, 47(7):13 (July 1984)
D. Guariello, "When Doctor's Orders Aren't the Best Medicine," *RN*, 47(5):19 (May 1984)
W. H. Roach, "Responsible Intervention: A Legal Duty to Act," *J. Nurs. Admin.* 10(7):18 (July 1980)
L. Stanley, "Dangerous Doctors: What to do when the MD is wrong," *RN*, 42:22 (March 1979)
Wickliffe v. Sunrise Hospital, Inc., 706 P. 2d 1383 (Nev. 1985)
Bivins v. Detroit Osteopathic Hospital, 258 N.W. 2d 527 (Mich. 1981)
Killeen v. Reinhardt and Glen Cove Community Hospital, 419 N.Y.S. 2d 175 (N.Y. 1979)
Hunsaker v. Bozeman Deaconess Foundation, 588 P. 2d 493 (Mont. 1978)
City of Somerset v. Hart, 549 S.W. 2d 814 (Ky. 1977)
Carlsen v. Javurek, 526 F. 2d 202 (8th Cir. 1975)
Toth v. Community Hospital at Glen Cove, 292 N.Y.S. 2d 440 (N.Y. 1968)
Arnold v. Haggin Memorial Hospital, 415 S.W. 2d 844 (Ky. 1967)
Goff v. Doctors General Hospital, 333 P. 2d 29 (Cal. 1959)

Physicians' Assistants

W. Regan, "Physicians' Assistants and Quality Patient Care," *Regan Report on Nursing Law,* 23(3):1 (Aug. 1982)

B. Bullough and C. Winter, "Physicians' Assistants and the Law," in *The Law and the Expanding Nurse Role,* B. Bullough (ed.), Appleton-Century-Crofts, New York, 1980, chapter 14

"Judge Rules PA Orders Not Legal Until Countersigned," *Amer. J. Nurs.,* 78:1143 (July 1978)

J. S. Rothberg, "Nurse and Physician's Assistant: Issues and Relationships," *Nurs. Outlook,* 21:154 (March 1973)

L. Wolper, "The Legal Status of the Physician's Assistant," *Hosp. Progr.,* 53:44 (Oct. 1972)

"Legal Implications Relative to Orders from Physicians' Assistants," *Kansas Nurse,* 47:1 (Aug. 1972)

S. J. Blumberg, "Tort Liability and the California Health Care Assistant," *Southern Cal. L. Rev.* 45:768 (1972)

Central Anesthesia Associates v. Worthy, 325 S.E. 2d 819 (Ga. 1985)

Polischeck v. United States, 533 F. Supp. 1261 (Pa. 1982)

Washington State Nurses Association v. Board of Medical Examiners, 605 P. 2d 1269 (Wash. 1980)

Reynolds v. Medical and Dental Staff, etc., 382 N.Y.S. 2d 618 (N.Y. 1976)

Observation and Diagnosis Errors

T. Fadden, "Nursing Diagnosis, A Matter of Form," *Amer. J. Nurs.,* 84(4):470 (April 1984)

J. Warren, "Accountability and Nursing Diagnosis," *J. Nurs. Adm.,* 13(10):34 (Oct. 1983)

J. Bruce and M. Snyder, "The Right and Responsibility to Diagnose," *Amer. J. Nurs.* 82(4):645 (April 1982)

C. Campbell, *Nursing Diagnosis and Intervention in Nursing Practice,* John Wiley & Sons, New York, 1978

Cignetti v. Camel, 692 S.W. 2d 329 (Mo. 1985)

Hippocrates Mertsaris v. 73rd Corp., 482 N.Y.S. 2d 792 (N.Y. 1985)

Poor Sisters of St. Francis v. Catron, 435 N.E. 2d 305 (Ind. 1982)

Utter v. United Hospital Center, Inc., 236 S.E. 2d 213 (W. Va. 1977)

Hiatt v. Groce, 523 P. 2d 320 (Kan. 1974)

Thomas v. Corson, 288 A. 2d 379 (Md. 1972)

Moore v. Guthrie Hospital, 403 F. 2d 366 (4th Cir. 1968)

Darling v. Charleston Memorial Hospital, 211 N.E. 2d 253 (Ill. 1965)

Wilmington General Hospital v. Manlove, 174 A. 2d 135 (Del. 1961)

Goff v. Doctors General Hospital, 333 P. 2d 29 (Cal. 1959)

Cooper v. National Motor Bearing Co., 288 P. 2d 581 (Cal. 1955)

Failure to Communicate

E. Bernzweig, "How a Communications Breakdown Can Get You Sued," *RN*, 48(12):47 (Dec. 1985)

M. Cushing, "Failure to Communicate," *Amer. J. Nurs.*, 82(8):1597 (Oct. 1982)

Ramsey v. Physicians Memorial Hospital, 373 A. 2d 26 (Md. 1977)

Krestview Nursing Home v. Synowiec, 317 So. 2d 94 (Fla. 1975)

Thomas v. Corso, 288 A. 2d 379 (Md. 1972)

Garafola v. Maimonides Hospital of Brooklyn, 279 N.Y.S. 2d 523 (N.Y. 1967)

Darling v. Charleston Memorial Hospital, 211 N.E. 2d 253 (Ill. 1965)

Improper Supervision

E. Bernzweig, "When a Nurse Doesn't Fit the Job," *RN*, 48(1):13 (Jan. 1985)

G. Pozgar, *Legal Aspects of Health Care Administration*, Aspen Systems Corp., Germantown, Md., 1983, pp. 80–81.

W. Regan, "Nursing Supervisors and Careless RN's," *Regan Report on Nursing Law*, 21(9):1 (Feb. 1981)

Carter v. Anderson Memorial Hospital, 325 S.E. 2d 78 (S.C. 1985)

Macy v. Presbyterian Intercommunity Hospital, 612 P. 2d 769 (Ore. 1980)

Valentin v. La Société de Bienfaisance Mutuelle, 172 P. 2d 359 (Cal. 1946)

Piper v. Epstein, 62 N.E. 2d 139 (Ill. 1945)

Medication Errors

D. Guariello, "Nursing Negligence," in D. Louisell and H. Williams, *Medical Malpractice*, Matthew Bender & Co., New York, 1983, § 16A.07

D. Mills, "Malpractice and the Administration of Drugs," *Medical Times*, 93:657 (June 1965)

Miller v. Hood, 536 S.W. 2d 278 (Tex. 1976)

Kallenberg v. Beth Israel Hospital, 357 N.Y.S. 2d 508 (N.Y. 1974)

Su v. Perkins, 211 S.E. 2d 421 (Ga. 1974)

Burns v. Owens, 459 S.W. 2d 303 (Mo. 1970)

Bernardi v. Community Hospital Association, 443 P. 2d 708 (Colo. 1968)

Habuda v. Trustees of Rex Hospital, Inc., 164 S.E. 2d 17 (N.C. 1968)

Larrimore v. Homeopathic Hospital Association of Delaware, 181 A. 2d 573 (Del. 1962)

O'Neil v. Glens Falls Indemnity Co., 310 F. 2d 165 (8th Cir. 1962)

Hallinan v. Prindle, 62 P. 2d 1075 (Cal. 1937)

Negligence in Treating Mentally Ill Patients

R. Reubin, "Spotting and Stopping the Suicide Patient," *Nurs. 79*, 9(4):82–85 (April 1979)

E. Schneidman, "Preventing Suicide," *Amer. J. Nurs.*, 65:111 (May 1965)

Stokes v. Leung, 651 S.W. 2d 704 (Tenn. 1983)

North Miami General Hospital v. Krakauer, 393 So. 2d 57 (Fla. 1981)

Abille v. United States, 482 F. Supp. 703 (Cal. 1980)
Delicata v. Bourlesses, 404 N.E. 2d 667 (Mass. 1980)
Horton v. Niagara Falls Medical Center (N.Y. 1976)
Dinnerstein v. United States, 486 F. 2d 34 (2d Cir. 1973)
Maben v. Rankin, 10 Cal. Rptr. 353 (Cal. 1961)
Gray v. United States, 199 F. 2d 239 (10th Cir. 1952)

Miscellaneous Acts of Negligence

Lambert v. Sisters of Mercy Health Corp., 369 N.W. 2d 417 (Miss. 1985)
Hughes v. St. Paul Fire & Marine Insurance Co., 401 So. 2d 448 (La. 1981)
Elizondo v. Tavarez, 596 S.W. 2d 667 (Tex. 1980)
Variety Children's Hospital v. Perkins, 382 So. 2d 331 (Fla. 1980)
Muller v. Likoff, 310 A. 2d 303 (Pa. 1973)
Burke v. Pearson, 191 S.E. 2d 721 (S.C. 1972)
Quinby v. Morrow, 340 F. 2d 584 (2d Cir. 1965)

Part Four
Intentional Wrongs
and
Consent to Treatment

Part 4

INTRODUCTORY NOTE

The prime focus of this course is nursing malpractice, where the nurse's liability is based on some negligent act or omission to act which causes injury to the patient. There are, however, related areas of nursing practice that involve acts of an intentional nature, and these frequently create legal problems for nurses. Because of the close relationship of these intentional acts to the unintentional (negligent) acts discussed in this course, we will devote this Part to a brief explanation of them. In the material that follows we will discuss several intentional torts and the problem of consent to medical or nursing treatment.

Assault and Battery

4-1   In Part 1 we pointed out that a tort may be either an intentional wrong or an unintentional wrong, but that in either case the wrong is vindicated by way of a civil action for damages against the person who caused it. We also noted that some *intentional* wrongs represent antisocial behavior that is also punishable under the criminal law. Assault and battery are examples of two intentional torts that often result in criminal charges, even though a civil action also may result.

True	False	
☐	☐	An act that constitutes an intentional tort also may constitute a crime.
☐	☐	An act must be either a tort or a crime, but cannot be both.
☐	☐	All torts involve intentional behavior.
☐	☐	Assault and battery are torts based on intentional conduct.

4-2   We begin our discussion of intentional torts with the torts of assault and battery, and will concern ourselves with the use of these terms in the civil law context only.

While the words "assault" and "battery" are often used as though synonymous, they are quite different in the legal sense. A *battery* is the unconsented and unlawful touching of another's person. (A touches B without B's consent.) An *assault* is the act of placing another person in fear of being touched without his consent—or, a threatened battery. (A tells B: "If you don't keep quiet, I'm going to give you an injection to calm you down.")

A patient who has been civilly assaulted

☐ has a legal basis for suing even if not physically touched

☐ has a legal basis for claiming assault and battery in a lawsuit

☐ has no legal basis for suing unless he or she has suffered some bodily harm

4-1	*True*	*False*
	☑	☐
	☐	☑
	☐	☑
	☑	☐

4-2   *has a legal basis for suing even if not physically touched*

4-3   What legal element is necessary for a civil assault to take place?

☐   the physical ability to cause harm

☐   the threat of harm

☐   actual harm

4-4   In the civil law context assault and battery refer to

☐   a single legal act

☐   two distinct legal acts

4-5   A battery (unauthorized or unconsented touching) may result even in the absence of intent to do harm. As a matter of fact, even a touching that is beneficial may constitute a battery if it was not authorized or consented to by the person physically touched.

What would be necessary for a doctor's successful defense in a civil action for battery arising out of his or her treatment of a patient?

☐   proof that the patient's condition improved

☐   proof that no harm resulted to the patient or that the harm was trivial

☐   proof that the patient authorized or consented to the treatment in question

4-3 *the threat of harm*	**4-4** *two distinct legal acts*	**4-5** ☐ ☐ ☑

4-6   A patient's consent to treatment has no legal effect on the doctor's or nurse's liability for negligence in carrying out the authorized procedure.

Indicate in which of the following cases a patient's suit claiming battery would probably be successful or unsuccessful.

Successful   *Unsuccessful*

☐   ☐   A patient consents to treatment with a diathermy machine. The diathermy is carelessly administered and the patient suffers extensive burns.

☐   ☐   A patient agrees orally to the taking of a blood sample. In the process, the nurse's hand slips and the needle injures P.

☐   ☐   In the course of a routine examination, without saying anything to the patient, the doctor lances a large boil on the patient's back.

☐   ☐   A patient agrees to removal of a polyp in his right ear. The doctor successfully removes a polyp from the patient's left ear instead.

4-7   In considering a nurse's liability for battery, the question of whether or not the specific nursing act benefited the patient

☐   is legally relevant

☐   may be legally relevant

☐   is legally irrelevant

4-6   *Successful*   *Unsuccessful*
☐   ☑
☐   ☑
☑   ☐
☑   ☐

4-7   *is legally irrelevant*

If you have any problem with this answer, turn to p. 188, Note A.

POINTS TO REMEMBER

1. Assault and battery, in addition to being the basis of criminal action, are recognized by the law as intentional torts that may give rise to civil actions for damages.

2. A civil assault is the act of placing another person in fear of being touched without his or her authorization or consent.

3. A civil battery is the actual unconsented touching of another's person.

4. A battery may result even if there is no assault, and an assault may result without any battery.

5. Even though an unauthorized touching proves beneficial, it is nevertheless considered unlawful and will give rise to legal liability in a civil action.

6. A patient's consent to a particular form of treatment has no effect on the doctor's or nurse's liability for negligence in providing that treatment.

THE CONCEPT OF CONSENT TO TREATMENT

An area of professional conduct that has become increasingly troublesome to doctors and nurses alike is that which stems from the legal requirement that a physician obtain a patient's consent to treatment. The doctrine of informed consent to medical treatment has been with us since the turn of the century. It is premised on the notion that all persons of adult years and sound mind have the fundamental right to decide for themselves whether, and the extent to which, they will allow other persons to violate their bodily integrity. Thus, in the absence of emergency or extenuating circumstances, a physician or surgeon must first obtain the consent of the patient (or of someone legally authorized to give it on the patient's behalf) before treating or operating on him or her. Failure by the physician to obtain such consent will give rise to possible legal action for battery, based on the unauthorized touching of the patient.

Much confusion has arisen in the legal literature with regard to the matter of consent due to a failure to distinguish between various types of consent-to-treatment issues. The problem is often less related to the scope or quality of the patient's consent than the fact that the consent was not obtained at all. In the material that follows, we will focus on several of the more important consent issues, including consents in connection with emergency situations, with the treatment of minors and incompetents, and operations extending beyond the one consented to.

The nurse becomes legally concerned—and sometimes enmeshed—in these cases not because of any primary responsibility to obtain the patient's consent, but because he or she is generally present at the time the proposed course of treatment is explained to the patient. Every nurse should understand that the law places the duty of informing the patient concerning the proposed treatment on the treating physician, not the nurse. As a practical matter, nurses are often asked to "get the patient's signature" on a standard consent form used by a hospital. Getting the patient's signature is no guarantee that he or she understands what is to happen, nor will it prevent the patient from later alleging that he or she was not adequately "informed" about the nature of the treatment or its alternatives. As a matter of fact, in nearly all malpractice cases alleging lack of informed consent, a document with the patient's signature on it has been offered as proof of the patient's legal consent. The courts invariably ignore these *pro forma* consent forms and ask instead, "What did the doctor actually tell the patient? What questions did the patient ask? How was consent really manifested?" These and other consent issues relevant to nursing practice are discussed in the material that follows.

4-8   An individual may, of course, give consent to the touching of his or her person, and if he or she does so, there is no legal battery. Sometimes this consent is given *expressly* (either by words or in writing), and sometimes it is *implied* by the surrounding circumstances. By way of illustration, when a person engages a physician to treat an ailment, he or she implicitly consents to all procedures that form a reasonable and customary part of that treatment.

A patient goes to her doctor's office for a routine annual physical. Which of the following procedures would she implicitly consent to merely by presenting herself for examination?

- ☐ taking of her pulse
- ☐ removal of a plantar wart
- ☐ taking of a blood sample

4-9   In the eyes of the law, the patient's consent to a particular type of treatment

- ☐ may be implied by the circumstances
- ☐ must be obtained in writing
- ☐ must be given verbally

> NOTE: The common law does not require a patient's *written* consent to treatment, but rather, his or her voluntary and informed consent, whether in writing or not.* The written consent form is merely proof of the fact that the patient signed a document presented to him or her that purportedly reflects the patient's consent to the treatment proposed. While its value in an evidentiary sense cannot be minimized, neither should the mere signing of the form lull the doctor or nurse into a false sense of security. Informed consent cases are proliferating at an amazing pace, and the prudent doctor and nurse will not naively assume that a consent form is a guarantee against liability.

* In Canada, several provincial legislatures have long made it a *statutory* requirement to obtain the patient's consent in writing where a surgical procedure is involved. More recently, several American states have enacted similar laws. Notwithstanding these statutory enactments, a patient may still sue the physician on the theory that he or she was not adequately informed concerning the proposed procedure, the written consent representing merely a rebuttable presumption that true consent was obtained, as under the common law.

4-8   ☑
           ☐
           ☑
	4-9 *may be implied by the circum-stances*

4-10   Even when a patient consents to a particular type of treatment, the consent extends only to all procedures that form a reasonable and customary part of that treatment or are otherwise necessary to repair unforeseen consequences of the treatment to which consent was given. Even an express verbal or written consent does not extend to wholly unrelated or unnecessary procedures.

P enters the hospital for removal of gallstones, and gives his written consent to the operation.

For which of the following might the operating surgeon be held legally liable for battery?

☐ for extending the incision 3 inches because of the unusual location of the gallbladder

☐ for removing the patient's normal appendix

☐ for removing a mole on the patient's abdomen

4-11

P goes to her doctor for treatment of an infection, and the doctor gives a penicillin injection. On receiving the injection, P develops symptoms of anaphylaxis, whereupon the doctor gives an injection of epinephrine.

Why would the doctor not be held liable for committing a battery in this situation?

☐ because penicillin and epinephrine are both injectable substances

☐ because the injection of epinephrine was a reasonably necessary procedure for dealing with the life-threatening circumstances

☐ because the doctor can always choose to employ any therapeutic procedure he or she deems best, once a patient's consent is obtained

---

4-10   ☐
            ☑
            ☑

4-11   *because the injection of epi-nephrine was a reasonably necessary procedure . . .*

4-12

P requests an immunization before going overseas and Nurse N gives a typhoid injection. In the process, the needle breaks off in the patient's arm, requiring the physician-employer of Nurse N to remove the needle surgically, leaving a scar.

A later lawsuit by P against the physician alleging battery

☐ will probably be successful

☐ will probably be unsuccessful

☐ may or may not be successful, depending upon the degree of negligence proved

---

4-13   It is not always appreciated that a person who has given his or her free and voluntary consent has the legal right to revoke or withdraw that consent at any time prior to the commencement of treatment. The physician or nurse who proceeds with treatment in reliance on the original consent will be held liable for battery if it is shown that he patient in fact withdrew his or her consent before treatment began.

P enters the hospital for a series of radiation therapy treatments. He gives his consent to the proposed treatment in writing. After the first treatment he experiences intense discomfort and pain, and tells the doctor and nurse he does not want to proceed with further treatment. Nevertheless, the doctor orders the second treatment and the nurse (with the aid of an orderly) forcibly takes P to the radiation therapy room. In the course of this second treatment, P sustains serious burns and he later sues for battery.

Check each of the following statements you believe to be true.

☐ P would prevail even though initially he consented to the entire series of treatments.

☐ Because of his written consent, P could not later verbally withdraw his consent.

☐ The subsequent injury is a key factor in determining liability for battery.

4-12   *will probably be unsuccessful*   **4-13**   ☑
                                                                      ☐
If you checked the wrong   ☐
box, turn to p. 188, Note B.

POINTS TO REMEMBER

1. If a person consents to the touching of his or her person, no civil battery has been committed.

2. Consent to medical treatment may be given expressly or implicitly. Consent given either way will be legally effective.

3. Consent given to a particular medical procedure is generally limited to the procedure in question and those related procedures necessary to repair unforeseen consequences of the authorized procedure.

4. Consent, once validly given, may be revoked by the patient either orally or in writing at any time prior to commencement of the procedure in question.

5. Written consent, in and of itself, is no more legally effective than oral consent or consent implied by law or by the patient's actions.

4-14

True	*False*	
☐	☐	A suit alleging battery can be successfully defended by showing the patient's consent was obtained.
☐	☐	A valid consent must always be in writing.
☐	☐	A written consent may be withdrawn only in writing.
☐	☐	A suit alleging battery will be successful only if some harm results to the patient.

Consent in Emergency Situations

4-15   The principles we have been discussing up to this point concern treatment of an elective or nonemergency nature. In an emergency, however, where the patient's life is threatened and it is impossible to obtain the consent of the patient or someone legally authorized to act on the patient's behalf, the law permits the necessary treatment to be undertaken without obtaining consent. In this specific situation the law *implies* the patient's constructive consent to all procedures necessary to save the patient's life.

The law implies a patient's constructive consent to treatment when

☐ the patient's condition has taken a turn for the worse

☐ the patient is unconscious and cannot give consent

☐ the patient's life is in danger and consent cannot be obtained from anyone authorized to give such consent

4-16   In an emergency situation, the law permits the doctor or nurse to proceed with treatment

☐ only if the patient is mentally incompetent

☐ only if the consent cannot otherwise be obtained

☐ only if the patient is an adult

4-14	*True*	*False*		**4-15** ☐	If you checked the 2d		**4-16** ☐
	☑	☐		☐	box, turn to p. 188,		☑
	☐	☑		☑	Note C.		☐
	☐	☑					
	☐	☑					

EXPLANATORY NOTES

Note A   (from Frame 4-7)

Whether or not an unconsented procedure proves to be beneficial to a patient is legally irrelevant. The law recognizes the absolute fundamental right of adult, competent patients to refuse any unauthorized invasion of their persons, even for admittedly beneficial procedures or essential surgery. Hence, knowing that a patient has categorically refused to undergo a certain procedure or course of treatment, a nurse must not risk legal liability by proceeding or participating in carrying out the procedure. This applies even if a doctor orders the nurse to do so. The proper course of action for the nurse in these circumstances is to call the matter to the attention of the nursing supervisor or a responsible hospital official.

Proceed to Frame 4-8.

Note B   (from Frame 4-12)

It should be noted that P consented to the immunization injection in the first place, and no later adverse result would alter the legal effect of this consent. The point to remember is that in a suit alleging *battery,* the critical element is proof of an unauthorized touching—not whether harm resulted from the procedure. Obviously, where harm does result, the patient is more likely to bring suit alleging *negligence* (malpractice) rather than *battery*. The example was intended to illustrate the distinction between the legal bases for these two causes of action.

Proceed to Frame 4-13.

Note C   (from Frame 4-15)

Unconsciousness does not necessarily signify that a patient is in immediate danger of death or other serious harm. Thus, under the given facts there may be no emergency at all. On the other hand, even if a true emergency exists, and the patient is unconscious, an attempt should be made to locate the patient's spouse, a close relative, or other authorized legal representative before proceeding with treatment. However, under no circumstances should treatment be delayed unduly in order to locate such a person. The law presumes "constructive consent" in this situation, and the nurse should have little fear of liability if he or she proceeds with treatment.

Proceed to Frame 4-16.

4-17   In which of the following situations would an emergency room nurse be justified in proceeding with treatment without obtaining consent, verbal or otherwise?

☐   An unconscious, profusely bleeding auto accident victim is brought in by ambulance.

☐   A 13-year-old child is brought to the emergency room after suffering a fractured arm while at school.

☐   A construction worker comes to the emergency room to have a boil lanced.

4-18   The rule permitting treatment without obtaining anyone's consent in an emergency situation applies whenever (1) there is immediate danger of death or serious bodily harm, and (2) the patient is physically or legally incapable of giving consent.

True   *False*
☐   ☐

4-19

A patient is under general anesthesia for removal of cancerous tissue in her stomach. During the operation, the surgeon discovers that the patient has a dangerously inflamed appendix.

Yes   *No*
☐   ☐   May the surgeon remove the appendix without obtaining anyone's consent?

☐   ☐   Would this situation fall within the emergency (constructive consent) rule?

☐   ☐   Could the surgeon be held liable for battery if he or she is negligent in removing the appendix?

4-17 *An unconscious, profusely bleeding auto accident victim . . .*	**4-18** *True*	**4-19** *Yes* *No* ☑ ☐ / ☑ ☐ / ☐ ☑

Consent for Treating Minors and Mental Incompetents

4-20   The law considers minors (i.e., persons legally under age) and mentally incompetent persons incapable of giving consent to treatment. Before treating a minor or a person of doubtful mental capacity, the necessary consent should be obtained from a duly authorized person—generally a parent, spouse, legal guardian, or person standing *in loco parentis* ("in place of the parent").

In a situation involving the treatment of a child or a person of doubtful mental competence, liability for unauthorized treatment will be avoided if

- ☐ the individual agrees to assume all responsibility for any possible harm
- ☐ the treatment in question is relatively simple in nature
- ☐ an authorized person consents to the treatment in question

---

4-21   Before undertaking nonemergency treatment on a minor child, the physician or nurse should make sure that the person who requests such treatment for the child is the child's

- ☐ next of kin or closest adult friend
- ☐ parent, legal guardian, or person standing *in loco parentis*
- ☐ teacher or spiritual adviser

4-22   In the previous frame, does the physician or nurse risk being sued for battery if he or she merely assumes the adult has the necessary legal authority to give consent to the treatment proposed without inquiring into the latter's authority?

Yes	No
☐	☐

4-20 *an authorized person consents to the treatment in question*	**4-21** *parent, legal guardian, or person standing* in loco parentis	**4-22** *Yes*

TREATING MATURE MINORS

Emancipated Minors

In most states, the age of majority is 18 years, such that persons under that age are considered legally incapable of giving or withholding consent to medical treatment. In these cases, the physician generally has been required to obtain the express consent of the minor's parent or legal guardian, provided no life threatening emergency is involved. As the law has evolved, however, there has been greater legal recognition of the status and rights of minors on matters relating to consent to medical treatment. Today, all jurisdictions have carved out areas in which mature minors are allowed to make medical decisions for themselves. For example, 14 states have laws permitting minors who are "emancipated" (i.e., minors who are married or clearly are no longer dependent on parents for their support or are otherwise under parental control) to consent to general medical treatment without parental approval. Five others specify age minimums in addition to the requirement of being emancipated. Thirty-four states allow minors to consent to medical care on their own if they are married, and another twenty-two states allow minors to consent to treatment if they are parents. Only eight states limit emancipated minor status to minors who are, or have been, pregnant.

Mature Minors

Another legal doctrine finding increasing acceptance in the legal community concerns the legality of consent given by a mature minor—someone who can and does make his or her own decisions on daily affairs, is mobile, independent, and intellectually able to appreciate the risks and benefits of proposed medical treatment. Thus far, only four states have incorporated the doctrine into their statutes, although courts in a few states have applied the concept under common law principles.

Treating Specific Conditions

Finally, every state has enacted legislation that enables minors to consent to treatment for specific medical conditions such as venereal disease, alcohol and drug abuse, birth control information, pregnancy care, and abortion. Many of these statutes include parental notice provisions that give the treating physician the option of notifying the parents, if he or she believes this to be advisable.

4-23   As just noted, in some jurisdictions a minor is authorized to give valid consent to medical treatment without parental approval if he or she is legally considered emancipated or is considered a mature minor. This can only be determined by careful questioning of the minor.

Choose from the brief facts presented below those situations *clearly* indicating the minor is capable of giving a valid consent to surgery or other nonroutine medical treatment.

☐   Bill is 16 and a student at a military prep school.

☐   Janice is 13, lives at home with her parents, and shows symptoms of being pregnant.

☐   Irene is 15, has a steady boyfriend, and is the school's top math student.

☐   Hank is 17, has his own apartment, and works full time as a gardener.

4-24

A 17-year-old woman, recently graduated from high school, comes to the office of a plastic surgeon for the purpose of having cosmetic surgery to remove a birthmark on her cheek. Before undertaking to treat this patient in any manner, the physician (or office nurse acting on the physician's behalf) should

☐   make sure the patient is intelligent enough to comprehend all the risks of the surgery before proceeding

☐   insist upon obtaining the consent of the patient's parents before proceeding

☐   determine whether the patient is emancipated or otherwise capable of giving proper consent before proceeding

---

4-23   ☐
☑
☐
☑

4-24   *determine whether the patient is emancipated or otherwise capable. . . .*

4-25   Check each of the situation(s) below in which the physician or nurse may assume adequate legal consent for treatment of the minor patient.

☐   A father brings his 10-year-old son to a clinic for a routine physical. While undergoing the physical, the boy objects to having his blood taken for analysis.

☐   A married, 17-year-old college student goes to a private physician for treatment of a disabling arthritic condition.

☐   Neither of the above.

NOTE: Obtaining proper legal consent where a minor patient claims to be legally emancipated or sufficiently mature to consent to treatment on his or her own can present a problem to busy medical/nursing personnel who seldom have the time to corroborate the minor's claim of independence from parental control. When in doubt, the wisest course of action is to temporarily postpone undertaking any clearly "elective" treatment until it is determined that the minor actually is emancipated or is sufficiently mature to be able to consent thereto under state law. Hospital-based nurses should consult with the hospital's legal counsel on the current status of consent laws in their respective states. Once the decision is made to proceed with treatment on the basis of the minor's consent alone, this decision and the surrounding circumstances should be fully documented in the patient's medical record.

After valid legal consent has been given, all the usual rules relating to consent apply. Thus, a minor can always withdraw his or her consent after it has been given, and the physician or nurse can be held liable for battery if he or she continues treatment thereafter. Note also, the rules relating to consent for minors in nonemergency cases do not apply where the minor patient's injury is life threatening and no person with authority to give valid legal consent (i.e., a parent, legal guardian, or person standing *in loco parentis*) is readily available. In that situation, the law implies the necessary consent.

4-25   ☑   If you did not
           ☑   check the 2nd box,
           ☐   turn to p. 202,
               Note A.

4-26   For many purposes the law presumes that a person is mentally competent until declared otherwise in a legal proceeding. This legal presumption is clearly applicable to persons seeking medical treatment.

A physician is confronted with a patient of adult years who seems to be of doubtful competence. Before proceeding, the physician should first

- ☐ ascertain the patient's legal status as to his or her mental competence
- ☐ determine the patient's mental status through test procedures
- ☐ obtain the patient's personal opinion of his or her mental competence

---

4-27

An elderly patient whose mental faculties appear to be affected by senility comes to a physician's office accompanied by his adult son. Cancer is diagnosed and the physician normally would recommend immediate hospitalization and the prompt commencement of chemotherapy. The physician asks the son in private whether his father has been declared mentally incompetent, and the son replies in the negative, but urges the physician to proceed with the treatment proposed. The father tells the doctor he is unwilling to undergo the chemotherapy.

Would the physician be on legally safe ground if he or she were to proceed with treatment in this case?

	Yes	*No*
	☐	☐

4-28   The physician in the above example would be justified in honoring the son's request to begin treatment only if

- ☐ the father was too confused to give his consent
- ☐ the son was a physician himself
- ☐ the son was the father's legal guardian

4-26 *ascertain the patient's legal status as to his mental competence*	**4-27** *No*	**4-28** *the son was the father's legal guardian*

POINTS TO REMEMBER

1. Consent is not legally required where immediate treatment is necessary to save the patient's life and consent cannot be obtained either from the patient or from a duly authorized legal representative.

2. The type of consent recognized in a medical emergency situation is called constructive consent, or consent implied in law.

3. Persons who are considered minors under state law* or who are adjudged mental incompetents are not legally capable of giving valid consent to medical treatment.

4. Minors who live apart from their parents, or who are married, frequently are considered in the eyes of the law to be emancipated, and capable of giving consent to medical treatment.

5. A number of states have enacted special laws pertaining to the rights of minors to give legal consent to specific types of medical treatment.

---

* In most states, a minor is anyone below the age of 18 (below the age of 21 in a few states) who has not been emancipated by marriage or some other special circumstance.

Informed Consent

4-29   We turn now to the subject of informed consent. The underlying concept of informed consent is a simple one: a patient's consent to a particular medical procedure is not legally effective unless the patient fully understands what he or she is consenting to. The mere signing of a consent form (valuable though this may be) does not necessarily mean the patient fully understood what he or she was consenting to. Failure to obtain the patient's informed consent will give rise to possible legal action for battery, based on the unauthorized touching of the patient, or an action alleging negligence, based on failure to adequately disclose the risks of treatment.

The failure to obtain a patient's informed consent is properly classified as

☐   tortious conduct

☐   unethical professional conduct

☐   criminal conduct

4-30   A patient's consent to treatment is said to be informed when

☐   he consents to the procedure in writing

☐   her physician has spoken to her about the proposed treatment

☐   he fully understands the nature of the treatment

4-31   From the legal standpoint, obtaining the patient's written consent to a particular course of treatment is legal proof that she understands the nature of the proposed treatment.

True   *False*
☐   ☐

4-29 *tortious conduct*	4-30 *he fully understands the nature of the treat-ment*	4-31 *False*

4-32   If a patient's informed consent to treatment has not been obtained, he is likely to prevail in a suit filed against all who participated in the treatment if he alleges

☐   assault and battery

☐   negligence or battery

☐   willful misconduct

4-33   The fundamental purpose of the informed consent requirement is to stop the practice of getting patients to consent to treatment in writing.

True   *False*
☐   ☐

4-34   Under what circumstances do you think a patient's informed consent to treatment would not be necessary?

☐   when at least two physicians agree that the patient's condition is terminal in nature

☐   under no circumstances, since the doctrine is rigidly applied to all medical situations

☐   only when the patient is unable to give consent and a medical emergency exists

---

4-35   The doctrine of informed consent recognizes the fundamental right of   ☐ the

doctor   ☐ the patient   to decide what course of treatment to undertake.

4-32 *negligence or battery*	**4-33** *False*	**4-34** ☐	**4-35** *the patient*
For amplification of this response, turn to p. 202, Note B.		☐ ☑	

4-36   As noted earlier, there are occasions when the patient's consent to treatment can be *implied* (such as when the patient needs immediate treatment in an emergency but is unable to consent, or when the patient's consent is clearly indicated by his or her actions). The patient may, of course, give his or her consent *expressly,* either verbally or in writing, and either way is considered legally effective so long as it can be later proved he or she fully understood the nature of the proposed treatment.

Indicate the type of legal consent demonstrated in the described situations.

Express	Implied	
☐	☐	An unconscious accident victim is treated for a cranial fracture.
☐	☐	A patient rolls up his sleeve to receive a vitamin injection.
☐	☐	A patient signs a consent form for a vasectomy.
☐	☐	A patient needing minor surgery tells the doctor to "go ahead."

4-37   In the eyes of the law, a patient's oral consent does not have the same legal effect as a consent given in writing.

True   *False*
☐   ☐

4-38   Neither express consent nor implied consent is legally effective when the patient is mentally incompetent.

True   *False*
☐   ☐

4-36 *Express*	*Implied*	**4-37** *False*	**4-38** *True*
☐	☑		
☐	☑		
☑	☐		
☑	☐		

4-39   For his or her consent to be effective, the patient must understand what is to be done and the essential nature of the choices available. Liability will result if the physician withholds any facts that are necessary to form the basis of an intelligent choice by the patient, or if the physician minimizes the known dangers of a procedure in order to induce the patient's consent.

As a general proposition, consent will be legally *ineffective* when

- ☐ the patient is given information that is ambiguous or vague
- ☐ the doctor denies the patient information because he or she believes it might cause the patient to refuse the treatment
- ☐ the doctor does not discuss the available options with the patient

---

4-40   A blanket consent form used by Hospital H authorizes the carrying out of "any medical or surgical procedure the treating physician deems necessary for the patient's welfare."

This type of consent form is

- ☐ generally upheld as a valid consent provided it is signed by the patient
- ☐ generally held to be invalid since it does not adequately describe the proposed treatment
- ☐ worse than using no consent form at all

4-39   ☑
☑
☑

4-40 *generally held to be invalid since it does not adequately describe the proposed treatment*

4-41

Doctor D chooses not to tell a terminal cancer patient of the risk of burns involved in cobalt irradiation, knowing the patient probably will decline the treatment. Based on the information given, the patient gives her written consent to the treatment, and thereafter sustains painful burns and scarring of her skin.

The patient sues the doctor for damages, alleging lack of informed consent.

What is the likely result?

☐ The doctor will prevail because a patient with a terminal condition is legally incapable of giving an effective consent.

☐ The patient will prevail because the doctor withheld information essential for her to give an informed consent.

☐ The doctor will prevail because only a physician can decide how to treat a patient with a terminal condition.

4-42   In the above example the patient's consent to the cobalt treatment

☐ was legally insufficient because she failed to ask about the risks involved

☐ was legally insufficient because it was obtained through deception on the doctor's part

☐ was legally proper because of the doctor's superior knowledge of the consequences of refusal of treatment

---

4-43   The result of the above lawsuit might be different if the risk of burns was too insignificant to bring to the patient's attention.

True   *False*
  ☐   ☐

4-41 *The patient will prevail because the doctor withheld . . .*	**4-42** *was legally insufficient because it was obtained through deception on the doctor's part*	**4-43** *True* For additional discussion, turn to p. 202, Note C.

THE NURSE'S ROLE IN OBTAINING THE PATIENT'S CONSENT

Even though a nurse may be capable of explaining a proposed medical or surgical procedure to a patient in such a manner that the patient will be fully "informed" about what is to be done, that is not the nurse's legal responsibility—it is the responsibility of the physician. As a matter of fact, the nurse who undertakes to provide such information to a patient not only runs the risk of being held liable to the patient for giving incorrect or incomplete information, but may well be accused of unprofessional conduct in interfering with the doctor-patient relationship.

This does not mean, however, that the nurse has absolutely no responsibility in dealing with the matter of consents. Quite the contrary, both the hospital and its nurse-employees have a duty to use reasonable care to ascertain whether the patient's consent (not just a signed consent form) has, in fact, been obtained. Thus, if the nurse becomes aware of the fact that a patient who has signed a consent form, or is being asked to sign one, (1) has been told nothing about the proposed procedure, (2) has not been adequately informed of all the material risks of the procedure by the physician, or does not appear to comprehend the significance of the information provided, or (3) indicates a genuine change of heart about proceeding with treatment, *the nurse has a legal obligation to notify the patient's physician or the nursing supervisor as soon as possible.*

Nurses are often asked to "get the patient's signature" on a surgical consent form, sometimes just prior to surgery, and this can present some tactical as well as legal problems where the operating surgeon has not adequately discussed the risks of surgery with the patient. From a practical standpoint, when a nurse asks a patient to sign a surgical consent form and it is clear that the patient has been given little or no information about the procedure or its risks by the operating surgeon, the nurse should immediately cease all efforts to get the patient's signature on the form. The nurse should also decline to answer the patient's questions about the procedure and its risks and instead advise the patient that this is the doctor's responsibility and that he or she will bring the matter to the doctor's attention, using language such as, "I'll tell Dr. Thompson about our conversation, and I'm sure he will want to talk with you about these matters." Obviously, the nurse should proceed to do so *promptly.*

Also, bear in mind that it is the nurse's continuing legal duty to observe the patient and recognize all critical factors relating to the treatment, including the patient's emotional state and degree of comprehension of what is about to be done with his or her body. Thus, even when a patient has been fully informed about a surgical procedure and has given written consent thereto, if there is any indication the patient does not want to proceed with the surgery, the nurse must bring this to the attention of the surgeon or nursing supervisor at once, and, if necessary, the surgical procedure should be postponed until the issue is satisfactorily resolved.

EXPLANATORY NOTES

Note A   (from Frame 4-25)

The second fact situation was given to illustrate the legal concept of emancipation. As noted in Frame 4-23, an emancipated minor is one who—though legally a minor because of age—either is married or has otherwise taken steps to emancipate himself or herself from parental control. Merely being a college student living away from home would not prove legal emancipation, but a married college student certainly would be considered emancipated and capable of giving legal consent to treatment. In a number of states laws have been enacted authorizing or validating consents by legal minors in specific situations (e.g., blood donation, abortion, receipt of contraceptive information, obstetrical care,etc). Prudent nurses should become familiar with the relevant laws in their states.

Proceed to Frame 4-26.

Note B   (from Frame 4-32)

While a patient may bring a suit alleging battery, more and more suits alleging lack of informed consent are being predicated on a theory of negligence—failure on the part of the physician to disclose to a patient what other reasonably prudent practitioners would normally disclose under the same or similar circumstances. The choice of legal theory can have a significant effect upon the type of proof necessary as well as the amount of damages that may be recovered. Although Frame 4-32 indicates the action will be one for negligence or battery, the reader should be aware that the trend of the law is toward viewing informed consent cases as a problem of negligence in physician-patient communications, rather than one of battery.

Proceed to Frame 4-33.

Note C   (from Frame 4-43)

Frames 4-41 to 4-43 illustrate the overall problem of informed consent. The mere fact that a patient may have a terminal condition does not vitiate the fundamental legal principle that *every* person has a right to decide what will or will not be done to his or her body, provided the patient is legally competent to make such decision. No physician can usurp this basic right, and the physician who uses deceptive tactics to gain a patient's consent will be held legally liable for so doing in a later lawsuit alleging lack of informed consent. The courts invariably side with the patient in cases of this nature.

Proceed to Frame 4-44.

POINTS TO REMEMBER

1. An informed consent is one that is given by a patient who fully understands what he or she is consenting to.

2. The mere signing of a consent form does not represent legal proof that the patient fully understood the nature of the proposed course of treatment.

3. In a medical emergency, where consent cannot be obtained from the patient or an authorized legal representative, formal consent to treatment is not necessary. The law implies constructive consent in these situations.

4. Informed consent may be reflected either orally or in writing, and both ways are legally effective. For purposes of proving that consent was given, however, it is generally considered advisable to obtain the patient's consent in writing.

5. For a consent to be an informed one, the patient must be told the nature of the proposed treatment, the alternative treatment(s) possible, and the relative risks of the proposed and alternative treatment(s).

6. Liability for battery or negligence will result if a physician minimizes the dangers of a procedure in order to obtain the patient's consent thereto.

7. Blanket consent forms are a poor way of obtaining consent, and rarely stand up in cases where the issue of informed consent is involved.

NOTE: The law is extremely unsettled with regard to *how much* information must be given to a patient in order to obtain a legally effective consent. In essence, every case must be judged on its own set of facts.

Generally, the patient must be told all the *inherent* risks of the proposed procedure, but need not be told about the *unexpected* risks that may arise after the procedure is underway. Similarly, disclosure must be made whenever the nature of the procedure is such that serious injuries may result (e.g., as in electroshock therapy or insulin shock therapy).

Since physicians must place the welfare of their patients above all else, they sometimes must choose between alternative courses of action, and the choice is seldom an easy one. On the one hand, a physician can explain to the patient *every* risk attendant upon the proposed procedure, no matter how remote, thereby possibly alarming the patient unduly where the risk may not warrant such all-out candor. On the other hand, the physician can regard each patient as a distinct problem and can choose to exercise discretion in discussing the potential risks of treatment with him, basing the scope of disclosure on what he or she believes to be consistent with the patient's mental and emotional state.

There are no fast and hard rules in this area of the law, which is clearly in a state of flux. However, the tendency of the courts in the more recent cases has been to require *more* rather than *less* disclosure, so the wise physician will avoid the tendency to preempt the patient's right to decide for himself or herself what to do.

In the final analysis, the problem of informed consent is simply a communication problem, and the doctor who maintains good rapport with a patient is generally the one who does not get into legal difficulty because of a failure to disclose essential information to the patient.

4-44   Based upon the preceding note, indicate whether you believe the following statements to be true or false.

	True	*False*	
	☐	☐	The details a physician has a duty to disclose to a patient about a proposed course of treatment may vary from case to case.
	☐	☐	The more likely the possibility of serious injury, the greater the legal responsibility of the physician to disclose the risk of injury.
	☐	☐	Misrepresenting the need for an operation is never legally justifiable.
	☐	☐	The likelihood of liability is reduced if the physician establishes good communication with the patient.

	4-44	*True*	*False*
		☑	☐
		☑	☐
		☑	☐
		☑	☐

CONSENT TO ABORTION, STERILIZATION, RECEIPT OF BIRTH CONTROL INFORMATION, AND TREATMENT OF VENEREAL DISEASE

It is not within the scope of this programmed course to discuss the underlying philosophical, moral, and religious issues pertaining to abortion, sterilization, birth control, and the like. However, these matters directly affect the activities of nurses and nursing students— primarily in the area of consent—and thus deserve mention at this point.

Abortion

The landmark Supreme Court decisions of *Doe v. Bolton,* 410 U.S. 179 (1973), and *Roe v. Wade,* 410 U.S. 113 (1973), held that during the first trimester of pregnancy (12 weeks) the state is without power to restrict or regulate abortions; hence, during this period the decision to undergo an abortion is strictly a matter between the pregnant woman and her physician. The Court further held that the consent of the pregnant woman's spouse to an abortion during the first trimester is not necessary and any state law requirement of such consent is unconstitutional.

The Supreme Court also ruled that during the second trimester (fourth to sixth month) the state may regulate the medical conditions under which an abortion is performed, but only to the extent that such regulations reasonably relate to the preservation and protection of the mother's health. Thus, the state may regulate the qualifications of the person who is to perform the abortion, the licensure of that person, the type of facility in which the abortion is to be performed, and the licensure of that facility. Beyond these limited matters, the state cannot otherwise interfere in the regulation of abortions, and later court cases have confirmed this position.

In the third trimester the Supreme Court held that a state may prohibit all abortions except those deemed necessary to protect the mother's life or health.

Since the Supreme Court decisions in 1973, most of the state legislatures have tried to impose various limitations on the availability of abortions both before and after the fetus has become viable. Many of these efforts have been invalidated by the Supreme Court, but other states have left their unconstitutional statutes untouched because a majority of legislators in those states either oppose freely available abortions or fear reprisals at the polls from anti-abortion constituents if they attempt to change their laws.

There is little doubt that the Supreme Court has not retreated from its interpretation of the Constitution in *Doe v. Bolton,* and *Roe v. Wade,* and reaffirmed the holding(s) therein as recently as 1983 in *City of Akron v. Akron Center for Reproductive Health, Inc.,* 103 S. Ct. 2481. Thus, unless an anti-abortion amendment to the U.S. Constitution is ratified, the rulings in the *Doe* and *Wade* cases will continue to be the law of the land and the current right of women to elect medically indicated abortions is protected.

It should be noted that the Supreme Court specifically recognized the right of physicians, nurses, and other hospital personnel to refuse to participate in abortion procedures, because of religious, moral, or personal reasons, without incurring any occupational redress or civil liability. Virtually all states now have a "conscience clause" in their statutes relating to abortion.

To the extent that nurses or nursing students choose not to participate in abortion procedures on grounds of conscience, they should make their position known in advance to their clinical instructor, head nurse, or other supervisory official. On the other hand, if they do not so object, they can feel secure in the knowledge that their participation in abortion procedures legally sanctioned by the Supreme Court will not subject them to civil or criminal liability simply by assisting therein.

Sterilization

When a pregnancy might seriously endanger a woman's life or health, it may be medically necessary to terminate her ability to conceive or her husband's ability to impregnate. Because of the medical necessity involved in these cases, the resulting sterility is deemed incidental to the basic medical objective. Therapeutic sterilizations of this nature are not against public policy, nor do they raise any unique legal questions for the medical and nursing personnel involved.

Legal questions do arise, however, when no therapeutic reason exists for removing a reproductive organ or for preventing impregnation. Many states have enacted special laws concerning contraceptive sterilizations, generally aimed at ensuring that both husband and wife fully comprehend the consequences of the procedure in question, and requiring their documented informed consent thereto. Sometimes the statute specifies a waiting period (e.g., 30 days) before the physician may perform the sterilization. The important point to note is that since sterilization affects the procreative function, both spouses have a legitimate legal interest that cannot and must not be ignored.

Ultimately, the legal problem boils down to the effectiveness of the consent obtained; and although it is the physician's responsibility to explain the procedure and its consequences, everyone who participates in the patient's care has a stake in the matter, because the aggrieved patient (or spouse) generally sues not only the doctor but everyone involved in his or her treatment.

Birth Control Information

The U.S. Supreme Court has ruled that many medical decisions, and especially those relating to procreation, involve the constitutionally protected right to privacy. As far back as 1965 the court held that a state law making the use of contraceptives a criminal offense was unconstitutional. *Griswold v. Connecticut,* 381 U.S. 479. Minors, too, have the constitutional right of privacy in childbearing decisions, and no state presently requires parental consent for contraceptive services to minors. As matters now stand, parents do not have a constitutional right to receive prior notice that their minor children are getting birth control information and supplies from family planning clinics or other authorized medical sources. Indeed, the Supreme Court's decision in *Planned Parenthood of Central Missouri v. Danforth,* 428 U.S. 52 (1976), made it clear that a state cannot even condition a minor's right to get a first trimester abortion on obtaining the parent's consent.

Treatment of Venereal Disease

Currently, all 50 states and the District of Columbia have laws allowing a minor to consent to diagnosis and treatment of venereal disease without prior parental consent. As noted earlier, some of these statutes give the physician discretionary authority to notify the parents, even over the minor's objection. Many of these state laws also authorize minors to consent to treatment for alcohol and drug abuse without need for parental consent. Legal counsel for the hospital in which the nurse is employed, or legal counsel for the state nurses association, are two good sources of information about these special statutes.

False Imprisonment

4-45   We turn now to another type of intentional tort—false imprisonment. In legal terms, false imprisonment is the unlawful restraint or detention of another person against his or her wishes. Actual force is not necessary to constitute a false imprisonment. All that is required is that there be a reasonable fear of force to restrain or detain the threatened individual. The potential to carry out the threat can be implied by words or gestures.

A charge of false imprisonment will not lie unless

☐ A threatens physical harm to B

☐ A threatens to harm B if B leaves a specified confined area

☐ A places B in a confined area

4-46

P, a 25-year-old male of Arab extraction who cannot speak English, is brought by ambulance to the hospital emergency room after receiving a stab wound while being mugged. After the wound is treated, P attempts to leave, but Nurse N quickly calls a uniformed security guard and tells him, "Watch this character for me until we find out who's going to pay his bill." P is detained for 3 hours in this manner until N finally gets around to calling an interpreter. Through the interpreter it is learned that P is the son of a Kuwaiti diplomat who, upon being called, agrees to pay the bill at once.

The fact that would lend the greatest legal support to a later claim of false imprisonment brought by P against Nurse N would be

☐ the assignment of the security guard to watch over P

☐ N's generally antagonistic attitude toward P

☐ N's delay in calling for an interpreter

4-45 *A threatens to harm B if B leaves a specified confined area*	**4-46** *the assignment of the security guard to watch over P*

4-47   Which of the following is *not* necessary for a charge of false imprisonment to be successfully made?

☐   actual force

☐   fear of bodily injury

☐   physical confinement

4-48   The nurse may be subject to legal liability for false imprisonment if he or she locks a patient in a room against the patient's will and with the threat of force. Most often, cases of this type relate to mentally ill persons, and the nurse engaged in psychiatric care should be particularly alert to his or her liability for false imprisonment.

Which of the following statements most accurately summarizes the foregoing?

☐   False imprisonment is a charge that will be brought whenever a patient is locked in a room.

☐   Liability for false imprisonment is a legal hazard only for nurses engaged in psychiatric care.

☐   Most false imprisonment lawsuits arise out of the confinement of mentally ill patients.

4-49   What is the common element in the intentional torts of assault and false imprisonment?

☐   physical injury

☐   threatened physical injury

☐   violent and abusive language

4-47 *actual force*	**4-48** *Most false imprisonment lawsuits arise out of . . . .*	**4-49** *threatened physical injury*

4-50

P had been a surgical patient at Hospital H. The day of her scheduled discharge she was asked to pay her bill, but she steadfastly declined, claiming that her postoperative care was terrible and that she would sue the hospital unless her bill was reduced. Supervisory Nurse S was sent to P's room to "persuade" her to make payment. After a fruitless discussion, Nurse S finally remarked: "If you think you're going to leave here without paying your bill, you're sadly mistaken. I'll give you just 5 minutes more to reconsider, and if you haven't changed your mind by the time I return, I'm going to sedate you with a needle and keep you sedated until you *do* change your mind." In fact, Nurse S had no intention of carrying out this threat, but P believed she would and remained in her room for nearly 5 additional hours until relatives came to get her.

P later brings a suit against S, charging false imprisonment. Which of the following will be the most likely result?

☐ S will be held liable for false imprisonment even though she never came near P with a hypodermic needle.

☐ S cannot be held liable for false imprisonment since the discussion in question did not relate to nursing care but to the hospital's finances.

☐ S cannot be held liable for false imprisonment because she had no intention of carrying out her threat.

4-51   If sued, Hospital H could not be held liable for Nurse S's conduct in this case.

True   *False*
☐   ☐

4-52   The basis of Nurse S's liability in this case would be

☐ the doctrine of *respondeat superior*

☐ the rule of personal liability

☐ the supervisor's liability for the acts of others

4-50 *S will be held liable for false imprisonment even though she . . . .*	**4-51** *False*	**4-52** *the rule of personal liability*

4-53   On what legal theory or rule of law would Hospital H be held liable, if at all?

☐   A hospital is liable for all harms caused by its supervisory personnel.

☐   A hospital is liable for harm resulting from the acts of its employees within the scope of their employment.

☐   A hospital is liable for harms caused by employees, but only if related to the care and treatment of patients.

4-54   If Nurse S actually had given P a sedative in the manner threatened

☐   S could be held liable for assault and battery, but not false imprisonment

☐   S could be held liable only for false imprisonment, as charged

☐   S could be held liable for assault and battery as well as false imprisonment

---

4-55   Being charged with false imprisonment is a professional hazard most likely to be
faced by

☐   supervisory nurses

☐   emergency room nurses

☐   psychiatric nurses

4-53 *A hospital is liable for harm resulting from the acts of its employees within the scope of . . .*	**4-54** *S could be held liable for assault and battery as well as false imprisonment.*	**4-55** *psychiatric nurses*

POINTS TO REMEMBER

1. False imprisonment is the unlawful restraint or detention of another person against his or her will.

2. Force is not essential to hold an individual liable for false imprisonment. The law merely requires proof of a reasonable fear of force on the part of the person restrained or detained.

3. Most false imprisonment cases in the medical setting involve locking up mentally ill patients in their rooms. For this reason, nurses engaged in psychiatric nursing should be alert to their exposure to false imprisonment claims by their patients.

4. Under the doctrine of *respondeat superior,* a hospital can be held liable for the conduct of a nurse-employee who unlawfully confines or detains a patient against his or her will.

SELECTED REFERENCES—PART 4

Unauthorized Treatment—Battery

L. Smith, "Battery in Medical Torts," *Cleveland-Marshall L. Rev.* 16:22 (1967)

Note, "Surgery Without Consent—Malpractice or Battery?" *Albany L. Rev.* 29:342 (1965)

Comment, "Physicians and Surgeons—Liability for Unauthorized Treatment," *North Dakota L. Rev.* 38:334 (1962)

G. McCoid, "A Reappraisal of Liability for Unauthorized Medical Treatment," *Minn. L. Rev.* 41:381 (1957)

Lojuk v. Quandt, 706 F. 2d 1456 (7th Cir. 1983)

Dale v. State of New York, 355 N.Y.S. 2d 485 (N.Y. 1974)

Stowers v. Wolodzko, 191 N.W. 2d 355 (Mich. 1972)

Bang v. Charles T. Miller Hospital, 88 N.W. 2d 186 (Minn. 1958)

Allen v. Giuliano, 135 A. 2d 904 (Conn. 1957)

Lacey v. Laird, 139 N.E. 2d 25 (Ohio 1956)

Caldwell v. Knight, 89 S.E. 2d 900 (Ga. 1955)

Mohr v. Williams, 104 N.W. 12 (Minn. 1905)

Need for Patient's Consent to Treatment

61 *Am Jur 2d,* PHYSICIANS, SURGEONS and OTHER HEALERS § § 152–161

W. Prosser, *Handbook of the Law of Torts,* 4th ed., West Publishing, St. Paul, 1971, pp. 165–166

Annotations, 88 ALR 3d 1008, 69 ALR 3d 1223 and 1250, 79 ALR 2d 1028, 56 ALR 2d 695

Dessi v. United States, 489 F. Supp. 722 (Va. 1980)

Scott v. Bradford, 606 P. 2d 554 (Okla. 1979)

Pegram v. Sisco, 406 F. Supp. 776 (Ark. 1976)

Bailey v. Belinfante, 218 S.E. 2d 290 (Ga. 1975)

Murray v. Vandevander, 522 P. 2d 302 (Okla. 1974)

Woods v. Brumlop, 377 P. 2d 520 (N. Mex. 1962)

Natanson v. Kline, 350 P. 2d 1093 (Kan. 1960)

Olmstead v. United States, 277 U.S. 438 (1928)

Schloendorff v. Society of New York Hospital, 105 N.E. 92 (N.Y. 1914)

Concept of Informed Consent to Treatment

D. Louisell and H. Williams, *Medical Malpractice,* Matthew Bender & Co., New York, 1983, § 22

E. Bernzweig, "Don't Cut Corners on Informed Consent," *RN,* 47(12):15 (Dec. 1984)

W. Regan, "Surgical Consent: RN Responsibilities," *Regan Report on Nursing Law,* 24(3):1 (Aug. 1983)

W. Ozzi, "Survey of the Law of Informed Consent," in *Legal Medicine, 1982,* C. Wecht (ed.), W. B. Saunders Co., Philadelphia, 1982, pp. 117–136

L. Besch, "Informed Consent: A Patient's Right," *Nurs. Outl.*, 27:32 (Jan. 1979)

S. Meisel, "The Exceptions to the Informed Consent Doctrine: Striking a Balance Between Competing Values in Medical Decisionmaking," *Wisc. L. Rev.*, 1979:413 (1979)

P. Simonaitis, "The Law of Informed Consent in All Jurisdictions," *Cal. Trial L. J.* 14:87 (Wint. 1974–75)

Annotation, 89 ALR 3d 12

Kinikin v. Heupel, 305 N.W. 2d 589 (Minn. 1981)

Babin v. St. Paul Fire & Marine Ins. Co., 385 So. 2d 849 (La. 1980)

Sard v. Hardy, 379 A. 2d 1014 (Md. 1977)

Small v. Gifford Memorial Hospital, 349 A. 2d 703 (Vt. 1975)

Wilkinson v. Vesey, 295 A. 2d 676 (R.I. 1972)

Cooper v. Roberts, 286 A. 2d 647 (Pa. 1971)

Canterbury v. Spence, 464 F. 2d 772 (D.C. Cir. 1972)

Cobbs v. Grant, 502 P. 2d 1 (Cal. 1972)

Withdrawal of Consent

Busalacchi v. Vogel, 429 So. 2d 217 (La. 1983)

Mims v. Boland, 138 S.E. 2d 902 (Ga. 1964)

Patient's Right to Undergo or Refuse Treatment

B. Eichler, "Nursing Home Residents' Right to Refuse Treatment," *J. Med. Soc. N.J.*, 82(5):359 (May 1985)

M. Fowler, "Appointing an Agent to Make Medical Treatment Choices," *Colum. L. Rev.*, 84:985 (1984) pp. 987–992

A. Davis, "An Obligation to Treat Vs. a Right to Refuse," *Amer. J. Nurs.*, 81(7):1370 (July 1981)

G. Bryn, "Compulsory Lifesaving Treatment for the Competent Adult," *Fordham L. Rev.*, 44:1 (1975)

R. Epstein and D. Benson, "The Patient's Right to Refuse," *Hospitals*, 47:38 (Aug. 16, 1973)

Annotation, 93 ALR 3d 67

Goedecke v. State, 603 P. 2d 123 (Colo. 1980)

Lane v. Candura, 376 N.E. 2d 1232 (Mass. 1978)

Saltz v. Perlmutter, 363 So. 2d 160 (Fla. 1978)

Suenram v. Society of Valley Hospital, 383 A. 2d 143 (N.J. 1977)

John F. Kennedy Memorial Hospital v. Heston, 279 A. 2d 670 (N.J. 1971)

Grannum v. Berard, 422 P. 2d 812 (Wash. 1967)

Implied or Constructive Consent to Treatment

Hernandez v. United States, 465 F. Supp. 1071 (Kan. 1979)

Banks v. Wittenberg, 266 N.W. 2d 788 (Mich. 1978)

Causey v. Dean, 280 So. 2d 251 (La. 1973)

Cobbs v. Grant, 502 P. 2d 1 (Cal. 1972)
Wells v. McGehee, 39 So. 2d 196 (La. 1949)
Barnett v. Bachrach, 34 A. 2d 626 (D.C. 1943)

Applicability of Consent Doctrine in Emergency Situations

Charter Medical Corp. v. Curry, 262 S.E. 2d 568 (Ga. 1979)
Bourgeois v. Davis, 337 So. 2d 575 (La. 1976)
Dunham v. Wright, 423 F. 2d 940 (3d Cir. 1969)
Smith v. Yohe, 194 A. 2d 167 (Pa. 1963)
Rogers v. Lumberman's Casualty Co., 119 So. 2d 649 (La. 1960)
Huffman v. Lundquist, 234 P. 2d 34 (Cal. 1951)
Jackovach v. Yocom, 237 N.W. 444 (Iowa 1931)

Minor's Authority to Consent to Medical Treatment

R. Cohn, "Minor's Right to Consent to Medical Care," *Med. Trial Tech. Q.,* 31:286 (Winter 1985)
R. Brown and R. Truitt, "The Right of Minors to Medical Treatment," *DePaul L. Rev,* 28:289 (1979)
M. Mancini, "Nursing, Minors, and the Law," *Amer. J. Nurs.* 78(1):124 (Jan. 1978)
Annotation, 25 ALR 3d 1439
Planned Parenthood of Central Missouri v. Danforth, 428 U.S. 52 (1976)
Ballard v. Anderson, 95 Cal. Rptr. 1 (Cal. 1971)
Lacey v. Laird, 139 N.E. 2d 25 (Ohio 1956)

Consents Given by Emancipated Minors

The Legal Status of Adolescents, U.S. Department of Health and Human Services, Washington, D.C., 1981
Comment, "Medical Care and the Independent Minor," *Santa Clara Lawyer,* 10:334 (1970)
Carter v. Cangello, 164 Cal. Rptr. 361 (Cal. 1980)
Younts v. St. Francis Hospital & School of Nursing, 469 P. 2d 330 (Kan. 1970)
Bach v. Long Island Jewish Hospital, 267 N.Y.S. 2d 289 (N.Y. 1966)
Inakay v. Sun Laundry Corp., 42 N.Y.S. 2d 344 (N.Y. 1943)
Kirby v. Gilliam, 28 S.E. 2d 40 (Va. 1943)

See also references in the preceding section

Minor's Right to Receive Birth Control Information

42 U.S.C. § 602(a)15) (f)
Carey v. Population Services, International, 431 U.S. 678 (1977)

Consent Required when Treating Incompetent Persons

Comment, "Legal Rights of the Mentally Retarded," *Southwestern L.J.* 35:959 (Nov. 1981)

W. Regan, "No-Code Orders and Incompetent Patients," *Regan Report on Hospital Law,* January, 1979, p. 1

Davis v. Hubbard, 506 F. Supp. 915 (Ohio 1980)

Matter of Quackenbush, 383 A. 2d 785 (N.J. 1978)

Northern v. State of Tennessee, 575 S.W. 2d 946 (Tenn. 1978)

In re Schiller, 372 A. 2d 360 (N.J. 1977)

Dale v. State of New York, 355 N.Y.S. 2d 485 (N.Y. 1974)

Long Island Jewish-Hillside Medical Center v. Levitt, 342 N.Y.S. 2d 356 (N.Y. 1973)

Farber v. Olkon, 254 P. 2d 520 (Cal. 1953)

See also references for Living Wills and Durable Powers of Attorney in Part 8

Consent for Abortion or Sterilization

B. J. George, "State Legislation Versus the Supreme Court: Abortion Legislation in the 1980's," *Pepperdine L. Rev.* 12:427 (1984)

Comment, "Accommodation of Conscientious Objection to Abortion: A Case Study of the Nursing Profession," *Brigham Young L. Rev.,* 1982:253 (1982)

Annotation, 62 ALR 3d 1097

Flateau v. Thom, 393 So. 2d 392 (La. 1980)

Bellotti v. Baird, 428 U.S. 132 (1979)

Beck v. Lovell, 361 So. 2d 245 (La. 1978)

Rothenberger v. Doe, 374 A. 2d 57 (N.J. 1977)

Wolfe v. Schroering, 541 F. 2d 523 (6th Cir. 1976)

Nurse's Right of Conscience

L. Rosen, "The Right to Refuse," *Today's OR Nurse,* 6(12):29 (Dec. 1984)

Kenny v. Ambulatory Centre of Miami, 400 So. 2d 1262 (Fla. 1981)

Swanson v. St. John's Lutheran Hospital, 597 P. 2d 702 (Mont. 1979)

Who Has the Duty to Obtain the Patient's Consent?

E. Bernzweig, "Don't Cut Corners on Informed Consent," *RN,* 47(12):15 (Dec. 1984)

M. Lysman, "Informed Consent and the Nurse's Role," *RN,* 42(9):50 (Sept. 1972)

G. Barbee, "Consents: The Nurse's Role in Obtaining and Using Them," *Hosp. Forum,* 9:23 (Sept. 1966)

Roberson v. Menorah Medical Center, 588 S.W. 2d 134 (Mo. 1979)

Cooper v. Curry, 589 P. 2d 201 (N. Mex. 1978)

Scaria v. St. Paul Fire & Marine Ins. Co., 227 N.W. 2d 647 (Wis. 1975)

Fiorentino v. Wenger, 227 N.E. 2d 296 (N.Y. 1967)

Liability for False Imprisonment

"Patient Sues Hospital for Unnecessary Restraint, Seclusion," *Ment. Dis. L. Rep.,* 4:93
  (Mar.–Apr. 1980)
Annotation, 4 ALR 4th 449
Patrick v. Menorah Medical Center, 636 S.W. 2d 134 (Mo. 1982)
Meier v. Combs, 263 N.E. 2d 194 (Ind. 1970)
Whitree v. State, 290 N.Y.S. 2d 496 (N.Y. 1968)
Maben v. Rankin, 358 P. 2d 681 (Cal. 1961)

Part Five
Regulation of Nursing and Scope of Nursing Practice

Part 5

INTRODUCTORY NOTE

Occasionally, significant conflicts occur when nurses are asked by their employers to perform tasks that extend beyond those permitted by the state nursing authority. Nurses who do carry out such tasks run the risk of severe penalty, including license revocation, in addition to incurring liability for any injury caused the patient.

In this part we discuss the issue of nurse licensure and the range of tasks a nurse is permitted to perform without exceeding the scope of practice authorized by law. We will also take up the question of how far the nurse can go without incurring legal liability when assuming more specialized functions in the treatment curriculum.

REGULATION OF THE PRACTICE OF NURSING

In this part, we will be discussing an issue of great importance—the legal scope of the nurse's authority to practice as a nurse. Before doing so, however, it would be appropriate to outline briefly the manner in which nurses are licensed, and how their professional activities are regulated by statute.

Every state requires that anyone who wishes to practice nursing within its jurisdiction shall be appropriately licensed before being permitted to do so. The state's authority to license nurses (as well as other professionals) includes the authority to define nursing practice, to establish qualifications for obtaining such license, to collect license fees, to establish standards of nursing practice, to exercise disciplinary authority over licensees and suspend or revoke their licenses, and other responsibilities relating to the practice of nursing deemed to be in the public interest. The statutory authority to carry out these responsibilities is given to the state nurse licensing board, an official body usually consisting of about 10 persons appointed by the governor of the state.

Under all the state laws, an applicant for a nursing license must pass a written examination and meet statutory educational requirements. Many state licensing boards have been using the national, standardized licensing examination, which is administered twice a year. Nurses already licensed in one state are generally allowed to obtain their licenses in another state without the necessity of taking a second examination, in accordance with so-called "reciprocity" statutes between the states. While graduates of Canadian nursing schools are accorded the same rights as graduates of American schools, nurses graduated from schools in other foreign countries generally must meet special educational and experience requirements before being allowed to apply for licensure in the United States.

A license to practice nursing is not a right, but a privilege, and it can be suspended or revoked by the state if the licensee does not continue to meet the state's licensing standards. The typical grounds for suspending or revoking a nurse's license include: unprofessional, dishonorable, immoral, or illegal conduct (both on the job or off-duty); habitual intoxication or drug addiction; physical or mental incapacity; and incompetence, negligence, or malpractice. Obviously, some grounds for revocation are easier to prove than others, e.g., conviction of a criminal act, or clear-cut cases of drug addiction or mental instability. Revocation on grounds of incompetence or malpractice is much more difficult to prove, and many licensing boards are less likely to initiate revocations based on those grounds than they are to take action after a nurse has been held liable for malpractice in a court action.

One thing should be made clear: the state's nurse practice act plays a major role in defining the term "nursing" or "the practice of nursing," and this, in turn, defines the scope of the nurse's legal authority within that state. As we shall discuss shortly, some major recent court cases have addressed that issue in detail, and, even though there are still areas of unresolved issues, the trend is definitely toward recognizing nursing as a separate and independent profession. This has great significance for nurses who have assumed new roles as clinical nurse-specialists and specialists in such areas of practice as surgery, anesthesiology, pediatrics, coronary care, intensive care, emergency care, renal dialysis, and hyperbaric oxygen therapy.

The following material discusses the legal principles applicable to nurses entering these expanded areas of patient care. Generically, they are called "scope of practice" issues, since they relate to the scope of the nurse's authority to legally undertake certain acts or procedures.

Scope of Nursing Practice

5-1   The fundamental issue underlying all scope of practice questions is whether a particular act or procedure carried out by a nurse is legally within or beyond the scope of his or her license to practice.* Since state laws vary with respect to what a nurse may or may not do, each case involving a scope of practice question must be viewed in the light of the applicable local law.

As a general proposition, scope of nursing practice questions are resolved

☐   essentially the same way from state to state, based upon common law principles

☐   differently from state to state, based upon the governing local statutes

☐   differently from state to state, based upon common law principles

---

5-2   In most instances, a nurse in State A   ☐ could   ☐ could not   be sure of his or her legal position on a scope of practice question arising in State B.

5-3   Scope of practice legal questions concern primarily the following area of nursing practice:

☐   the degree of care with which a nurse executes a nursing procedure

☐   the patient's right to be treated by a doctor instead of a nurse

☐   the nurse's legal authority to carry out a particular assigned procedure

---

* Nursing care rendered by a nurse who is *unlicensed* raises a different question entirely. Most state nurse practice acts make practicing without a license a crime, punishable by a fine and/or imprisonment. These laws generally exempt nursing care rendered by family members, neighbors, and domestic help. Here we are concerned only with the conduct of duly licensed nursing personnel.

5-1 *differently from state to state, based upon the governing . . .*	**5-2** *could not*	**5-3** *the nurse's legal authority to carry out a partic-ular . . .*

5-4   Not only is there little uniformity among the states regarding the definition of nursing practice, but their statutes generally describe authorized nursing functions in broad, general areas with few specifics. Medical practice acts, on the other hand, are generally rather clear. By and large, they define the practice of medicine in terms of the physician's authority to diagnose, treat, and prescribe. Moreover, the physician not only may do these things himself or herself, but may direct the carrying out of a specific procedure by a nurse under his or her direct orders or supervision.

The problem with most state statutes defining the practice of nursing is that

☐   they are too vague with respect to what a nurse may or may not do

☐   they are too specific with respect to what a nurse may or may not do

☐   they are not as authoritative as medical practice acts

5-5   The problem described in the above frame   ☐ is   ☐ is not   the same with respect to state statutes defining the practice of medicine.

5-6

Doctor D, licensed professional Nurse N, and licensed practical Nurse L, are licensed to practice in the same state. Assuming that each is a reasonably competent practitioner, indicate whether the following statements are true or false.

True	*False*	
☐	☐	Doctor D can delegate to Nurse N the carrying out of a medical function under D's supervision without violating the state medical practice act.
☐	☐	Nurse N can delegate the same function to Nurse L without violating the state nurse practice act.

5-4 *they are too vague with respect to what a nurse may or may not do*	**5-5** *is not*	**5-6** *True* *False*
		        ☑ ☐
		        ☐ ☑

5-7   Numerous areas of medical and nursing practice overlap one another, so that the same act may be considered the practice of medicine when performed by a physician and the practice of nursing when performed by a nurse. It is these overlapping areas that create legal problems for nurses who have assumed expanded responsibilities in highly technical areas of patient care.

Select from the list below those areas of medical or nursing practice that are *most likely* to raise legal questions about the nurse's scope of practice.

☐   giving anesthesia

☐   initiating IV therapy

☐   removing sutures

☐   giving vaccinations

5-8   We are concerned here with legal problems arising out of the delegation of specific medical tasks. What fundamental rule of liability applies to the conduct of nurses who are directed to carry out medical tasks assigned to them?

☐   The nurse will avoid liability for harm to the patient provided the order came from a duly licensed physician.

☐   The nurse will be held liable for harm to the patient if the nurse undertook the task without knowing how to execute it competently.

☐   The nurse will avoid liability for harm to the patient provided he or she is properly licensed as a professional nurse.

5-9   In and of itself, the carrying out of a procedure by a nurse that is described as a medical function in the state medical practice act is sufficient to hold the nurse liable for exceeding the scope of his or her license to practice nursing.

<table>
<tr><td></td><td>*True*</td><td>*False*</td></tr>
<tr><td></td><td>☐</td><td>☐</td></tr>
</table>

| 5-7 ☑ ☑ ☐ ☐ | 5-8 *The nurse will be held liable for harm to the patient . . .* | 5-9 *False* |

5-10   Unless legally sanctioned by statute, nurses may not make medical diagnoses or initiate medical treatment on their own without running the risk of being held to have exceeded the scope of their license to practice. However, in medical emergencies, where a physician is not present and cannot be quickly summoned, nurses may initiate such procedures as they deem necessary, whether or not medical in nature, in order to save patients' lives.

The emergency treatment rule noted above is *most closely* related to

☐   the standard of care rule

☐   the informed consent rule

☐   the Good Samaritan rule

5-11

P, an adult male, is admitted to the emergency room of Hospital H at 1:30 A.M. semiconscious with a foreign body in his throat. No doctor is present and Nurse N directs an attendant to summon the on-call physician at once. Without waiting for the physician's arrival, however, Nurse N immediately attempts to manually extricate the foreign object, but without success. Noticing P's increasingly cyanotic condition, Nurse N performs a tracheotomy, which opens the air passage and keeps the patient alive until the physician finally arrives.

Under the described circumstances, Nurse N's conduct

☐   was perfectly proper and within the law

☐   extended well beyond the practice of nursing and would be grounds for revocation of N's license

☐   was sufficiently flagrant to warrant the bringing of a malpractice suit by Patient P

5-12   In the preceding example assume that, notwithstanding Nurse N's actions, the patient died. In what respect, if any, would the legal consequences of Nurse N's conduct be different from that noted above?

☐   Nurse N would be charged with manslaughter.

☐   Nurse N's license to practice nursing would be summarily revoked.

☐   The legal consequences would be the same.

5-10 *the Good Samaritan rule*	**5-11** *was perfectly proper and within the law*	**5-12** *The legal consequences would be the same.*

5-13   An act normally viewed as a medical function may be viewed as within the scope of nursing practice

☐   provided the patient does not suffer injury as a result thereof

☐   if the nurse was directed to carry out the procedure by a physician

☐   if the nurse had been specially trained to carry out the procedure in question

---

5-14   In the hospital, nursing home, and occupational health setting, numerous medical functions are delegated to nurses (usually nurse-specialists) by means of "standing orders." The object of these orders is to anticipate and deal with critical emergency situations and to legitimize the nurse's execution of clearly prescribed medical functions before the physician arrives. The courts have long recognized the legal validity of this type of delegated authority.

> Nurse N is a specialist in coronary care assigned to the coronary care unit of Hospital H. Standing orders for coronary patients in the CCU call for administering prescribed drugs and for administering precordial shock to terminate life-threatening arrhythmias. One evening, the alarm in the CCU indicates that Patient P's heart has gone into ventricular fibrillation. Without first contacting a physician, Nurse N attempts to stabilize P by injecting lidocaine intravenously, and when this doesn't succeed, Nurse N administers precordial shock. Despite these efforts, P dies.

True	False	
☐	☐	N's conduct constitutes the unauthorized practice of medicine.
☐	☐	P's estate can hold Nurse N liable for having performed medical acts instead of first calling a physician.
☐	☐	Both Hospital H and Nurse N acted completely within the law in the described circumstances.
☐	☐	But for the emergency, and the standing orders, N's actions clearly would be beyond the scope of nursing practice.

5-13 *if the nurse was directed to carry out the procedure by a physician*	**5-14** True False ☐ ☑ ☐ ☑ ☑ ☐ ☑ ☐

5-15   It may be stated as a general rule that when faced with a life-threatening situation, a nurse

- ☐ should do everything possible to assist the patient short of performing a clear-cut medical act
- ☐ should do whatever is reasonably calculated to save the patient's life
- ☐ should exert all efforts to locate a physician as quickly as possible

---

5-16   A nurse who initiates medical treatment without a physician's order or approved standing orders in a nonemergency situation, and who injures the patient in the process, runs the risk of

- ☐ being sued for malpractice
- ☐ being disciplined by the state licensing authority
- ☐ being discharged by his or her employer

5-17   In which of the following instances has the nurse acted within the scope of his or her legal authority?

- ☐ Patient A (while hospitalized) experiences symptoms that might be attributable to either acute indigestion or a coronary occlusion. Nurse A makes a diagnosis of acute indigestion and provides the customary nursing care for that condition.
- ☐ Patient B is scheduled to be released from the hospital following the amputation of a limb, but his depressed mental condition prompts Nurse B to probe for underlying causes. Nurse B diagnoses his condition as a fear of being unable to obtain gainful employment and arranges for him to receive appropriate psychological counseling to cope with his depressive reaction.
- ☐ Patient C seeks aid from occupational health Nurse C for a painful puncture wound received on the job. Nurse C diagnoses the injury as a superficial surface wound only, treats it with antiseptic and a bandage, and sends the patient back to her job.

5-15 ☐	**5-16** ☑	**5-17** ☐
☑	☑	☑
☐	☑	☐

THE EXPANDED ROLE OF NURSES: *SERMCHIEF v. GONZALEZ*

If nursing is to flourish as a distinct professional endeavor, it is inevitable that nurses will continue to seek out and assume more important responsibilities for patient care; that is exactly what has been happening, at least in the United States. At the forefront of this movement are those nurses who, as a result of education and training, have become proficient in various forms of advanced nursing practice. Most of them work in the hospital setting (generally called clinical nurse-specialists) while others work in ambulatory settings (generally called nurse-practitioners). At least 40 states have modernized and expanded their nurse practice acts during the past 15 years, many of them specifically recognizing the right of nurses to engage in specialized areas of practice. Even in the eight states that have no statutory provisions for advanced nursing practice, nurses with specialty training are generally permitted to engage in such practice under the broad definition(s) of nursing contained in their respective state nurse practice acts.

Missouri is one of the states whose nurse practice act does not specifically authorize advanced nursing practice, and it was there that a case of major significance to professional nurses was decided by the Missouri Supreme Court in 1983. In *Sermchief v. Gonzalez,* 660 S.W. 2d 683, two nurse-specialists employed by a rural Missouri family planning clinic performed a variety of sophisticated diagnostic and treatment functions, including performing breast and pelvic exams, taking Pap smears and gonorrhea cultures, performing blood serology, inserting IUDs, fitting diaphragms, and prescribing and administering oral contraceptives. All these functions were performed pursuant to written standing orders and protocols issued by five physicians working for the clinic. The orders, incidentally, were specifically directed to the two nurses in question and to no one else.

The state's medical licensing board (called the Board of Registration for the Healing Arts) threatened to initiate proceedings to punish the nurses for practicing medicine without a license. The board also took steps to revoke the licenses of the physicians for aiding and abetting the unauthorized practice of medicine. The nurses and the physicians countered with a suit seeking a declaratory judgment on the issue, and when the trial court ruled that the acts of the nurse did, in fact, constitute the unlawful practice of medicine, the case was appealed directly to the Missouri Supreme Court.

The court's task was to interpret the language of the Missouri nurse practice act, which contained a definition of professional nursing practice that had been substantially broadened in 1975. Although the statute enumerated the wide variety of functions a professional nurse could engage in, it did not specifically mention nurse-specialists or nurse-practitioners as such. One of the court's principal conclusions was that the legislature had revealed "a manifest desire to expand the scope of authorized nursing practices." An equally important conclusion was that the legislature's formulation of an open-ended definition of professional nursing eliminated the requirement that a physician directly supervise nursing functions. Specifically, the court ruled that the acts performed by the two nurses—pursuant to standing orders and treatment protocols—fell within the legislative standard as set forth in the Missouri statute. The court further recognized that the act of making a diagnosis is not solely within the province of physicians, and that nurses can make diagnostic judgments and can institute treatment in accordance with such standing orders and protocols.

Sermchief has been hailed as a significant victory for professional nurses seeking greater recognition of their expanding roles as specialists. Nevertheless, it did not resolve all of the issues surrounding the authority to engage in specialized fields of nursing practice. Without doubt, critical legal liability and scope of practice problems will continue to arise whenever a nurse assumes patient-care functions that (1) traditionally have been held to be within the province of physicians, (2) are not subject to standing orders, or (3) are not generally recognized as legitimate nursing functions by accredited professional organizations. On the other hand, the judicial trend (at least in the United States) is definitely toward recognizing the gradual expansion of nursing practice into specialty areas, and nurse-specialists in states that have legitimized such practice by statute are not likely to suffer any unusual exposure to legal liability while so engaged.

In Canada, the situation is totally different. The surplus of physicians, particularly family physicians and general practitioners, has sounded the death knell for the nurse-practitioner movement, and there is little expectation that it will be revived at any time in the foreseeable future. In fact, the last major educational program for nurse-practitioners in Canada was discontinued in 1983.

SELECTED REFERENCES—PART 5

The Expanded Role of Nurses

B. Bullough, *The Law and the Expanding Nursing Role,* 2d ed., Appleton-Century-Crofts, New York, 1980

"Nurse Practitioners Fight to Restrict Their Practices," *Amer. J. Nurs.,* 78:1285 (Aug. 1978)

C. De Angelis and W. Curran, "The Legal Implications of the Extended Roles of Professional Nurses," *Nurs. Clin. N. Amer.,* 9:403 (Sept. 1974)

B. Du Gas, "Nursing's Expanded Role in Canada," *Nurs. Clin. N. Amer.,* 9:523 (Sept. 1974)

Sermchief v. Gonzalez, 660 S.W. 2d 683 (Mo. 1983)

Fraijo v. Hartland Hospital, 160 Cal. Rptr. 331 (Cal. 1979)

Scope of Practice

M. Kelly and T. Garrick, "Nursing Negligence in Collaborative Practice: Legal Liability in California," *Law, Medicine & Health Care,* 12:260 (Dec. 1984)

M. Wolff, "Court Upholds Expanded Practice Roles for Nurses," *Law, Medicine & Health Care,* 12:26 (Feb. 1984)

"Tennessee Board of Nursing Revokes Non-certified Midwife's RN License," *Amer. J. Nurs.,* 79:574 (April 1979)

W. T. Eccard, "A Revolution in White—New Approaches in Treating Nurses as Professionals," *Vanderbilt L. Rev.* 30:839 (1977)

R. Hall, "The Legal Scope of Nurse Practitioners under Nurse Practice and Medical Practice Acts," in *The New Health Professionals,* Aspen Systems, Rockville, Md., 1977

Arkansas State Nurses Association v. *Arkansas State Medical Board,* 677 S.W. 2d 293 (Ark. 1984)

Magit v. Board of Medical Examiners, 366 P. 2d 816 (Cal. 1961)

Chalmers-Francis v. Nelson, 57 P. 2d 1312 (Cal. 1936)

Frank v. South, 194 S.W. 375 (Ky. 1917)

Part Six
Proving the Nurse's Liability

Part **6**

INTRODUCTORY NOTE

The procedural aspects of law, while of secondary concern to the nurse, cannot be ignored entirely. The injured patient who wishes to sue a nurse for malpractice faces a number of procedural obstacles, and even though there may be a substantial *medical* basis for bringing the suit, the patient will not be successful unless he or she can overcome these *legal* procedural obstacles.

In Part 6 the basic elements of a lawsuit, the role of the Court and the jury, the question of burden of proof, and several of the more important legal doctrines which apply in the trial of malpractice cases in the United States will be discussed. Although the fundamental legal principles of malpractice law are the same both in Canada and the United States, there are many differences between the two countries in the way malpractice cases are prosecuted in the courts. For example, juries are customary in malpractice cases in American courts but decidedly not customary in Canadian courts.

Because of these procedural differences, Part 6 is based solely on the law as it applies in American courts. Many (if not most) of the principles discussed will be equally applicable in Canada, however, and therefore of interest to the Canadian nurse.

Who Can Sue and Be Sued

6-1   The complaining party in a malpractice suit is called the "plaintiff," and may or may not be the injured patient himself or herself since, under certain circumstances, the law permits such a suit to be brought by the injured person's spouse, parent, or appointed legal representative. As a *general rule,* however, the plaintiff in a malpractice suit is usually the injured patient.

Which of the following persons, under appropriate circumstances, might legally bring a malpractice suit against a nurse?

☐ the injured patient

☐ the patient's spouse

☐ the patient's legal guardian

☐ all the above

6-2   The formal term used in referring to the complaining party in a malpractice suit is

☐ complainer   ☐ litigant   ☐ plaintiff.

6-3   Under what circumstances do you think a malpractice suit might be brought by someone other than the patient?

☐ if the patient is hospitalized

☐ if the patient is deceased

☐ if the patient is unable to afford a lawyer

6-1 *all the above*	**6-2** *plaintiff*	**6-3** ☐ If you checked the 1st or ☑ 3rd box, see p. 240, ☐ Note A.

6-4   Does the law *require* that a malpractice suit be brought only by the injured patient?

Yes   *No*
☐   ☐

6-5   The responding or answering party in a lawsuit is called the "defendant." Where the suit involves nursing malpractice, the defendant is usually the nurse himself or herself although the plaintiff *may,* in some cases, have the right to sue the nurse's employer as well as the nurse.

Nurse N is employed by a private physician. In the course of her work she negligently injures a patient while taking a blood sample.

Who *could be* the defendant in a lawsuit brought by the patient?

☐ only Nurse N

☐ both Nurse N and her employer

☐ only Nurse N's employer

6-6   A single lawsuit may involve multiple plaintiffs and defendants, and more than one legal issue. For example, the plaintiff may sue a hospital and one of its nurses, alleging different types of negligence against each of the defendants.

Which of the following (if any) are true?

☐ There can be more than one defendant in a lawsuit involving a nurse's malpractice.

☐ A lawsuit against a hospital and a nurse may involve malpractice as well as ordinary negligence.

☐ There may be several plaintiffs in a lawsuit against a single defendant.

☐ None of the above.

6-4 *No*	**6-5** *both Nurse N and her employer*	**6-6** ☑
		☑
		☑
		☐

Elements of a Malpractice Suit

6-7   Every nursing malpractice suit includes the following basic elements: (1) a claim that the nurse owed the patient a special duty of care, (2) a claim that the nurse was required to meet a specific standard of care in carrying out the nursing act or function in question, (3) a claim that the nurse failed to meet the required standard of care, and (4) a claim that harm or injury resulted, for which compensation is sought.

The preceding list of basic elements does not refer to any particular class of nurses. What is the significance of this observation?

☐   Different principles of law apply to registered nurses, practical nurses, and nursing students.

☐   The same principles of law apply whether the defendant is a registered nurse, a practical nurse, or a nursing student.

☐   Some classes of nurses are immune from suit entirely.

6-8   One of the basic elements of every malpractice suit is that the defendant nurse owed the patient a special duty of care.

What would be the best way for a plaintiff to prove this?

☐   by showing the nurse's general competence and experience as a nurse

☐   by proving the existence of a nurse-patient relationship

☐   by proving the nurse's employment status at the time of the incident

---

6-7   *The same principles of law apply whether the defendant is a registered nurse, a practical nurse, or a nursing student.*

6-8   *by proving the existence of a nurse-patient relationship*

6-9   Another basic element of every nursing malpractice suit is a claim that the nurse failed to meet the required standard of care in carrying out a specific nursing act or function. This is generally the most disputed issue in the entire case since it relates to the fundamental question of negligence.

In a nursing malpractice case, which of the following issues would be considered the most significant?

☐ the degree to which the defendant conformed or deviated from the applicable standard of care

☐ the nature and severity of the plaintiff's injuries

☐ whether the nurse won or lost other malpractice cases

6-10   What do we mean when we say that a nurse failed to meet the required standard of care in a given situation?

☐ The nurse showed little interest in treating the patient.

☐ The nurse did not do what other reasonably prudent nurses would have done under the same or similar circumstances.

☐ The nurse did not have the educational background and training necessary to carry out the nursing function in question.

6-11

A patient sues Nurse N, claiming that the nurse bullied her constantly while she was in the hospital and generally made her hospital stay an unpleasant experience.

What *significant* element of a malpractice suit is missing in this case?

☐ no special duty of care shown

☐ no standard of care shown

☐ no compensable harm shown

6-9 ☑ ☐ ☐	**6-10** ☐ ☑ ☐	**6-11** ☐ If you checked the wrong ☐ answer, turn to p. 240, ☑ Note B.

EXPLANATORY NOTES

Note A   (from Frame 6-3)

As a rule, a malpractice suit would be brought by someone other than the injured patient only if the patient was no longer alive or had been declared legally incompetent. In that case, a court-appointed legal representative would be the complaining party. A patient can legally file a lawsuit when he or she is hospitalized even though the actual trial of the case might have to be delayed until the patient is out of the hospital.

With respect to the patient who is unable to afford a lawyer, this would not be a legal basis for permitting someone else to bring the lawsuit in his or her behalf, assuming this to be a valid argument in the first place. Actually, it is not, since most personal-injury lawyers do not require payment of legal fees in advance and will generally handle a malpractice case on a contingent-fee arrangement under which the plaintiff agrees to pay the lawyer an agreed percentage of the amount actually recovered, provided there is a recovery. Otherwise, the patient pays no legal fee whatsoever.

Proceed to Frame 6-4.

Note B   (from Frame 6-11)

The really *significant* element missing from the given example is the absence of any compensable harm or injury to the patient. From the standpoint of the law, displeasure, disgust, anger, and other similar subjective states of mind are not a sufficient basis for bringing a lawsuit. On *rare* occasions, where a particularly unnerving experience due to a nurse's negligent conduct has resulted in psychic trauma to the patient, the courts have permitted a recovery, but only where the psychic trauma has produced fairly severe physiological effects. Generally speaking, however, a nurse will not be held liable unless his or her negligence is the direct cause of injury to the patient.

Note carefully, however, that bullying tactics on the part of a nurse and other similar behavior may be an important *psychological* mechanism leading to a later malpractice suit. This point is examined more thoroughly in Part 7 of this course.

Proceed to Frame 6-12.

POINTS TO REMEMBER

1. The complaining party in a malpractice suit is called the plaintiff. Usually the plaintiff is the injured patient although the law also permits other persons to bring such a suit.

2. The answering party in a malpractice suit is called the defendant. Usually the defendant is the nurse himself or herself although in some instances the law permits the suit to be brought against the nurse's employer as well as the nurse.

3. The basic elements of every nursing malpractice suit are (1) a claim that the nurse owed the plaintiff a special duty of care, (2) a claim that the nurse was required to meet a specific standard of care in carrying out the nursing function in question, (3) a claim that the nurse's failure to meet the required standard of care resulted in harm or injury to the plaintiff, and (4) a claim for money damages to compensate the plaintiff for the harm or injury sustained.

4. The most significant legal element in a nursing malpractice case is whether or not the defendant nurse failed to meet the required standard of care. The degree to which the nurse meets the required standard of care or deviates from it is the basis of the fundamental question of negligence (or malpractice).

6-12   The following are the elements of every nursing malpractice suit:

A. A special duty of care owed to the plaintiff by the nurse defendant

B. The specific standard of care applicable to the nursing function in question

C. The nurse's departure from the applicable standard of care (i.e., his or her negligence)

D. Compensable harm or injury resulting from the nurse's negligent conduct

Indicate which of the above elements are essential if a plaintiff is to win a malpractice case against a nurse.

A	B	C	D
☐	☐	☐	☐

6-13   The plaintiff's attorney's summation to the jury includes the statements quoted below. Referring again to the items listed in Frame 6-12, indicate which legal element shown there corresponds with each statement below.

☐ "As several witnesses have testified, it is standard nursing practice in this state to report all unusual symptoms and reactions of the patient to the treating physician."

☐ "Because of her depressed state of mind, the plaintiff unfortunately attempted to take her life and, in the process, suffered permanently disabling injuries."

☐ "The defendant was a registered nurse who was specifically assigned to care for the plaintiff while she was at the hospital."

☐ "The medical record clearly shows that the defendant made no mention to the treating physician of the plaintiff's strange behavior."

NOTE: A little later in this part we will discuss in some detail the subject of defenses to the allegations made by plaintiffs in malpractice suits. We shall first, however, address other matters pertaining to the litigation process.

6-12 A ☑	**6-13** B
B ☑	D
C ☑	A
D ☑	C

Questions of Fact and Law

6-14 At the trial of a malpractice action some of the elements listed in Frame 6-12 are considered questions of fact and others are considered questions of law. The importance of the distinction is that questions of fact are *normally* left to the *jury* to decide while questions of law are *always* left to the *Court* (the trial judge). Not all cases are tried before juries since the parties may waive trial by jury in a civil proceeding. When there is no jury, the Court will decide the factual as well as the legal questions presented by the parties.

In the *usual* malpractice action all questions of fact are resolved by

☐ the Court ☐ the jury.

6-15 The Court will decide all questions, both those of law and fact, when

☐ the jury agrees to this process

☐ the complexity of the case requires

☐ there is no jury

6-16 Before a jury is permitted by the Court to hear any evidence on disputed questions of fact, the Court itself must decide that the defendant nurse owed the plaintiff a special duty of care. *The finding of a nurse-patient relationship is the way this is normally accomplished,* and if the Court so finds, the case will proceed on the remaining legal issues. However, if the Court determines that a nurse-patient relationship did *not* exist, it will immediately dismiss the plaintiff's case without further proceedings.

To the plaintiff, proving the existence of a nurse-patient relationship is

☐ important but not essential

☐ important and essential

☐ unimportant

when bringing a malpractice suit against a nurse.

6-14 *the jury*	**6-15** *there is no jury*	**6-16** *important and essential*

General-duty Nurse N has a casual conversation about the merits of cosmetic surgery with the wife of a patient hospitalized for severe angina. Based on this conversation, the wife, who has been contemplating such surgery for a long time, decides to proceed with a face lift. The surgery turns out poorly and she later brings suit against both the plastic surgeon and Nurse N.

At the trial, the issue of Nurse N's legal relationship to the plaintiff wife would be

☐ a question of fact   ☐ a question of law,   to be decided by   ☐ the judge   ☐ the jury.

6-18   The most important question of fact for the jury to decide in a nursing malpractice case is whether the defendant nurse failed to conform to the required standard of care. In cases in which no jury is present, the Court decides this crucial issue of fact in addition to all questions of law.

If the jury in a malpractice case was to decide that the plaintiff failed to prove that the nurse deviated from the applicable standard of care, the jury would have decided

☐ a question of law

☐ a question of fact

which would

☐ for all practical purposes decide the case in the nurse's favor

☐ still leave many other equally important issues of law and fact to be resolved

---

6-17 *a question of law*

the judge

6-18 *a question of fact*

for all practical purposes decide the case in the nurse's favor

6-19   It was stated earlier that the standard of care is *normally* considered a question of fact for the jury to decide. There are circumstances, however, under which the jury is not permitted to decide this question. One example is when a statute prescribes the applicable standard of care. In this situation the Court will so rule as a matter of law, leaving it to the jury to determine only whether the prescribed standard (the statute) was or was not violated.

A state or provincial statute that prescribes a particular type of conduct on the part of a nurse is an example of   ☐ a statutory standard of care   ☐ statutory negligence.

6-20

A practical nurse employed by a general hospital is sued by a former patient, who alleges in his complaint that the nurse negligently gave him an injection of morphine and that, in any event, the nurse was not legally authorized to give injections of narcotic drugs.

At the trial of this malpractice case, which of the following would be questions of fact for the jury to decide and which would be questions of law for the Court to decide?

Fact	*Law*	
☐	☐	Did the nurse violate the state statute which relates to the administration of narcotic drugs by giving the injection in question?
☐	☐	Is the state statute regarding the licensure of practical nurses applicable in this case?
☐	☐	Did the nurse's actions give rise to a nurse-patient relationship?
☐	☐	Was the nurse negligent in the manner in which he gave the plaintiff the injection of morphine?

6-19 *a statutory standard of care*

6-20	*Fact*	*Law*
	☑	☐
	☐	☑
	☐	☑
	☑	☐

Legal Precedents

6-21   Over the years, many court decisions have been handed down involving numerous types of nursing activities and functions. Once a common-law decision has established the standard of care for a particular activity or function, it is referred to by later courts in cases involving similar facts. Such decisions are called "legal precedents." They not only serve as guidelines to the courts in deciding future cases but establish authoritative guidelines for future conduct of nurses in carrying out specific nursing activities and functions.

Indicate *two* important effects of a court decision that lays down a specific rule of law (e.g., a standard of care) in a case involving a particular nursing activity or function:

☐   The decision gives the Court added prestige and an opportunity to display its wisdom in a technical field of law.

☐   The decision becomes an authoritative guide to future nursing conduct on the part of nurses.

☐   The decision lends stability to the judicial process by serving as a guideline for deciding future similar cases.

☐   The decision automatically decides other malpractice cases involving nurses in that particular nursing activity or function.

6-22   Is a legal precedent in a malpractice case an example of statutory or common law?

Statutory law   *Common law*
☐   ☐

6-21   ☐
            ☑
            ☑
            ☐

6-22   *Common law*

If you selected the wrong answer, you should reread Frames 1-4 through 1-9.

Judicial Notice

6-23   When a Court determines that a particular prior decision or a particular statute applies to the facts of the case at hand, it takes "judicial notice" thereof, which means that it officially recognizes the earlier court decision or the statute as controlling.

If in the course of a malpractice case the Court takes judicial notice of a prior court decision, what is the legal effect of this action?

- ☐ The case under consideration will be decided without regard to the earlier court case.

- ☐ The case under consideration will be decided exactly the same way as the earlier case.

- ☐ The case under consideration will be decided in accordance with the legal principles decided in the earlier case.

6-24

A patient files suit against a nurse for malpractice, alleging negligence in the nurse's manner of carrying out a particular nursing function. The state in which the suit is brought has never had a similar case before its courts, and there is no state statute regulating the activity in question.

Under these facts, which of the following statements would be true?

- ☐ There is no legal standard of nursing care in this situation, so the Court has nothing it can judicially notice.

- ☐ The Court will judicially notice the lack of an existing legal standard of nursing care.

- ☐ The Court will take judicial notice of the novel facts presented and decide the case by itself.

6-23 ☐ ☐ ☑	**6-24** ☑ If you did not select the cor- ☐ rect answer, turn to p. 254, ☐ Note A.

6-25   The decision in a case of this type will probably establish a judicial precedent with respect to the applicable standard of care for the nursing technique in question.

	True	*False*
	☐	☐

6-26   In which *two* of the following instances would a Court most likely take judicial notice of a standard of care already applicable to the case under consideration?

☐ when the case under consideration presents novel facts involving a gap in the existing rules of law regarding the standard of care

☐ when the case under consideration involves a nurse who has been sued in several prior malpractice cases

☐ when the case under consideration involves a nurse's violation of a statute that prescribes or prohibits a particular nursing function or responsibility

☐ when the case under consideration involves the same type of nursing function or responsibility adjudicated in an earlier court case in the same state

---

6-27   The way in which a Court officially rules that a particular statute or prior legal decision is controlling in a malpractice case is to

☐ request briefs from each of the parties

☐ submit the matter to the jury for their concurrence

☐ take judicial notice thereof

6-25 *True*	**6-26** ☐ ☐ ☑ ☑	**6-27** *take judicial notice thereof*

POINTS TO REMEMBER

1. At a jury trial, questions of fact are normally left to the jury to decide while questions of law are left to the Court. When there is no jury, the Court decides both the factual and the legal questions presented by the case.

2. A preliminary legal question is whether the defendant nurse owed the plaintiff any special duty of care. If the Court finds that a nurse-patient relationship existed between the parties, the case will proceed; otherwise, the Court will dismiss the suit without further proceedings.

3. While the standard of care is normally a fact question for the jury to decide, when a statute prescribes the governing standard of care, the Court will so rule as a matter of law, leaving it to the jury to determine only whether the statute was in fact violated.

4. Common-law court decisions in malpractice cases provide authoritative guidelines for the future conduct of nurses in carrying out the specific nursing functions which were the subject of these suits. They also serve as legal precedents in deciding future similar cases.

5. The way a Court officially rules that a statute or a prior court decision is controlling in a malpractice case is to take judicial notice thereof.

Burden of Proof

6-28   One of the most important rules of evidence applied in a malpractice case is the rule that the plaintiff has the burden of proving that the defendant nurse was negligent. In other words, until the plaintiff can satisfactorily *prove* the defendant's negligence, he or she is legally presumed to be free from liability (i.e., not negligent). If the plaintiff cannot meet this burden of proof, he or she will lose the case.

When a malpractice case is brought against a nurse, there is an initial presumption of law that the nurse

☐   was negligent

☐   was neither negligent nor free from negligence

☐   was free from negligence

6-29   This initial presumption of law has the following effect:

☐   It places a burden on the plaintiff to prove the nurse's negligence.

☐   It places a burden on the nurse to prove the absence of any negligence on his or her part.

☐   It places a burden on the Court to see that both parties to the suit introduce substantial evidence on the question of negligence.

6-30   Why does the burden-of-proof rule give the defendant nurse an initial courtroom advantage?

☐   because the defendant nurse does not have to prepare a defense

☐   because the defendant nurse is generally blameless and has the jury's sympathy

☐   because the defendant nurse does not have to prove his or her freedom from negligence, while the plaintiff must affirmatively prove the nurse's negligence

6-28 *was free from negligence*	**6-29** *It places a burden on the plaintiff. . . .*	**6-30** *because the defendant nurse does not have to prove his or her freedom from negligence. . .*

6-31   Why is the rule relating to the plaintiff's burden of proof so important in a malpractice suit?

☐   because it effectively relieves the defendant of all liability for his or her negligent conduct

☐   because it assures the orderly presentation of evidence at the trial

☐   because the plaintiff's inability to meet the burden of proof will result in the plaintiff's losing the case

---

6-32

Patient P sues Nurse N for an act of alleged malpractice while he was a hospitalized patient. P claims N failed to take adequate precautions to see that he did not fall out of his bed following a subtotal gastrectomy. The undisputed evidence showed that P fell out of bed and severely injured his hip, although when he was discovered on the floor, the side rails of his bed were up (i.e., in proper position).

Based on the above facts alone, the standard of care in this case would be   ☐ a question of fact   ☐ a question of law.

6-33   Would P's injury, sustained in the manner described above, be legal proof of N's negligence?

Yes   *No*
☐   ☐

6-34   Which two of the following items will P have to prove?

☐   N's professional background and experience

☐   a nurse-patient relationship between N and himself

☐   N's failure to take adequate precautions

6-31 ☐	6-32 *a question of fact*	6-33 *No*	6-34 ☐
☐			☑
☑			☑

6-35   In order to sustain the burden of proof in a malpractice case, the plaintiff must prove his or her case by a "preponderance of the evidence." This means that the plaintiff must introduce enough credible (believable) evidence to persuade the jury (or Court) that all the essential allegations of his or her complaint are *more probably true than not*. If the evidence is evenly balanced on both sides or favors the defendant more than the plaintiff, the latter has not sustained the burden of proof and will lose the case.

Which of the following comes closest to describing what is meant by a preponderance of the evidence?

☐ evidence beyond all reasonable doubt

☐ evidence more likely true than not

☐ evidence convincing to more than half of the jurors

6-36   Three scales of justice are illustrated below. Symbolically, in which of the illustrations below has the plaintiff (P) failed to meet the burden of proof in his or her suit against the defendant (D)? (The blocks on each scale represent the relative weight of the evidence presented by each party.)

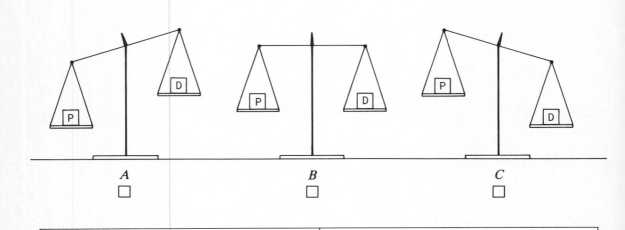

| *A* | *B* | *C* |
| ☐ | ☐ | ☐ |

6-35 *evidence more likely true than not*	**6-36** *B and C*

6-37   To meet the burden of proof, the plaintiff must present convincing evidence in his or her favor on the following fundamental issues:

1. The existence of a special duty of care owed the plaintiff by the defendant nurse

2. The specific standard of care applicable to the nursing function involved in the case

3. The nurse's departure from the applicable standard of care

4. The nature and extent of damages suffered as a result of the nurse's negligent conduct

The failure to sustain the burden of proof on any one of the first three issues will ordinarily result in the plaintiff's losing the case. The plaintiff must always prove he or she has suffered some damages, but even if the plaintiff cannot prove *all* the alleged damages, he or she may still win the case.

Which *two* of the following would be *essential* items for the plaintiff to prove in a malpractice case against a nurse?

☐   the accreditation status of the hospital in which the nurse was employed

☐   the existence of a nurse-patient relationship

☐   the nurse's age, place of schooling, and date of licensure

☐   the amount of the plaintiff's future anticipated loss of earnings as a result of the injury

☐   the act or omission that constituted negligent conduct on the part of the nurse

---

6-38   The plaintiff in a malpractice suit is able to prove the nurse's negligence without difficulty.

If the plaintiff claims a total of $20,000, comprised of $2,000 for medical expenses, $1,000 for wage loss, and $17,000 for pain and suffering, but is able to prove only the first two items, what will be the result?

☐   The case will be dismissed for lack of proof of all claimed damages.

☐   The plaintiff will recover the full amount of the damages claimed.

☐   The plaintiff will recover all provable expenses plus an additional amount for pain and suffering, as determined by the jury.

6-37   ☐
       ☑
       ☐
       ☐
       ☑

6-38   ☐   If you are uncertain about the
       ☐   correct answer, turn to p.
       ☑   254, Note B.

EXPLANATORY NOTES

Note A   (from Frame 6-24)

When no prior court decision or statute applies to a particular nursing function, the concept of judicial notice does not come into play—at least not with respect to the standard of care applicable to that function. There are, of course, many other legal issues presented in a court case, and a Court may be required to judicially notice a variety of matters during the course of a trial so that time will not be wasted in having them proved repetitiously. For example, Courts are required to take judicial notice of the statutes and judicial decisions applicable within their respective jurisdictions. Courts are also required to take judicial notice of widely accepted scientific facts, mortality tables, and a multitude of other established facts. The doctrine of judicial notice is a legal extension of the rules of common sense and common knowledge, and is designed to expedite the proceedings at the trial.

Proceed to Frame 6-25.

Note B   (from Frame 6-38)

Although the text did not discuss the matter, pain and suffering are considered a compensable item of damages in every malpractice suit where liability of the defendant is established. As a matter of fact, damages awarded for pain and suffering generally comprise the major portion of a malpractice suit and the amount awarded is generally left to the jury to decide. In recent years, malpractice recoveries have kept pace with general inflationary trends and it is not uncommon for an award to be in excess of $100,000, with some awards totaling several hundred thousand or even a million dollars where injuries have been devastating.

The plaintiff's case will not be dismissed, therefore, merely because of an inability to precisely prove the value of his or her pain and suffering. On the other hand, no one can predict with any certainty what a jury will allow for this rather speculative element. In practice, when a jury award seems out of proportion to the injury sustained (as happens on occasion), the Court will set the verdict aside as excessive, in which event the case may either be retried or an appeal may be taken by the plaintiff.

Proceed to Frame 6-39.

POINTS TO REMEMBER

1. It is a fundamental rule of evidence in every malpractice case that the plaintiff has the burden of proving the defendant's liability throughout the case. This results from the basic legal proposition that the defendant is presumed to be free from liability until proved otherwise.

2. The plaintiff's inability to sustain the burden of proof on the question of the defendant's alleged negligence will cause the plaintiff to lose the case.

3. The plaintiff must prove his or her case by a preponderance of the evidence in order to win. A preponderance of the evidence is sufficient, believable evidence to persuade the jury (or Court) that the allegations of the complaint are more probably true than not.

4. In every nursing malpractice case the plaintiff must prove (1) the existence of a special duty of care owed him or her by the nurse, (2) the particular standard of care applicable in the case, (3) the nurse's failure to meet the standard of care (i.e., the nurse's negligence), and (4) the nature and extent of damages sustained due to the nurse's negligence.

6-39   Another essential issue that the plaintiff must prove by a preponderance of the evidence is that he or she suffered some compensable harm or injury as a result of the defendant's conduct. Negligent conduct that does not cause any harm or injury reducible to monetary terms will not give rise to legal liability.

A month after she has been discharged from the hospital, Patient P is informed by her physician: "There was a mix-up one day while you were at the hospital. It seems that Nurse Simpson gave you the wrong medication, but we learned about it in time and your present condition shows that you suffered no harm."

P goes to a lawyer the following day to ask whether the above facts are sufficient to entitle her to bring suit against Nurse Simpson.

Which of the following responses by the lawyer expresses the legal position most accurately?

☐   "You've got a good case because the doctor has already admitted that Nurse Simpson was negligent, and the doctor's admission is sufficient to hold the nurse liable for damages."

☐   "I would be happy to take your case since the nurse was clearly negligent, but unless we can prove you have sustained damages, there is no point in filing suit."

☐   "The fact that you know something went wrong while you were at the hospital is enough proof of legal harm, and we should have little difficulty in recovering a substantial amount by way of damages."

6-40   The preceding case *best* illustrates the following:

☐   Negligent conduct that does not cause any harm will not give rise to legal liability.

☐   The chance of winning a malpractice case is practically assured if one has a doctor as a witness.

☐   A nurse can be sued for negligence even though the patient may not have been aware of the nurse's negligence at the time.

6-39 *"I would be happy to take your case since the nurse was clearly negligent, but unless. . . ."*	**6-40** *Negligent conduct that does not cause any harm will not give rise to legal liability.*

6-41   The process of deciding whether the plaintiff has met the burden of proving the defendant's negligence (by a preponderance of the evidence) requires the jury to weigh the evidence presented by both sides. What counts is not the *number* of witnesses produced by one side as against the other but rather the *quality, relevance,* and *persuasive character* of the evidence, and the members of the jury must evaluate all this evidence on the basis of their own general experience and knowledge of human affairs.

Which of the following statements is correct?

☐ It is generally recognized in malpractice litigation that the party who presents the greatest number of witnesses is most likely to win the case.

☐ In a malpractice case it is for the Court to decide as a matter of law whether or not the plaintiff has sustained the burden of proof.

☐ In a malpractice case it is the express function of the jury to sift and weigh all the evidence presented and to decide whether the burden of proof has been met.

6-42   Since members of the jury must evaluate all the evidence presented in a malpractice case on the basis of their individual experiences and knowledge of human affairs, it is reasonable to say that

☐ the outcome of a malpractice case is impossible to forecast with any degree of certainty

☐ the outcome of a malpractice case is nearly always predictable once all the evidence is presented

☐ members of a jury seldom differ in their evaluation of the truthfulness of witnesses or the weight to be attached to their testimony

6-41 ☐	**6-42** *the outcome of a malpractice*
☐	*case is impossible to forecast*
☑	*with any degree of certainty*

NOTE: As we have seen, under our system of justice the plaintiff has the burden of proving all the essential elements of his or her malpractice case, and if the plaintiff cannot sustain that burden, he or she will lose. In other words, the defendant nurse can win merely by disputing the plaintiff's primary allegations and forcing the plaintiff to prove, for instance, that the nurse failed to meet the applicable standard of care, or that he or she owed no particular duty to the plaintiff. This burden is never easy in a malpractice case, which is one reason why most of these cases are won by the defendants, notwithstanding all the attention given by the media to plaintiff's victories involving huge sums of money.

As we shall see in the discussion that follows, sometimes the defendant nurse can assert one or more affirmative legal defenses to the plaintiff's malpractice claim in addition to merely refuting the primary allegations made; when these defenses apply, they can be quite effective. An important point to note: when a defendant asserts one of these defenses in the course of a malpractice trial, he or she has the burden of proving that defense by a preponderance of the evidence—a reversal of roles with respect to who has the obligation or burden to go forward with proof.

Contributory Negligence

6-43   One of the standard defenses in any malpractice action (as it is in any negligence action) is the defense of contributory negligence, which may be stated as follows: When a patient's failure to exercise reasonable care aggravates an injury initially caused by a nurse's negligence, the patient will *not* be permitted to recover damages in some American states and Canadian provinces (i.e., the nurse will not be held liable under these circumstances).

In view of the rule of contributory negligence, a nurse who admits to an act of malpractice may avoid liability by showing that

☐   the patient was aware of the negligent conduct at the time it was committed

☐   the patient either caused or contributed to his or her own injury

☐   the patient made unreasonable demands upon the nurse's time

6-43   *the patient either caused or contributed to his or her own injury*

6-44

Patient P is hospitalized for elective surgery. The day before the operation he sustains an injury to his foot caused by his own negligence in getting out of bed.

Why would the rule of contributory negligence not apply in this case?

☐ because the patient had not yet undergone surgery

☐ because the patient did not exercise reasonable care

☐ because there was no negligence on the part of another person to which the patient's negligence could contribute

---

6-45   When the defense of contributory negligence is established and proved by the defendant, it constitutes a *complete defense* to the plaintiff's claim. In effect, the defendant will win the case by proving that the injury received (or aggravated) was the plaintiff's own fault.

Patient P had been hospitalized for a leg fracture, requiring that her leg be placed in a cast. Nurse N gave P specific instructions about leaving the cast alone. Nevertheless, P pushed a traction weight down with her leg until the weight became useless, and also attempted to remove the cast with a table knife. When her leg became permanently disabled, P sued Nurse N for the resulting damages.

Based on the foregoing, which of the following would be the most likely result?

☐ P could recover full damages against Nurse N for failing to supervise her more closely.

☐ P could not recover any damages against Nurse N because P's conduct aggravated the fracture and subsequent disability.

☐ P could recover damages against Nurse N only for the additional disability she suffered while hospitalized.

6-44 *because there was no negligence on the part of another person to which the patient's negligence could contribute*

6-45 *P could not recover any damages against Nurse N. . . .*

6-46   Failure of the patient to follow the doctor's or nurse's orders or instructions is the usual ground for raising the defense of contributory negligence. And so long as patients are physically and mentally able to understand and follow such instructions, their failure to use reasonable care for their own safety will prevent them from recovering damages from the doctor or nurse in a malpractice action.

> P, a 45-year-old male machinist, suffered a cut while at work. Occupational health Nurse N sutured the wound and advised P he would need a tetanus antitoxin shot. Because her own supply of the antitoxin was exhausted, N (in accordance with standing orders) instructed P to get a tetanus shot from his personal physician immediately. P went home instead, and did not contact his physician. Several days later, P developed tetanus and died.

Should or should not P's estate prevail in its claim for damages against Nurse N, and for what reason?

☐ Should not—because P's failure to follow N's instructions was the primary factor leading to his death

☐ Should—because P had a right to expect Nurse N to follow up on her instructions and make sure that P got his tetanus shot

☐ Should—because Nurse N had no right to refer P to his own doctor to get a tetanus shot

---

6-47   Why would the defense of contributory negligence not apply to a person who was unconscious when the treatment was rendered?

☐ because the law allows no defense to a claim brought by a person who was unconscious while undergoing treatment

☐ because an unconscious person cannot contribute to his or her own injuries

☐ because the law presumes medical or nursing negligence where an unconscious person suffers injury

6-46 *Should not—because P's failure to follow N's instructions was . . .*	**6-47** ☐	
	☑	
	☐	

COMPARATIVE NEGLIGENCE VERSUS CONTRIBUTORY NEGLIGENCE

As previously discussed, when the rule of contributory negligence comes into play, the plaintiff's claim is defeated in its entirety. Because of the obvious inequities that have resulted from this harsh rule, the defense of contributory negligence has been greatly limited, and in some states entirely nullified, by the adoption of the doctrine of comparative negligence. Under this doctrine, when a plaintiff brings a tort suit seeking to recover damages for the allegedly negligent acts of the defendant, the degree of negligence of both plaintiff and defendant are compared, and the damages awarded to the plaintiff (if any) are apportioned according to the relative degrees of negligence found.

Thus far, 37 states have enacted comparative negligence statutes, and there is a clear trend toward the comparative negligence rule in all states. The doctrine of comparative negligence has been adopted by: Alaska, Arkansas, California, Colorado, Connecticut, Florida, Georgia, Hawaii, Idaho, Illinois, Kansas, Louisiana, Maine, Massachusetts, Michigan, Minnesota, Mississippi, Montana, Nebraska, Nevada, New Hampshire, New Jersey, New Mexico, New York, North Dakota, Oklahoma, Oregon, Pennsylvania, Rhode Island, South Dakota, Texas, Vermont, Washington, West Virginia, Wisconsin, and Wyoming.

Assumption of Risk

6-48   A second legal defense to a malpractice suit is the doctrine of assumption of risk. Simply stated, this doctrine says that when a patient understands all the risks of unpreventable adverse results of treatment and knowingly consents thereto, he or she cannot prevail in a later malpractice claim alleging that an adverse result he or she was informed of was attributable to negligence.

P, a diabetic, is warned in advance of surgery that her condition is susceptible to unavoidable infection. She authorizes the surgeon to proceed, and when postoperative infection does occur, her leg must be amputated.

Did P assume the risk of surgery in this case?

Yes	*No*
☐	☐

6-49   If P decides to sue the surgeon, what, if anything can she legally recover in the way of damages?

☐   nothing at all

☐   only her actual out-of-pocket expenses

☐   all losses suffered, including her pain and suffering

6-50   Patients do not assume the risks of treatment unless

☐   they do not want the doctor to refuse their case

☐   they fear they may not recover from the illness

☐   they know what the risks are

6-48 *Yes*	**6-49** *nothing at all*	**6-50** *they know what the risks are*

6-51   The doctrine of assumption of risk is closely related to the doctrine of informed consent. And, just as is the case with informed consent, a patient who has been informed of possible adverse results of treatment never assumes the risks of *negligent* treatment.

> Patient P is told by his doctor that radiation therapy is the preferred mode of treatment for his condition. In describing the therapy, the doctor tells P about the possibility of radiation burns, but P nevertheless decides to proceed. Through an error in calibration, P receives an overdose of radiation and is severely burned.

P   ☐ would be   ☐ would not be   within his rights to bring a malpractice claim against the doctor because

☐   he did not assume the risk of being burned

☐   he assumed the risk of being burned

☐   he did not assume the risk of negligent use of the equipment

---

6-52   A patient may assume the risks of treatment if he or she chooses to proceed in spite of being warned *against* being treated.

> P comes to Doctor D's office without an appointment to have her ears irrigated to remove excessive wax. Since the doctor is not there, P asks Nurse N to perform the procedure. N tells P he is not qualified to perform the irrigation procedure but, at P's insistence, he agrees to perform the procedure. In the process N causes P's eardrum to be ruptured.

P's later malpractice claim against Nurse N will probably

☐   succeed, because N carried out the procedure negligently

☐   fail, because P knew N was not qualified to perform the procedure and willingly assumed the risk of possible injury

☐   fail, because there was no nurse-patient relationship in effect

---

6-51   *would be*

      he did not assume the risk of negligent use of the equipment

6-52   ☐
      ☑
      ☐

Emergency

6-53   As noted earlier in this course, the law takes the surrounding circumstances into consideration whenever a malpractice claim is brought against a doctor or nurse. Thus, the fact that treatment was given in a life or death emergency may provide a complete defense to a suit claiming negligence in treatment if it can be shown that the urgent circumstances required a relaxed standard of care.

> A patient is brought to the emergency room choking on a bone in his throat. Emergency room Nurse N attempts to remove the bone, but is unsuccessful. Noticing the patient's cyanotic condition, Nurse N performs a tracheotomy and breathing is restored, but in the process, she injures the patient's vocal chords.

Yes No

☐ ☐ Is this the type of emergency that would provide a good defense to a malpractice suit against Nurse N?

☐ ☐ Was Nurse N justified in performing the tracheotomy under the circumstances described?

☐ ☐ Would Nurse N have been justified in performing the tracheotomy if a doctor was available in 15 minutes?

☐ ☐ Has Nurse N run the risk of losing her license for performing the tracheotomy in the described circumstances?

6-54   The legal defense of emergency will be effective in a nursing malpractice case only when the defendant nurse can prove that

☐ there were insufficient nurses on duty to assist when the emergency arose

☐ the treatment in question was a matter of life or death

☐ the emergency circumstances were brought about by the patient's own willful conduct

---

6-53	Yes	No
	☑	☐
	☑	☐
	☑	☐
	☐	☑

6-54   *the treatment in question was a matter of life or death*

NOTE: We have just reviewed the three most significant legal defenses available to a defendant in a malpractice case. In addition to these defenses based on the merits of the case, there are certain *procedural defenses* that might also come into play. The first of these is the defense of statute of limitations. Every lawsuit seeking money damages must be brought within a specified period after the incident giving rise to the cause of action occurred. The period is always prescribed by statute and is thus commonly referred to as the "statute of limitations." Since the statutory periods within which malpractice claims must be brought vary from state to state, they are not detailed here. The nurse's legal defense counsel will know when (and how) to invoke the defense of statute of limitations when it is applicable.

Another procedural defense relates to the doctrine of governmental immunity; as noted earlier in this course, nurses who are employed by the Veterans Administration and by the United States Public Health Service enjoy immunity from suit for any acts of malpractice that occur while on duty. The fellow-servant doctrine is another procedural defense that might be asserted by an occupational health nurse who is sued by a coworker seeking to recover damages from the nurse for aggravation of an on-the-job injury normally covered only by workers' compensation. As mentioned above, the nurse's lawyer will know when and how to invoke any of these legal defenses once the lawsuit has been instituted.

We return now to the trial process itself, covering briefly those areas of trial practice that are of relevance to nurses who may be sued.

POINTS TO REMEMBER

1. Unless the plaintiff has sustained some compensable harm, the defendant cannot be held liable in a malpractice case.

2. Weighing the evidence in a malpractice case is the function of the jury, which must decide whether the plaintiff has met the burden of proof on all essential factual issues.

3. Some jurisdictions permit a defendant to assert the legal defense of contributory negligence if it can be shown that the plaintiff's own failure to exercise reasonable care contributed to or aggravated an injury caused by a nurse's negligence. When this defense is applicable, it is a complete bar to any recovery of damages by the plaintiff.

4. When a patient is fully informed of all the risks of unpreventable adverse results of treatment, and accepts them, legally he or she assumes those risks and cannot later prevail in a malpractice suit seeking to recover damages arising out of a risk he or she assumed.

5. A patient never assumes the risk of negligent treatment, even when the patient is informed of, and has agreed to assume, specified risks of unpreventable adverse results.

6. When treatment is given in a life or death emergency, the law relaxes the normal standard of care, and the plaintiff will not be allowed to recover damages for injuries arising out of those emergency circumstances.

Directed Verdicts

6-55   As noted earlier, questions of fact ordinarily are left to the jury to decide, but on rare occasions a Court may "direct a verdict" in favor of the plaintiff or the defendant. When this occurs, the case is removed from consideration by the jury and is decided solely by the Court.

The Court is legally *required* to direct a verdict in favor of one party or the other when *both* of the following occur: (1) There is no substantial dispute in the evidence as to what events took place, and (2) the conclusion whether the nurse was negligent or not is so clear and obvious that reasonable minds could not arrive at a different conclusion.

Consider the following case:

Patient P sues Nurse N for malpractice. In her suit P claims only that Nurse N gave her an oral medication that caused her to suffer an allergic reaction. N admits these allegations but claims he was in no way negligent.

Which of the following best explains why the Court would be inclined to direct a verdict in N's favor in this case?

☐   The Court is ordinarily more inclined to believe the defendant than the plaintiff in a malpractice suit involving an adverse reaction to medication.

☐   The facts are not in dispute, and since N is legally presumed to be free from negligence, the Court must rule in N's favor in the absence of proof of specific negligent conduct.

☐   Many people react adversely to medications and the Court, aware of this fact, will rule in N's favor to avoid unnecessary speculation on the part of the jury about what caused P's reaction.

NOTE: In actual practice a directed verdict for the plaintiff is extremely rare in a malpractice case; occasionally, though, a Court will direct a verdict in favor of a defendant where the plaintiff's evidence is so weak as to warrant the dismissal of the case.

6-55   *The facts are not in dispute, and since N is legally presumed to be free from negligence, the Court must rule in N's favor in the absence of proof of specific negligent conduct.*

Need for Expert Testimony

6-56   In a nursing malpractice case the key question of whether the nurse acted with reasonable care ordinarily is a matter that requires the opinions of *expert witnesses*. This is so because members of the jury are lay persons and cannot be expected to know of their own accord what nursing skills or procedures should have been followed in the case at hand. Accordingly, the plaintiff must introduce the testimony of one or more experts to prove the applicable standard of care and thereby help the jury decide what a reasonable nurse would have done in the given situation.

Why is the question of whether or not a nurse acted in a reasonable manner usually not left to the jury to decide?

☐   because members of a typical jury often are unreasonable in their own lives and therefore cannot be expected to judge fairly what is reasonable conduct on the part of others

☐   because members of a jury often are confused when confronted with novel fact situations, particularly those that relate to the acts of medical personnel

☐   because members of a jury are lay persons and therefore do not have an adequate basis for arriving at a judgment with regard to the professional conduct of a nurse

---

6-57   The expert witness is someone who qualifies as an expert by demonstrating that he or she has expert knowledge of the particular subject area of the lawsuit and advanced professional training, extensive practical experience, or a combination of the two.

Which two of the following persons would logically qualify as experts in a nursing malpractice case arising out of the administration of an anesthetic?

☐   an occupational health nurse

☐   an anesthesiologist

☐   a hospital administrator

☐   a nurse-specialist in anesthesiology

6-56   *because members of a jury are lay persons and therefore do not have an adequate basis for arriving at a judgment . . .*

6-57   *an anesthesiologist*

a nurse-specialist in anesthesiology

6-58

A malpractice suit is filed against a pediatrician's office nurse for leaving an unconscious child in the pediatrician's office unattended.

Which of the following would qualify as an expert witness in a case of this type?

- ☐ a pediatric nurse-specialist
- ☐ an experienced office nurse
- ☐ a pediatrician
- ☐ all the above

6-59   Since the jury ordinarily is not permitted to decide the issue of a nurse's alleged negligence without some expert testimony concerning the applicable standard of care, if no expert testimony on this issue is introduced by the plaintiff, the Court must direct a verdict in favor of the defendant nurse.

Patient P sues Nurse N for negligence in administering x-ray therapy that resulted in scalp burns. At the trial P seeks to prove N's negligence by introducing evidence of his injuries and of the good working condition of the x-ray machine that was used. N defends by claiming that P was fully informed of the potential risks involved and consented to the proposed course of treatment. N further claims that in any event there was no evidence to show she acted without reasonable care in giving the x-ray therapy.

The Court directs a verdict in N's favor. Which of the following reasons explains why?

- ☐ because N more than adequately proved she acted with reasonable care
- ☐ because P failed to prove by expert testimony that N's conduct did not constitute reasonable care
- ☐ because N's conduct could not be held negligent where the patient was fully informed of the risks involved

---

6-58 *all the above*

6-59   ☐   If you checked the last box,
            ☑   turn to p. 273, Note A.
            ☐

6-60   Expert testimony is not required where the alleged negligence involves something so common or ordinary that even a lay person would know that the injury could result only from negligent conduct. This determination is made by the Court.

Indicate in each of the following cases whether an expert witness would be needed by the plaintiff (P) to prove Nurse N's alleged negligence.

Expert needed	No expert needed	
☐	☐	P claims N negligently placed on his body an excessively hot heating pad, resulting in a severe burn.
☐	☐	P claims N erroneously gave her medication that was intended for another patient.
☐	☐	P claims N improperly administered an anesthetic agent.
☐	☐	P claims N failed to raise the side rails of his bed, permitting him to fall.

6-61   Which of the following best expresses the rule regarding the need for expert testimony?

☐   Expert testimony is always required in a malpractice case, and a plaintiff who fails to introduce such testimony will lose his or her case.

☐   The jury is permitted to decide, on the basis of all the evidence submitted, whether expert testimony is or is not needed in order for the plaintiff to win his case.

☐   Whether or not expert testimony is needed will depend upon the facts of each case, with the Court deciding whether the jury will be permitted to decide the issue of negligence without expert testimony.

6-60	*Expert needed*	*No expert needed*
	☐	☑
	☐	☑
	☑	☐
	☐	☑

6-61   *Whether or not expert testimony is needed will depend upon the facts of each case. . . .*

Doctrine of *Res Ipsa Loquitur*

6-62   As noted earlier, in the usual nursing malpractice case the plaintiff has the burden of proving the defendant's negligence by a preponderance of the evidence. Sometimes, however, the plaintiff cannot possibly meet this burden due to unusual circumstances surrounding the injury; in these instances the legal doctrine known as *res ipsa loquitur* ("the thing speaks for itself") comes into play. When the doctrine is applicable in a given case, the usual rule regarding burden of proof is modified and the jury is permitted to find the defendant negligent without any expert testimony on the part of the plaintiff.

Under ordinary circumstances the jury in a malpractice case is permitted to find the defendant liable for malpractice only on

☐   the defendant's admission of negligent conduct

☐   the testimony of expert witnesses

☐   specific instructions from the trial judge

6-63   Which of the following accurately describes the procedural advantage that results when the doctrine of *res ipsa loquitur* comes into play?

☐   Plaintiff does not have to introduce expert testimony to prove the defendant's negligence.

☐   Defendant does not have to introduce evidence proving his or her freedom from negligence.

☐   Evidence of the defendant's negligence can be dispensed with entirely.

6-62   *the testimony of expert witnesses*

6-63   *Plaintiff does not have to introduce expert testimony to prove the defendant's negligence.*

6-64   We come now to the special circumstances that will permit the doctrine of *res ipsa loquitur* to be applied in a nursing malpractice case:

1. The injury must be of a type that does not ordinarily occur unless someone has been negligent.

2. The conduct that caused the injury must have been under the exclusive control of the nurse.

3. The patient must not have contributed to his or her own injury.

Consider the following illustrative case:

The parents of a 1-year-old infant bring a malpractice suit against Nurse N, claiming damages for burns sustained by the infant while under N's care. The plaintiffs are able to prove that N placed a heat lamp near the infant's crib and that when the infant was next observed, she had been severely burned by the heat lamp that had fallen into her crib. Plaintiffs seek to invoke *res ipsa loquitur.*

Yes   *No*

☐   ☐   Was the injury one that ordinarily would not occur unless someone was negligent?

☐   ☐   Was the cause of the injury within the exclusive control of the defendant nurse?

☐   ☐   Did the patient contribute to her own injury?

☐   ☐   Should the doctrine reasonably apply in this case?

6-65   Keeping in mind the first requirement of *res ipsa loquitur*—that the injury must be of a type that ordinarily does not occur unless someone has been negligent—in which of the following situations might the doctrine reasonably be applied?

☐   fracture of an anesthetized patient's arm during surgery for removal of his gall bladder

☐   injury to a patient resulting from the leaving of a foreign object in the patient's body during surgery

☐   injury to a patient resulting from a fall out of bed

☐   injury to a patient resulting from administration of the wrong drug or wrong dosage form of a drug

6-64   *Yes*   *No*
☑   ☐
☑   ☐
☐   ☑
☑   ☐

6-65   ☑   If you are in doubt about any
           ☑   of these answers, turn to p.
           ☐   273, Note B.
           ☐

EXPLANATORY NOTES

Note A   (from Frame 6-59)

This last item raised an entirely new issue, and perhaps your unfamiliarity with the subject of consent to treatment caused you to select the wrong answer. You must always bear in mind that the general rule regarding burden of proof requires the plaintiff to prove the applicable standard of care by one or more expert witnesses. Thus, a Court is *required* to direct a verdict when no such expert testimony is introduced. In the given example P did not introduce any expert testimony, and the Court had no choice but to direct a verdict in N's favor on that ground alone.

But what about this matter of P's consent to the x-ray therapy? Would that in itself be a sufficient basis for denying P a recovery? The answer is No, at least not without more facts than given in the example. A patient's consent to treatment may prevent a later claim by the patient that he or she was given unauthorized treatment (the technical tort known as battery), but it would *not* absolve a nurse of any *negligence* while giving such treatment.

Proceed to Frame 6-60.

Note B   (from Frame 6-65)

The doctrine of *res ipsa loquitur* has been applied in many different types of cases but only where the injury was produced in such a manner as to leave little doubt that someone was negligent. The doctrine is widely applied in cases involving foreign objects left in a patient's body during surgery. It has also been applied in cases of burns or other injuries suffered by a patient while under anesthesia or otherwise unconscious, infections caused by unsterile instruments, and injuries from defective diathermy apparatus or other electrical equipment. In the cited examples, only the first two are clearly within the category of unusual types of injuries that normally do not occur unless *someone* is negligent. The remaining examples might or might not be due to negligence but, in any event, are not considered the sort of occurrences that raise an *inference* of negligence since they might involve contributory negligence on the part of the patient or might occur even if no one was negligent.

Proceed to Frame 6-66.

6-66   The doctrine of *res ipsa loquitur* does not become operative automatically. The plaintiff generally urges the Court to permit the doctrine to apply in the case. If the Court decides that the doctrine should be applied, it will instruct the jury that the circumstances under which the injury occurred raise a presumption or inference of the defendant's negligence. The presumption is rebuttable, however, which means that it may be contradicted or disproved. Thus, when *res ipsa loquitur* is applied in a given case, the burden shifts to the defendant to prove that he or she was *not* negligent.

When we say that the doctrine of *res ipsa loquitur* permits an *inference* of negligence on the part of the nurse, what do we mean?

☐   The nurse is considered liable whether or not he or she can show proof of due care.

☐   The circumstances under which the injury occurred are considered evidence of the nurse's negligence, which the nurse must disprove.

☐   The nurse's negligence is a purely legal question to be decided by the Court.

NOTE: You should be aware of the fact that the doctrine of *res ipsa loquitur* is not recognized in all jurisdictions. Moreover, this is an area of law that is rapidly undergoing transition, and hence only the broad outlines of the doctrine will be touched upon in this course. However, because the doctrine has such far-reaching consequences to a nurse when it is applied in a given case, you should be at least familiar with the fundamental legal concept involved.

6-66   *The circumstances under which the injury occurred are considered evidence of the nurse's negligence, which the nurse must disprove.*

POINTS TO REMEMBER

1. When the evidence is not in dispute and reasonable minds could not arrive at a different conclusion, the Court is required to direct a verdict (as a matter of law) in favor of the prevailing party.

2. The plaintiff is ordinarily required to introduce the testimony of expert witnesses to prove the standard of care and whether or not the defendant nurse conformed to that standard of care. Expert testimony is required because a jury of lay persons cannot be expected to know from their own experience what a reasonable nurse would do in a given situation.

3. When the plaintiff presents no expert testimony in a case requiring such testimony, the Court must direct a verdict for the defendant.

4. Expert testimony is not required to prove negligent conduct involving something within the knowledge or experience of most lay persons. The Court decides whether or not expert testimony is required in any given case.

5. The doctrine of *res ipsa loquitur* comes into play when a plaintiff sustains injury under circumstances that make it difficult or impossible to prove *how* the injury was sustained or *who* was legally responsible.

6. The Court decides whether the doctrine of *res ipsa loquitur* will apply in any given case. When *res ipsa loquitur* is applied, the jury is permitted to infer that the defendant nurse was negligent without the need for any expert testimony.

Res ipsa loquitur can apply only when the following elements are present:

a. The injury is of a type that ordinarily does not occur unless someone has been negligent.

b. The conduct causing the injury is under the exclusive control of the defendant.

c. The patient did not contribute to his or her own injury.

SELECTED REFERENCES—PART 6

Elements of Malpractice Suit

D. Louisell and H. Williams, *Medical Malpractice,* Matthew Bender & Co., New York, 1983, §§ 8.04–8.07
Restatement (Second) Torts, § 281
M. Hemelt and M. Mackert, *Dynamics of Law in Nursing and Health Care,* Reston Publishing, Reston, Va., 1978, pp. 13–18
D. Guariello, "Can You Be Sued Without Cause?" *RN,* 47(2):19 (Feb. 1984)
Annotation, 13 ALR 2d 11

Questions of Fact and Law

75 *Am Jur 2d,* TRIAL, §§ 320–321
Annotation, 71 ALR 2d 331
St. Petersburg v. Austin, 355 So. 2d 486 (Fla. 1978)
Hamilton v. Hardy, 549 P. 2d 1099 (Colo. 1976)
Capella v. Baumgartner, 494 F. 2d 36 (5th Cir. 1974)
Ferrarra v. Galluchio, 152 N.E. 2d 249 (N.Y. 1958)
Leonard v. Watsonville Community Hospital, 305 P. 2d 36 (Cal. 1956)

Legal Precedents

G. Wise, "The Doctrine of Stare Decisis," *Wayne L. Rev.* 21:1043 (July 1975)
Annotations, 121 ALR 210, 93 ALR 964
Exxon Corp. v. Butler, 585 S.W. 2d 881 (Tex. 1979)
Adkins v. St. Francis Hospital, 143 S.E. 2d 154 (W. Va. 1965)

Judicial Notice

75 *Am Jur 2d,* TRIAL, § 320
29 *AM Jur 2d,* EVIDENCE, §§ 14–122
Stone v. Sisters of Charity, 469 P. 2d 229 (Wash. 1970)
Daiker v. Martin, 91 N.W. 2d 747 (Iowa 1958)
Agnew v. City of Los Angeles, 218 P. 2d 66 (Cal. 1950)

Burden of Proof

29 *Am Jur 2d,* EVIDENCE, §§ 124, 127, 128, 130
D. Louisell and H. Williams, *Medical Malpractice,* Matthew Bender & Co., New York, 1983 § 14.03
Guilbeau v. St. Paul Fire & Marine Ins. Co., 325 So 2d 395 (La. 1976)
Pederson v. Dumouchel, 431 P. 2d 973 (Wash. 1967)
Beaudoin v. Watertown Memorial Hospital, 145 N.W. 2d 166 (Wis. 1966)

Contributory Negligence as a Defense

Comment, "Contributory Negligence in Medical Malpractice," *Cleveland State L. Rev.*
    21:58 (Jan. 1972)
Annotation, 100 ALR 3d 723
Haynes v. Hoffman, 296 S.E. 2d 216 (Ga. 1982)
Moon v. United States, 512 F. Supp. 140 (Nev. 1981)
Mackey v. Greenview Hospital, Inc., 587 S.W. 2d 249 (Ky. 1979)
Ferrara v. Leventhal, 392 N.Y.S. 2d 920 (N.Y. 1977)

Assumption of Risk as a Defense

Annotation, 50 ALR 2d 1043
Smith v. Hospital Authority, 287 S.E. 2d 99 (Ga. 1981)
Olson v. Molzen, 558 S.W. 2d 429 (Tenn. 1977)
Charrin v. Methodist Hospital, 432 S.W. 2d 572 (Tex. 1968)
DeBlanc v. Southern Baptist Hospital, 207 So. 868 (La. 1968)
Tunkl v. Regents of the Univ. of California, 383 P. 2d 441 (Cal. 1963)

Directed Verdicts

75 *Am Jur 2d*, TRIAL, § 463
Bryan v. Luverne Community Hospital, 217 N.W. 2d 745 (Minn. 1974)
Larson v. Harris, 231 N.E. 2d 421 (Ill. 1967)
Roberts v. Gale, 139 S.E. 2d 272 (W. Va. 1965)
Ahola v. Sincock, 94 N.W. 2d 566 (Wis. 1959)
Thomas v. Merriam, 337 P. 2d 604 (Mont. 1959)
Leonard v. Watsonville Community Hospital, 305 P. 2d 36 (Cal. 1956)
Seneris v. Haas, 291 P. 2d 915 (Cal. 1955)

Need for Expert Testimony

2 *Am Jur Trials*, Selecting and Preparing Expert Witnesses, p. 585
J. Taylor, "Serve As An Expert Witness? Read This First," *RN*, 47(4):21 (April 1984)
Annotations, 77 ALR 2d 1186, 27 ALR 2d 1263
Biundo v. Christ Community Hospital, 432 N.E. 2d 1293 (Ill. 1982)
O'Connor v. Bloomer, 172 Cal. Rptr. 128 (Cal. 1981)
Parker v. Knight, 267 S.E. 2d 222 (Ga. 1980)

Doctrine of *Res Ipsa Loquitur*

W. Prosser, *Handbook of the Law of Torts,* 4th ed., West Publishing, St. Paul, 1971, § 39

D. Louisell and H. Williams, *Medical Malpractice,* Matthew Bender & Co., New York, 1983, § 14.08

Annotations, 36 ALR 3d 1235, 9 ALR 3d 1350, 9 ALR 3d 1327, 72 ALR 2d 410

Morgan v. Children's Hospital, 480 N.E. 2d 464 (Ohio 1985)

Parks v. Perry, 314 S.E. 2d 287 (N.C. 1984)

Jones v. Harrisburg Polyclinic Hospital, 437 A. 2d 1134 (Pa. 1981)

Stevens v. Union Memorial Hospital, 424 A. 2d 1118 (Md. 1981)

White v. McCool, 395 So. 774 (La. 1981)

Spidle v. Steward, 402 N.E. 2d 216 (Ill. 1980)

Hanrahan v. St. Vincent Hospital, 516 F. 2d 300 (Iowa 1975)

Ybarra v. Spangard, 154 P. 2d 687 (Cal. 1944)

Part Seven
Principles of Malpractice Claims Prevention

Part 7

INTRODUCTORY NOTE

If malpractice claims arose *solely* due to errors in nursing practice, there would be no need for a separate part of this course dealing with the subject of malpractice claims prevention. To *prevent* malpractice claims, nurses would simply render the best possible nursing care to their patients as consistently as possible. But the fact of the matter is that malpractice suits also arise from several other causes, including sociological and psychological causes.

Teaching you about the various sociological and psychological causes of malpractice suits will be the function and aim of Part 7 of this course. It is hoped that when you have completed this part, you will have gained new insights into the fundamental bases of patient dissatisfaction and will know ways to reduce the causes of such dissatisfaction and the lawsuits generated thereby.

Malpractice Claims Prevention

7-1   Every nurse involved in direct patient care should regard malpractice claims prevention as an integral part of daily nursing responsibilities for two fundamental reasons: (1) All affirmative measures taken to minimize the occurrence of malpractice claims will minimize the nurse's exposure to personal liability, and (2) such measures will simultaneously result in higher-quality patient care.

The subject of malpractice claims prevention is something the nurse should want to know

☐   primarily to obtain continuing education credits

☐   as a part of everyday nursing responsibilities

☐   primarily to enable him or her to obtain a license to practice

---

7-2   The concept of malpractice claims prevention implies that the nurse

☐   can take affirmative steps to prevent malpractice claims from arising

☐   can avoid personal liability for his or her negligent conduct

☐   can obtain financial protection to help pay damages in malpractice claims brought against him or her

---

7-3   Is the following statement true or false?

There is a direct relationship between improved patient care and the subject of malpractice claims prevention.

True   *False*
☐   ☐

7-2 *as a part of everyday nursing responsibilities*	**7-2** *can take affirmative steps to prevent malpractice claims from arising*	**7-3** *True*

7-4   Nurses should want to prevent malpractice claims if for no other reason than to avoid the psychological disadvantages that generally accompany such claims. A malpractice suit represents an attack on the professional judgment and integrity of the nurse, and no matter how competent he or she is, the nurse who is challenged in this manner is bound to suffer anxiety and nervous tension while the case is in process.

Which of the following statements *best* expresses the foregoing?

☐   Malpractice claims are psychologically disturbing to the nurse primarily because he or she may have to pay damages to the injured party.

☐   Although malpractice claims often create psychological disadvantages for nurses who are professionally incompetent, they rarely affect competent nurses in this manner.

☐   Because their professional reputations are at stake when they are sued for malpractice, all nurses experience the psychological tensions that customarily accompany such suits.

7-5   What would be the *best* way for nurses to avoid the psychological disadvantages that accompany malpractice claims?

☐   They should increase the amount of their malpractice insurance.

☐   They should do what they can to prevent such claims from arising.

☐   They should lobby for legislation outlawing malpractice claims.

> NOTE: Malpractice claims and suits against nurses have increased considerably within the recent past, and all indications are that they will continue to grow in frequency in the future. Essential to any program of malpractice claims prevention is a basic understanding of the general and specific factors that influence *all* malpractice claims. Some of these factors are directly related to the quality of physical care given, while others represent sociological or psychological influences. All these factors will be discussed in the material that follows.

7-4   ☐
          ☐
          ☑

7-5 *They should do what they can to prevent such claims from arising.*

Causes of Malpractice Suits

7-6   One of the important sociological reasons why malpractice suits are becoming more frequent is the public's growing interest in medicine and awareness of medical facts. Discussions of medical topics appear daily in family magazines. Television programs dealing with medical subjects likewise have educated the public in many areas of medical practice. One of the unfortunate side effects of all this has been the tendency to underrate the dangers and overrate the benefits of medical care, leading to expectations that may not be fulfilled.

Which of the following *best* explains the sociological basis for the increasing number of malpractice suits?

☐   Malpractice suits are on the increase as a direct result of the effects on the public of magazine articles and television programs dealing with medical subjects.

☐   Malpractice suits have become more numerous due to the public's increasing familiarity with medical subjects and the erroneous expectations they often acquire from the mass media with regard to medical cures.

☐   Malpractice suits have increased as the public has become more conscious of lowered standards of medical care.

7-7   The public's attitude toward health professionals has changed considerably within recent years. As the public has become more sophisticated, its attitude has shifted from one of great respect and near reverence for those engaged in the healing arts to a more realistic view that doctors and nurses are fallible human beings who can and should be held legally responsible for their negligent conduct.

All other things being equal, the physician or nurse in practice today faces a threat of being sued for malpractice which

☐   is probably no greater than

☐   is probably greater than

☐   is probably smaller than

the threat of being sued faced by the physician or nurse practicing 20 years ago.

7-6 ☐ ☑ ☐	**7-7** *is probably greater than*

7-8   Answer yes or no to the following questions.

Yes   No

☐   ☐   Is the increase in malpractice suits due exclusively to changes in social attitudes?

☐   ☐   Could the fact that more lawyers now specialize in handling malpractice cases be a sociological factor behind the growing number of malpractice suits?

☐   ☐   As the public becomes more aware of the fact that physicians and nurses generally maintain malpractice insurance coverage, is it reasonable to conclude that the public will become less reluctant to sue a physician or nurse for malpractice?

7-9   Notwithstanding the sociological factors behind malpractice suits that have just been mentioned, *there can be no malpractice suit without some unfavorable medical result*. In Part 3 we saw examples of different types of negligent nursing conduct. When harm results from such conduct, the event invariably focuses the injured patient's thinking on a malpractice claim.

As a basic cause of malpractice suits, unfavorable medical results are

☐   more significant than

☐   no different than

☐   less significant than

the various sociological causes of malpractice suits.

7-8 Yes No	**7-9** *more significant than*
☐ ☑	
☑ ☐	
☑ ☐	

7-10   Unless a nurse's negligence results in some harm or injury to the patient, there can be no malpractice claim.

True   *False*

☐   ☐

7-11   When we refer to an unfavorable medical result as the basis of a malpractice suit, what do we mean?

☐ The patient and nurse have had one or more serious arguments, leading to a breakdown in their relationship.

☐ The nurse's conduct has resulted in some objective physical harm to the patient.

☐ The patient's condition has steadily worsened, notwithstanding proper care and treatment by the patient's physician and attending nurse.

7-10 *True*

If you checked the wrong answer, turn to p. 289, Note A.

7-11 ☐
          ☑
          ☐

POINTS TO REMEMBER

1. Malpractice claims prevention should be an integral part of the nurse's daily patient care responsibilities because the same steps taken to avoid malpractice claims are those that result in better patient care.

2. When a nurse is sued for alleged malpractice, the psychological disadvantages generally outweigh any possible financial loss.

3. Malpractice suits are attributable to medical, sociological, and psychological causes, each of which plays an important part in the patient's ultimate decision to sue.

4. A major sociological cause of malpractice suits is the public's tendency to overrate the curative power of medicine and to underrate the dangers and limitations of medical treatment. This tendency has been greatly fostered by means of the various media of communications.

5. As a result of greater public awareness of medicine and medical facts (including its awareness of malpractice claims insurance), there is far less hesitancy today about suing a physician or nurse for malpractice.

6. Sociological factors have combined with other causes of malpractice suits to bring about a decided increase in the number of such suits within recent years.

7-12   One point should be made perfectly clear: Not *every* unfavorable medical result is preventable, nor is *every* such result automatically the basis of legal liability. The law does not expect the nurse to be a guarantor against harm to the patient. It merely requires that the nurse exercise the degree of care other reasonably prudent nurses would exercise under similar circumstances in caring for their patients.

> Patient P enters the hospital for elective surgery, which proves to be uneventful. Postoperatively, he suffers an infection which extends his hospital stay an additional 3 weeks. He consults a competent lawyer for advice about the chances of success in a lawsuit against the medical personnel involved in his case while at the hospital.

What is the lawyer most likely to tell him?

☐ "Postoperative infection is an untoward medical event that may or may not be due to negligence. Under these facts you do not appear to have the basis for a lawsuit, but I'll inquire further into the matter."

☐ "Even if we cannot prove the postoperative infection was due to someone's negligence, the hospital and medical staff can be sued because you suffered the infection while under their care."

☐ "Postoperative infection is always attributable to someone's negligence, and you can therefore recover damages for the harm suffered in this case."

7-13   Which of the following unfavorable medical results, in and of itself, would reasonably be the basis of legal liability, and which of them would not?

Basis for liability	*No basis for liability*	
☐	☐	The patient was given 6 ounces of paraldehyde instead of 6 drams, due to a nurse's failure to check the physician's questionable handwriting.
☐	☐	The patient died from cardiac arrest during a cesarean delivery.
☐	☐	The patient suffered two broken teeth during the course of a laryngoscopy.
☐	☐	The patient suffered burns from a heat lamp placed too close to her bed.

7-12 ☑
☐
☐

7-13 *Basis* *No basis*
☑   ☐   If you missed more than one
☐   ☑   of these, turn to p. 289, Note
☑   ☐   B.
☑   ☐

EXPLANATORY NOTES

Note A   (from Frame 7-10)

Negligent conduct, in and of itself, does not establish legal liability on the part of the nurse. The courts do not recognize tort claims where there has been no injury to the plaintiff, no matter how offended the plaintiff may be. To illustrate, a patient enters the hospital for surgery and the operation proves to be entirely uneventful. He later learns that the nurse-anesthetist was unlicensed to practice in the state in question and immediately files suit against her for damages. Unless he can prove her conduct was in some way harmful to him, he cannot possibly prevail. As a matter of fact, the Court will most likely direct a verdict in the nurse's favor. The same result would occur if the unlicensed nurse had been negligent but no harm resulted from her negligence.

To repeat: Negligent conduct that creates no harm does not give rise to legal liability.

Proceed to Frame 7-11.

Note B   (from Frame 7-13)

Of all the unfavorable medical events listed, only the cardiac arrest during childbirth cannot reasonably be attributable to someone's negligence. Were we given more facts, even *that* incident might be the basis of liability against someone (e.g., the anesthetist). However, all the remaining events are explainable *only* as the product of negligent conduct on someone's part, and each could be the basis of liability against the responsible party.

Proceed to Frame 7-14.

7-14   The basis of every malpractice suit is some unfavorable medical result in the treatment process, but not every unfavorable medical result affords a basis for a malpractice suit.

True   *False*

☐   ☐

7-15   From the standpoint of physical care of the patient, nurses can do many things to forestall the possibility of malpractice suits. Select from the following list those things a nurse can and should do that might reasonably prevent a later malpractice suit.

☐   accurately record and report all significant facts relating to the patient's condition

☐   follow the physician's instructions without question

☐   determine whether a patient's needs can be safely carried out by another nurse

☐   administer medications prepared by other nurses

☐   safeguard the patient against falls

☐   diagnose the patient's ailment in the physician's absence

☐   clarify instructions whenever they are in doubt

7-14   *True*

7-15   ☑
           ☐
           ☑
           ☐
           ☑
           ☐
           ☑

7-16   Nursing is the core of the many activities that center on the hospitalized patient. In view of the frequency of nurse-patient contacts in the hospital setting, hospital nurses should be constantly aware of the malpractice claims potential of any improperly executed nursing functions. From the viewpoint of malpractice claims prevention, nothing is more effective than scrupulous attention to the requirements of good nursing practice.

Hospital nurses are more likely to be sued for acts of malpractice than other categories of health personnel because

☐   they are known to carry large amounts of malpractice insurance

☐   they have more patient contacts than other health personnel

☐   they make more professional errors than other health personnel

---

7-17   Which category of nurses should pay the *most* attention to the requirements of good nursing practice?

☐   hospital nurses

☐   private-duty nurses

☐   occupational health nurses

☐   public health nurses

☐   school nurses

☐   office nurses

7-16 *they have more patient contacts than other health personnel*	**7-17** ☐ None of the boxes should ☐ have been checked. The ☐ question was purposely de- ☐ signed to emphasize the fact ☐ that *all* nurses should pay at- ☐ tention to the requirements of good nursing practice, no matter where or for whom they work.

NOTE: Thus far we have examined some of the sociological and direct medical causes of malpractice suits. We now turn to a less obvious but extremely important cause of many malpractice suits: the patient's *psychological* dissatisfaction with the nursing care received.

7-18   A malpractice suit against a nurse often is merely the final stage of a deteriorating nurse-patient relationship. Whether or not the patient will resort to this dramatic way of showing dissatisfaction with the nurse will depend on a number of psychological factors, the most important of which are the patient's personality and the nurse's personality, particularly the way these two interacted during key treatment situations.

In analyzing the causes of malpractice claims, it is not often realized that psychological factors

☐   play only a minor role as causes of such claims

☐   are the principal causes of such claims

☐   are extremely important causes of such claims

7-19   A malpractice claim is always founded on some unfavorable medical result, but whether a particular result will trigger a suit against a nurse will depend in large part on

☐   the patient's prior attitude toward the nurse

☐   the patient's prior experience in courtroom cases

☐   the patient's knowledge of medicine and related matters

7-18 *are   extremely   important causes of such claims*

7-19 *the patient's prior attitude toward the nurse*

7-20   The tone of the nurse-patient relationship is determined by the daily interaction of the patient's personality and the nurse's personality.

Which of the following would be evidence of a poor nurse-patient relationship?

- ☐ The nurse and the patient's physician continually argue over the patient's nursing needs in the patient's presence.

- ☐ The nurse and the patient neither like nor respect each other.

- ☐ The nurse and the supervisor disagree on how the patient should be treated.

7-21   If malpractice claims are founded in part upon the interaction of the patient's and the nurse's personalities, then the role played by the nurse's personality in precipitating malpractice claims can be described as

- ☐ essentially neutral and, at most, secondary

- ☐ critical and more significant than all other factors

- ☐ decidedly influential but secondary to direct medical factors

---

7-22

True	*False*	
☐	☐	It is fair to state that a malpractice claim will result whenever there is an unfavorable medical event causing harm or injury to the patient.
☐	☐	It is fair to state that a malpractice claim will result whenever there is a breakdown in the nurse-patient relationship.

7-20		**7-21**		**7-22**	*True*	*False*	
	☐		☐		☐	☑	If you checked the wrong answer to either statement, turn to p. 306, Note A.
	☑		☐		☐	☑	
	☐		☑				

POINTS TO REMEMBER

1. A malpractice suit cannot be brought unless there has been some unexpected or unfavorable medical result directly related to a nurse's negligence.

2. Since the law does not require the nurse to be a guarantor against harm to the patient, not every unfavorable medical result will necessarily be grounds for a malpractice suit. Malpractice will exist only if the occurrence was preventable in the exercise of reasonable care by the nurse.

3. From the viewpoint of malpractice claims prevention, nothing is more effective than giving the highest-quality nursing care in accordance with recognized practices and procedures.

4. Psychological factors play an extremely important role as determinants of malpractice suits. More often than not a patient's decision to sue, although triggered by some adverse medical result, is one way the patient can obtain revenge for what he or she considers unsatisfactory treatment (in the psychological sense) on the part of the nurse.

5. Since malpractice claims are founded in part upon the daily interaction between the nurse and patient, the nurse's personality plays a significant role in the fostering or prevention of malpractice claims.

6. Because the psychological component can greatly influence a patient to sue or not to sue a nurse, all nurses should become familiar with the principles of patient psychology.

7-23   Careful study has shown that most nursing malpractice suits can be traced to patients' general dissatisfaction with the way they received care from the nurses they eventually sued. In order to understand the root causes of patient dissatisfaction and how to prevent it, a nurse must learn the fundamental principles of patient psychology.

Which of the following statements *best* summarizes the above paragraph?

☐   Patient dissatisfaction frequently leads to malpractice claims against nurses.

☐   A nurse's knowledge of patient psychology can uncover many of the causes of patient dissatisfaction and possibly prevent later malpractice claims.

☐   A knowledge of patient psychology is important to the nurse in carrying out everyday nursing responsibilities, but it is not likely to prevent malpractice claims from arising.

7-24   It may be stated as a fundamental rule that the less personal the relationship, the more likely the patient will think of suing for damages when something eventually goes wrong in the treatment process. Most patients want to be regarded as individuals and not as impersonal objects of medical treatment.

Which type of nurse is *most likely* to be sued for an act of malpractice, following some untoward medical event?

☐   the nurse who is generally efficient but always impersonal

☐   the nurse who is both efficient and friendly

☐   the nurse who is generally careless but always helpful

7-23 ☐ ☑ ☐	**7-24** *the nurse who is generally efficient but always impersonal*

7-25   Quality nursing care is more than just caring *for* the patient; it is caring *about* him as well. Although it may seem too obvious to state, all patients want to be treated with dignity and respect. Considerably more attention should be given to the interpersonal and emotional aspects of patient care, and the nurse should never forget that the patient's emotional and psychological needs are as important as physical comfort and safety.

Which of the following statements best summarizes the foregoing?

☐ Quality nursing care is concerned solely with the patient's physical needs and safety.

☐ Nurses place too much emphasis on ways of satisfying their patients' emotional needs.

☐ Nurses who pay attention to their patients' emotional needs thereby give recognition to an important aspect of patient care.

7-26   Three nursing students are discussing ways to prevent malpractice claims.

Nurse A: "The surest way to prevent malpractice claims is to be careful in meeting the patient's physical requirements."

Nurse B: "The surest way to prevent malpractice claims is to satisfy the patient's emotional needs."

Nurse C: "The surest way to prevent malpractice claims is to recognize the patient as a human being who has emotional as well as physical needs and to treat both in a competent manner."

Which of these nursing students is more nearly correct?

Nurse A   *Nurse B*   *Nurse C*
☐   ☐   ☐

7-25 *Nurses who pay attention to their patients' emotional needs thereby give recognition to an important aspect of patient care.*

7-26 *Nurse C*

Psychological Aspects of Patient Care

7-27   A basic understanding of the psychological aspects of patient behavior is important to the nurse not only from the standpoint of malpractice claims prevention but from the standpoint of stimulating and encouraging the patient's participation in the treatment process, thereby hastening his or her recovery.

Name two principal benefits to the nurse from a knowledge of patient psychology:

☐ prevention of malpractice claims

☐ greater intellectual achievement

☐ greater respect by the medical staff

☐ improved patient care

☐ lower malpractice insurance costs

7-28   The current emphasis on patient-centered treatment is based on the philosophy that the nurse should interact with the patient as a human being, instead of simply doing things for (or *to*) the patient in a stereotyped fashion. The patient is encouraged to understand and participate in his or her care, thereby assuming a degree of responsibility for the outcome of that care. With the focus on the patient rather than the task, the interaction between nurse and patient becomes more personal, less businesslike, and more satisfying to patient and nurse alike.

What does the patient-centered approach emphasize?

☐ prompt completion of the nursing task by enlisting the patient's help

☐ more nursing commands and less discussion with the patient, to prevent patient anxiety

☐ greater understanding by the patient concerning the treatment to be undertaken and how he or she can effectively participate therein

---

7-29   An underlying assumption of the patient-centered approach to nursing is that

☐ the patient wants to and should be encouraged to participate in his or her care

☐ the patient's cooperation is relatively insignificant in the treatment process

☐ the patient's participation in the treatment process tends to interfere with necessary nursing functions

7-27 *prevention of malpractice claims*
 	
 improved patient care
	7-28 ☐
	      ☐
	      ☑
		7-29 ☑
		      ☐
		      ☐

7-30   From the point of view of malpractice claims prevention the key to the success of the patient-centered approach is

☐ the ability to enlist the patient's help in performing necessary nursing functions

☐ the development of a more wholesome, therapeutic interaction between patient and nurse

☐ the opportunity given the nurse to experience more satisfying emotional relationships with patients

---

7-31   Since most patients react strongly to threats (real or implied) to their individuality, maturity, and adulthood, any procedure that requires them to be submissive is bound to give rise to feelings of helplessness, anxiety, and (to differing degrees) antagonism. On the other hand, when the patient is adequately informed of the procedure and encouraged to participate in it, feelings of helplessness diminish and the patient becomes a willing and cooperative partner in the therapeutic relationship.

A nurse informs a youthful maternity patient expecting her first child that standard hospital procedures require all maternity patients to get a predelivery enema.

What would be the best way to cope with the patient's apparent apprehensiveness?

☐ Assure her that the procedure is a routine one, generally safe, and in any event *necessary* in accordance with hospital policy.

☐ Say as little as possible to her since the more information she acquires, the more her anxiety is likely to increase.

☐ Give her a chance to express her reaction to the procedure and then explain how her conscious cooperation in relaxation and retention of the enema will have more effective results.

7-30   *the development of a more wholesome, therapeutic interaction between patient and nurse*

7-31   ☐ If you selected the wrong answer, turn to p. 306, Note B.
☐
☑

7-32   The nurse's ability to develop effective interpersonal relationships with patients requires a conscious effort. The nurse's words and actions must convey genuine interest and warmth so that the patient gets a feeling of real caring. Insincere mouthings intended merely to give the impression of the nurse's interest can prove to be more harmful than no conversation at all.

Nurse A begins her conversation with a patient as follows:

"I'm supposed to tell you about the barium enema you are scheduled for today."

Nurse B begins his conversation with a patient as follows:

"Good morning, Mr. Smith. I see that you're scheduled to undergo a barium enema, which is a simple diagnostic procedure. I'll be happy to tell you whatever you want to know about it."

What does Nurse A's introductory statement immediately reveal?

☐   She is genuinely concerned about keeping the patient posted on the treatment he is to undergo.

☐   She is making a routine explanatory statement that conveys neither warmth nor personal interest.

☐   She shows a sincere personal interest in the patient and his welfare.

7-33   What psychological effect is generally associated with addressing a patient by name, as Nurse B did in the example above?

☐   The patient's personal identity is recognized, and he feels that he has been treated with respect.

☐   The patient generally feels her personal privacy has been invaded.

☐   The patient generally does not care one way or another.

7-32 *She is making a routine explanatory statement that conveys neither warmth nor personal interest.*

7-33 *The patient's personal identity is recognized, and he feels that he has been treated with respect.*

POINTS TO REMEMBER

1. Most malpractice suits are traceable to the patient's psychological dissatisfaction with the nursing care received.

2. The less personal the nurse-patient relationship, the greater the likelihood that the patient will think of suing the nurse should something go wrong in the treatment process.

3. All patients want to be treated with dignity and respect, and the intelligent nurse will always give appropriate recognition to patients' emotional needs as well as their physical needs.

4. Understanding patient attitudes and behavior will not only prevent malpractice suits but will stimulate the patient's participation in his or her treatment.

5. By definition, patient-centered treatment focuses on the patient rather than the task, and this personal approach is calculated to be more beneficial to patient and nurse alike.

6. Patients should be encouraged to participate in their care to the greatest extent practicable, thereby assuring a more wholesome therapeutic relationship between patient and nurse.

7. Nurses should consciously try to develop effective interpersonal relationships with their patients and should demonstrate by their words and actions that they not only care for but care about their patients.

7-34   Hostility is a very common reaction to something that is viewed as a threat, and the hospital atmosphere has a tendency to heighten the anxiety and insecurity of many patients, making them extremely uncooperative and difficult to care for. Understanding the causes of hostility and helping the hostile patient to identify what he or she perceives as a threat will not only bring about a better therapeutic relationship but will greatly reduce the malpractice threat to the nurse that the hostile patient always presents.

Hostility in the hospital setting is

☐   something all patients exhibit

☐   a trait exhibited by relatively few patients

☐   a rather common type of behavior

7-35

Patient P is scheduled to undergo surgery for amputation of her left leg. She is worried about the loss of this important organ as well as her future chances of employment and shows her concern by being hostile to all who attend her. One day she tells Nurse N, "You're a miserable nurse. Nothing you do is right."

What is the best way for Nurse N to react to this hostile patient?

☐   He should react no differently than in any other similar situation. If he feels anger or hostility toward the patient, he should tell her so.

☐   He should help the patient identify the cause of her hostility and patiently explore with her ways of dealing with the stressful situation.

☐   He should first defend himself against the attack made on him and then make it clear to the patient that her behavior is disrupting the hospital routine.

7-34 *a rather common type of be-havior*	**7-35** *he should help the patient identify the cause of her hos-tility and patiently explore with her ways of dealing with the stressful situation.*

> NOTE: Nurses who react to hostility by defending their own actions are not much help to patients and may even aggravate an already hostile attitude. Experienced nurses will always direct their responses to the patients' problems and assure them (in a sincere way) that they care and want to help. Under no circumstances should nurses take advantage of the situation by giving vent to their *own* feelings of hostility, toward either difficult patients or other patients.

The Suit-Prone Patient

7-36   There is one type of patient who is more likely than any other to bring suit for malpractice when something goes wrong in the treatment process. This individual is often referred to as the "suit-prone" patient. Because this person's psychological makeup breeds resentment and dissatisfaction in *all* phases of life, he or she poses a serious malpractice threat to all health personnel involved in his or her treatment. Nurses should learn to recognize the symptoms of suit-prone patients and make appropriate allowance for their emotional needs.

What can the nurse do, if anything, to cope with the suit-prone patient?

☐   The nurse should leave this patient alone as much as possible.

☐   The nurse might possibly protect herself or himself against suit by a suit-prone patient by paying special attention to this patient's psychological needs.

☐   There is little or nothing a nurse can do to cope with a person who is suit-prone.

> NOTE: Before proceeding with the discussion of the suit-prone patient, it should be made clear that *not every patient is suit-prone, nor should all patients be regarded as potential litigants*. The fact is, patients who are suit-prone are probably in the minority, but they can create serious problems for conscientious nurses and, for that reason, should be dealt with carefully. The key to doing this, as noted above, is to learn how to spot suit-prone patients in the first place, and then deal with them appropriately.

7-36   ☐
       ☑
       ☐

7-37   The concept of suit-prone means that this type of person frequently chooses to express dissatisfaction or resentment by filing a lawsuit against the person who is the object of this dissatisfaction.

Which of the following would *best* describe patients who are suit-prone?

☐   They have an intimate knowledge of the law and are familiar with courtroom procedures.

☐   They have a genuine appreciation for the law and legal proceedings.

☐   Their preferred method of dealing with persons who antagonize them is to file lawsuits against them.

7-38   What is the threat to nurses posed by suit-prone patients?

☐   Their conduct is generally violent, which raises the constant threat of physical harm to a nurse.

☐   Their need to blame others whenever things do not go as expected may encourage them to sue a nurse for malpractice.

☐   Their lack of personal concern for their health and general indifference to treatment may retard their rate of recovery.

7-37   *Their preferred method of dealing with persons who antagonize them is to file lawsuits against them.*

7-38   ☐
          ☑
          ☐

7-39   The attitudes of suit-prone patients reflect a basic immaturity that is revealed in *all* aspects of their lives. They are insecure persons and express this insecurity by being hostile and uncooperative. Perhaps the thing that characterizes them best is their need to shift blame to other persons as a way of coping with their own inadequacies.

Which of the following personality traits would a suit-prone patient generally *not* possess?

- ☐ a well-defined sense of personal responsibility

- ☐ dependency and a generally insecure nature

- ☐ immaturity and avoidance of responsibility

7-40   Which of the following statements *most accurately* reflects the attitude of the suit-prone patient toward physicians and nurses?

- ☐ "I don't like medical people to begin with, and I'll get even with any one of them who treats me in a high-handed way."

- ☐ "Most doctors and nurses are nice people, and since they are bound to make mistakes occasionally, I make the usual allowances for their failings."

- ☐ "Undergoing medical treatment provides a nice change from my usual activities, and I never worry about things going wrong."

7-39 *a well-defined sense of per-sonal responsibility*

7-40 ☑
☐
☐

7-41   Suit-prone patients, by their very nature, are likely to be uncooperative patients. They frequently fail to state their complaints accurately and will not follow a prescribed therapeutic regimen. They react to their feelings of inferiority and insecurity by being difficult and negative in their dealings with medical personnel.

Which of the following traits would indicate to the nurse that a patient is probably suit-prone? (Select two.)

☐   The patient argues and is generally disagreeable.

☐   The patient is understanding and cooperative.

☐   The patient is a fault-finder and critic.

7-42   Studies have shown that the institutional structure of the typical hospital has a tendency to stimulate even greater dissatisfaction and resentment on the part of suit-prone patients than they normally display. The patients' enforced passivity, coupled with the invasion of their bodily privacy and control over their own actions, intensifies their feelings of inferiority, insecurity, and frustration.

Which of the following reactions might be expected to occur as a consequence of a patient's hospitalization? (Select two.)

☐   The patient generally receives more attention and hence is inclined to be more agreeable.

☐   The patient is required to be obedient, cooperative, and uncomplaining, all of which tends to make him or her more frustrated.

☐   The patient's enforced passivity tends to heighten his or her sensitivity and emotional reaction to any real or fancied slights by doctors or nurses.

7-43   It is well established that a suit-prone patient will sue for malpractice whenever he or she suffers some compensable harm or injury at the hands of a physician or nurse.

True   False
☐   ☐

7-41 ☑	**7-42** ☐	**7-43** *False*
☐	☑	
☑	☑	If you checked True, turn to p. 306, Note C.

EXPLANATORY NOTES

Note A   (from Frame 7-22)

Both of these statements are false. Even if some unfavorable medical event occurs, a patient may or may not decide to sue the offending nurse, depending upon a variety of factors. One of the most important of these is the way the patient believes he or she has been treated—emotionally as well as physically—prior to the incident in question. Looking at the other side of the coin, no matter how poorly patients believe they have been treated (both emotionally and physically), they cannot successfully bring malpractice suits unless they can prove some compensable harm. The important psychological bases for malpractice suits are discussed in the following frames.

Proceed to Frame 7-23.

Note B   (from Frame 7-31)

Most studies have revealed that the most successful relationship between patient and nurse occurs when there is mutual planning and consent. It can be disastrous for the nurse to assume an authoritarian role and place the patient in a position of being a recipient of care he or she may neither understand nor want. The failure to communicate with the patient generally results in *greater* anxiety on the part of the patient, not the reverse. All in all, it seems reasonably well established that encouragement of the patient's participation in matters such as administration of the predelivery enema has produced more effective results than when the patient was assigned a more passive role.

Proceed to Frame 7-32.

Note C   (from Frame 7-43)

Generally speaking, suit-prone patients will *not* sue for malpractice unless they have been badly treated—in the emotional sense—prior to the act of malpractice. Recognizing suit-prone patients, therefore, and making proper allowance for their emotional needs in an intelligent manner can effectively eliminate one of the principal causes of malpractice suits. Dealing with persons who have unusual emotional needs calls for patience and genuine understanding on the part of the nurse. It is a challenge to which all nurses should rise, knowing that success will make their chosen career a much more satisfying one from every point of view.

Proceed to Frame 7-44.

POINTS TO REMEMBER

1. Since hostility is a common reaction of many patients to the various threats posed by the hospital atmosphere, the nurse should try to help the hostile patient identify the source of his or her hostility and then come to grips with the stress-producing situation.

2. Nurses should never permit their own feelings of hostility to override their primary responsibility to the patients. Their responses should always be therapeutically oriented.

3. Some patients are particularly suit-prone as a result of built-in personality defects that are typified by dissatisfaction and resentment in all phases of their lives. Suit-prone patients pose the greatest malpractice threat to practicing nurses; nurses should learn to recognize their symptoms and make appropriate allowances for their emotional needs.

4. Suit-prone patients are immature, dependent, uncooperative, and frequently hostile. Their hallmark is their inability to be self-critical, and they invariably shift blame to other persons as a way of coping with their own inadequacies.

5. Treating a suit-prone person is hazardous under the best of circumstances, so the nurse must be especially alert to the problems this type of patient presents, in order to avoid a later malpractice claim.

NOTE: How should you cope with suit-prone patients? First and foremost, you should make a conscious effort to *know* these patients, not simply as ill persons, but as human beings. This means cheering them up when they are obviously depressed or fearful, showing interest and sympathy in their pain and suffering, and expressing appreciation when they are cooperative. A genuine atmosphere of *attentiveness, patience,* and *understanding* will foster the respect and confidence necessary to help bring about these patients' ultimate recovery.

7-44   In what way can a nurse be sensitive to a patient's latent or expressed fears?

☐   by being impersonal and objective

☐   by being sympathetic and attentive

☐   by letting him talk but not getting involved

7-45   If a patient is already suit-prone, any evidence that the nurse's sympathy and concern on his or her behalf are false will probably

☐   make the patient respect the nurse a little more

☐   not affect the patient at all

☐   reinforce the patient's suit-prone nature

7-44   *by being sympathetic and attentive*

7-45   *reinforce the patient's suit-prone nature*

7-46   Any adverse nursing incident is sufficient for the suit-prone patient to conclude that malpractice has occurred. At that point, however, the patient's decision to sue the nurse may depend not so much upon the adverse medical event itself but upon how well the patient believes he or she has been dealt with by the nurse in the psychological sense—that is, the degree of understanding, sympathy, and respect the patient has received from the nurse *prior* to the time of the incident.

In which of the following cases would the otherwise suit-prone patient probably *not* sue the nurse?

☐   A.   The nurse (acting on the doctor's orders) tells the patient he must get up and walk for 15 minutes. The patient tells the nurse he feels faint, nauseated, and slightly dizzy. The nurse insists he must walk anyway, and while so doing he falls and injures himself.

☐   B.   The nurse is summoned to the patient's bedside, and when he arrives the patient asks several vague questions and engages him in general small talk. Although the nurse is busy, he chats amiably with the patient and then leaves. Later that day the nurse negligently injures the patient while giving an injection.

☐   C.   The nurse is about to give the patient the second dose of a medicine when the patient reminds her that the first dose reacted very badly. "Never mind," says the nurse, "according to the chart you're supposed to get the second dose now, and I'm here to see that you get it." The second dose results in a more severe reaction than the first.

7-47   It is poor nursing practice to make special adjustments in a patient's care simply because the patient is known to be suit-prone.

True   *False*
☐   ☐

7-46   *A*   *B*   *C*
           ☐   ☑   ☐

7-47   *False*

If you checked True, turn to p. 314, Note A.

7-48

Mrs. P is 38 years old, a widow, and an active career woman. She has no children and only distant relatives. During her hospitalization for removal of an ovarian cyst, she exhibits all the traits and symptoms of the suit-prone patient (anger, resentment, dissatisfaction, un-cooperativeness, etc.), and all the floor nurses are aware of this. Mrs. P. shows extreme concern for her physical health, and whenever a nurse is near she regularly complains of numerous vague symptoms. The three nurses who have been caring for her react to these complaints as follows:

Nurse A shows signs of annoyance and remarks, ''Now, now, Mrs. P. It isn't as bad as all that. You are just upset about your operation, but you have nothing to worry about.''

Nurse B listens carefully to Mrs. P's complaints and then remarks, ''Don't worry, Mrs. P, I'm sure there's nothing seriously wrong, but I will make a note on your chart and tell Doctor D when he comes to see you.''

Nurse C shows little interest in Mrs. P's complaints and (acting on her own) administers a sedative to keep Mrs. P from bothering the nursing staff.

Which nurse reacted to Mrs. P in the professional manner calculated to help the patient the most as well as to minimize the risk of a later malpractice suit?

Nurse A	*Nurse B*	*Nurse C*
☐	☐	☐

7-49   The fundamental reason why a nurse should be attentive, patient, and understanding in caring for patients is to forestall the possibility of later malpractice suits.

True	*False*
☐	☐

7-48   A   B   C
        ☐   ☑   ☐

7-49   *False*

7-50   Nursing psychiatric patients calls for the utmost in patience, judgment, and intelligence on the part of the nurse since the basic personality disturbances of mentally ill persons are greatly heightened in the hospital atmosphere. With respect to this class of patient, therefore, special attention is necessary in order to forestall the possibility of a later malpractice claim.

The significant threat to the nurse that psychiatric patients present is

☐   they are more likely to complain about a nurse's services to the physician or nurse-supervisor

☐   they will probably make the nurse's life miserable

☐   they are more likely to sue a nurse for an act of malpractice

---

7-51   Since the suit-prone patient is one who (by definition) has unusual emotional needs, it follows that a mentally ill patient

☐   can be treated with considerably less attention to his or her emotional needs

☐   is probably not suit-prone at all

☐   is probably the most suit-prone patient of all

7-52   The nurses who are least likely to be sued by their patients, even though they may commit acts of malpractice, are

☐   the nurses who get along well with their nursing supervisors and with the hospital medical staff

☐   the nurses who are sensitive to all their patients' physical and emotional needs

☐   the nurses who keep up with the latest techniques in nursing practice through postgraduate courses

7-50 *they are more likely to sue a nurse for an act of malpractice*	**7-51** *is probably the most suit-prone patient of all*	**7-52** *the nurses who are sensitive to all their patients' physical and emotional needs*

NOTE: In the material that follows, we discuss briefly the problems associated with suit-prone nurses. Before doing so, however, it should be made clear that *most nurses do not fall within that category,* and this should not be inferred simply because the topic is discussed.

The Suit-Prone Nurse

7-53   Some nurses have great technical competence but nevertheless find it difficult to establish warm relationships with others. They may show their uneasiness with close person-to-person contacts by being authoritarian, aloof, or so busy with the mechanics of nursing care that they have little time for meaningful human interaction. It should be recognized that such personality patterns on the part of nurses may be important causes of later malpractice suits.

From the human relations standpoint, the success of the nurse-patient relationship requires the nurse to develop which of the following abilities?

☐   the ability to interact favorably with patients on a personal level

☐   the ability to accomplish all his or her nursing tasks with the greatest degree of proficiency

☐   the ability to successfully manage patients by appropriate directions, orders, and discipline

7-54

Nurse N has a fine record as a nurse who can initiate and carry out the most complex nursing procedures with technical perfection. Psychologically she is rigid and does not relate well to other persons. Although she gives the impression of one who "knows it all," she is extremely sensitive to criticism and reacts to criticism either by becoming verbally offensive or by stalking out of the room to show her displeasure.

What does Nurse N have in common, if anything, with the patient who is suit-prone?

☐   She has nothing in common with him.

☐   She has an insecure personality.

☐   She has the tendency to shift blame to others.

☐   She is probably just as suit-prone as he is.

7-53 *the ability to interact favor-ably with patients on a per-sonal level*	**7-54** ☐ If you did not check the last ☑ box, turn to p. 314, Note B. ☑ ☑

7-55   Under what circumstances would Nurse N be in *greatest* jeopardy, from the standpoint of her malpractice liability?

☐   when she is working under close supervision

☐   when she is caring for a suit-prone patient

☐   when she is carrying out standing orders

7-56   What two steps should Nurse N take to minimize her malpractice liability potential?

☐   She should learn the fundamentals of patient psychology and put them into practice as much as possible.

☐   She should devote more time to recognition and understanding of her own personality problems and make appropriate adjustments to enable her to relate more effectively to her patients.

☐   She should try to become more technically proficient in order to reduce the likelihood of errors.

7-57   All other things being equal, a nurse who has a reputation for being tough and inflexible and for going ''by the book'' is

☐   more likely

☐   less likely

☐   neither more nor less likely

to be sued for malpractice than a nurse who is more flexible and agreeable.

7-55 *when she is caring for a suit-prone patient*	**7-56** ☑ ☑ ☐	**7-57** *more likely*

EXPLANATORY NOTES

Note A   (from Frame 7-47)

The point that has been stressed throughout this discussion of psychological factors is that special attention *must* be paid to the patient who is suit-prone. In fact, it is one of the few things a nurse can do to prevent a later malpractice suit by such a person. Paying special attention to suit-prone patients means being aware of the way they react to illness, their attitude toward doctors and nurses, and their hidden fears and antagonisms. It means cheering them up when they are obviously depressed or fearful, showing interest and sympathy in their pain and suffering, and expressing appreciation for their efforts to cooperate in the recommended course of treatment. The worst mistake a nurse can make is to be insensitive to the suit-prone patient's unusual psychological needs. Indifference to the patient only adds fuel to a preexisting feeling of resentment, setting the stage for a later lawsuit.

Proceed to Frame 7-48.

Note B   (from Frame 7-54)

It may seem far-fetched to refer to a nurse as suit-prone, but the fact is that some nurses (certainly not the majority) are just that. Suit-prone nurses cannot admit to themselves their own limitations of training and experience and, when confronted by dissatisfied patients, generally respond to the situation by neglecting the patient (rejection) or by dismissing the complaints as trivial (ridicule). In an attempt to bolster their own faltering egos, suit-prone nurses refuse to accept responsibility for whatever may have gone wrong and tend to react to the situation by losing emotional control. Being more preoccupied with their own image, they tend to regard the patients as symbols of their own failure and punish them by total indifference to their emotional needs. In so doing, they completely distort the nurse-patient relationship and become prime targets for a patient's later desire for revenge. Thus, they are just as suit-prone as suit-prone patients even though they are the ones who are sued rather than the ones who initiate the suit.

Proceed to Frame 7-55.

POINTS TO REMEMBER

1. To cope with suit-prone patients the nurse should make a genuine effort to know and understand them as individuals. The nurse should be attentive, patient, and understanding.

2. The more rigid and impersonal a nurse is, the more likely that he or she will be sued by a suit-prone patient.

3. Whether or not a suit-prone patient will in fact sue the nurse, even after an adverse nursing incident, will depend upon how well the patient believes he or she was treated by the nurse (in the psychological sense) prior to the incident.

4. Since the suit-prone patient is one who is dependent, insecure, and socially immature, persons who are mentally ill and have intensified emotional problems are probably the most suit-prone of all.

5. Nurses who cannot take criticism and who do not relate well to other persons are sure targets for the suit-prone patient. Accordingly, they should make a sincere effort to learn more about their own personality limitations and make necessary adjustments therein to prevent unwanted malpractice suits.

RISK MANAGEMENT IN THE HOSPITAL

Throughout this discussion emphasis has been placed on the things the individual nurse can do to prevent malpractice suits. There are a number of other measures, however, that can and should be taken in the hospital setting that concern not just the individual practitioner but the hospital as a whole. Taken collectively, these measures form part of the hospital's *risk management plan,* designed to identify the risks of potential accidents and injuries to patients (and staff as well) and thereby to improve the quality of patient care.

A well-functioning hospital risk management program will include at the very least the following:

1. Some form of in-house complaint mechanism by which patients and/or their family members can make management aware of inadequacies in treatment (by doctors as well as nurses), demeanor of personnel, potentially harmful practices, billing problems, and so forth. Many hospitals now employ patient advocates or ombudsmen on a full-time basis to work directly with patients and their families in resolving reported grievances promptly, both to increase patient satisfaction and to forestall possible later litigation.

2. The continuous collection and evaluation of data concerning specific patient grievances and negative health care outcomes in general. In most cases, this data is collected in the form of incident reports filed by staff members—frequently nursing personnel—as these grievances and outcomes are brought to their attention. A good incident reporting program will alert both medical and administrative staff to those areas that need improvement, and is thus closely tied to item 3.

3. Mechanisms to evaluate the quality of medical care throughout the institution, including medical audit, nursing audit, utilization review, and tissue committees. This process includes the formulation and implementation of corrective actions designed to reduce all potential causes of injuries to patients, whether or not they give rise to malpractice claims.

4. Special education programs for hospital medical, nursing, and technical personnel designed to anticipate and prevent all potential causes of medical injury, as well as programs dealing with the legal aspects of patient care and ways of improving rapport with patients.

A good hospital risk management program will also include a number of other elements and areas of responsibility to ensure the safety of patients, whether in the emergency room, the surgical suite, the recovery room, the corridors, or anywhere else in the hospital. Usually, a hospital will establish a special risk management committee, comprised of representatives from each of the hospital's major departments and chaired by someone with expertise in the field of risk management who normally acts as coordinator and basic strategist for implementing corrective measures.

The importance of a formal hospital risk management program cannot be over-emphasized, especially in an era when malpractice suits against all providers of health care are on the increase. Nurses who are employed in the hospital setting will make it their business to become familiar with the hospital's incident-reporting system and other risk management procedures. Of course, they will also make it their business to understand the importance of malpractice insurance protection, a subject covered more fully in Part 8.

SELECTED REFERENCES—PART 7

Malpractice Claims Prevention

E. Bernzweig, "How a Communications Breakdown Can Get You Sued," *RN*, 48(12):47 (Dec. 1985)

M. Cushing, "First, Anticipate the Harm," *Amer J. Nurs.*, 85(2):137 (Feb. 1985)

M. Knight, "Our Safety Net Keeps Patients From Falling," *RN*, 48(12):9 (Dec. 1985)

D. Guariello, "Nursing Malpractice Litigation: Toward Better Patient Care," *Trial*, 18:78 (Oct. 1982)

S. Perry, "Managing to Avoid Malpractice," *J. Nurs. Admin.*, 8:43 (Aug. 1978)

H. Hassard, "Professional Liability Claims Prevention," *J.A.M.A.*, 163:1267 (1957)

E. Bernzweig, "Liability for Malpractice—Its Role in Nursing Education," *J. Nurs. Educ.*, 8:33 (April 1969)

See also, Risk Management references below

Psychological Aspects of Patient Care

D. Kivi, "Did He Say It Was OK To Use His First Name?" *RN*, 48(4):13 (April 1985)

C. Kasch, "Interpersonal Competence and Communication in the Delivery of Nursing Care," *Adv. Nurs. Sci.*, 6(2):71 (Jan. 1984)

D. Armstrong, "The Fabrication of Nurse-Patient Relationships," *Soc. Sci. Med.*, 17(8):457 (Aug. 1983)

D. Louisell and H. Williams, *Medical Malpractice,* Matthew Bender & Co., New York, 1983, § 5.08–5.09

F. Abdellah, I. Beland, et al., *New Directions in Patient Centered Nursing,* Macmillan, New York, 1973

E. Bernzweig, "Soothing Patient Psyche May Prevent Lawsuit," *Mod. Hosp.*, 112(2):83 (Feb. 1969)

R. Blum, *The Management of the Doctor-Patient Relationship,* McGraw-Hill Book Co., New York, 1960

Suit-Prone Patients

E. Bernzweig, "How to Spot the Suit-prone Patient," *RN*, 48(6):63 (June 1985)

A. Miller, "Nurse-Patient Dependency—Is It Iatrogenic?" *J. Adv. Nurs.*, 10(1):63 (Jan. 1985)

D. Barash, "Defusing the Violent Patient—Before He Explodes," *RN*, 47(3):34 (March 1984)

P. Brink, "The Patient as Victim," *Amer. J. Nurs.*, 84(7):964 (July 1984)

D. Gannon, "On Being a Patient: Hate, Love, and Nurses," *Med. J. Aust.* 140(8):486 (April 1984)

J. Groves, "Taking Care of the Hateful Patient," *N. Engl. J. Med.*, 299:366 (Aug. 17, 1978)

C. Levinson, "Beware the Malpractice Plaintiff," *J. Amer. Dent. Assn.,* 62:343 (March 1961)

R. Blum, *The Psychology of Malpractice Suits,* Study made for the California Medical Association, San Francisco, chap. 4. (March 1957)

Kakligian v. Henry Ford Hospital, 210 N.W. 2d 463 (Mich. 1973)

The Suit-Prone Nurse

E. Bernzweig, "When the Nurse is Her Own Worst Enemy," *RN,* 48(7):53 (July 1985)

S. Hardin, "Nonverbal Communication of Patients and High and Low Empathy Nurses," *J. Psychosoc. Nurs. Ment. Health Serv.,* 21(1):14 (Jan. 1983)

P. Schuster, "Preparing the Patient for a Barium Enema: A Comparison of Nurse and Patient Opinions," *J. Adv. Nurs.,* 7(6):523 (Nov. 1982)

B. Duldt, "Anger: An Occupational Hazard for Nurses," *Nurs. Outl.,* 29(9):510 (Sept. 1981)

Arnold v. Haggin Memorial Hospital, 415 S.W. 2d 844 (Ky. 1967)

Duling v. Bluefield Sanitarium, Inc., 148 S.E. 2d 754 (W. Va. 1967)

Incident Reports and Risk Management

C. Jacobs, *Hospital Risk Management and Malpractice Liability Control,* InterQual, Chicago, 1980

B. Brown, *Risk Management for Hospitals,* Aspen Systems Corp., Germantown, Md., 1979

Patient Safety Manual, American College of Surgeons, Chicago 1979

S. Salman, "Incident Reporting/Key Loss Control Program Ingredient," *Hosp. Health Care Section Safety Newsletter,* National Safety Council (Aug. 1976)

W. Curran, "The Medical Malpractice Problem: Patterns of Risk and Methods of Prevention," *Amer. J. Pub. Health,* 61:394 (Feb. 1971)

Kay Laboratories v. District Court, 653 P. 2d 721 (Colo. 1982)

Part Eight
Miscellaneous Legal Matters

Part 8

INTRODUCTORY NOTE

The prime objective of this programmed course is to teach nursing students and graduate nurses about their legal liability for malpractice, so the course content has been structured accordingly. There are a number of other legal problem areas, however, that do not pertain to nursing malpractice per se but nevertheless directly relate to the daily activities of nurses. Awareness of these problem areas is of particular importance to the nursing student, whose familiarity with the underlying issues and how to cope with them is generally minimal.

The material that is presented in Part 8 is intended to bridge this information gap in a nonprogrammed format so that it can be a quick-reference source of help when dealing with these non-malpractice issues. The inherent limitations of both time and space do not permit discussion of still other legal problems that affect the nurse's patient care activities, so nurses who are faced with specific legal problems should not hesitate to contact the hospital's legal counsel or the legal counsel for their state or local nursing association.

MEDICAL RECORDS

In part 3 of this course it was pointed out that one of the nurse's fundamental legal responsibilities is the duty to keep accurate records of the patient's physical and mental condition. The necessity for maintenance of accurate and complete medical records should be evident to all who work in the field of medicine. Such records are an integral and vital adjunct in patient care, providing the connecting links in the chain that extends from the patient's initial treatment for a medical complaint to his or her discharge from treatment after receiving the maximum benefits of care.

Medical records that are kept in a careful manner not only assist in the treatment of the patient—their primary and fundamental purpose—but incidentally aid materially in the defense of any claim, should a malpractice suit later be instituted. To be of any real value in serving either purpose, all entries in medical records should be clear and legible.

Bearing in mind the fact that medical records may one day be subpoenaed for use in litigation, physicians and nurses must guard against inserting gratuitous or defamatory statements in the patient's chart that might later prove embarrassing in court. Thus, the prudent nurse will avoid the temptation to include in the chart remarks concerning (1) the patient's personality traits or idiosyncracies (unless such remarks are relevant to the patient's treatment), (2) personal views to the effect that the patient is a malingerer or potential litigant, or (3) gratuitous admissions of legal liability with respect to untoward medical or nursing events.

Contents

The patient's medical record (or chart) is a written account of his or her illness and course of treatment by all members of the health care team during the patient's stay in the hospital, or by the physician in private practice providing treatment on an outpatient basis. Generally speaking, the medical record has two distinct parts. The first, usually prepared on the patient's admission, merely details the information necessary to identify the patient and to indicate the primary reason for his or her admission. The second part of the record is both dynamic and historic in that it details the clinical history of the patient's course of treatment. The information in this part of the patient's medical record is commonly prescribed by state licensing authorities, supplemented by the hospital's own rules and regulations. Normally it includes the patient's physical history, admitting diagnosis, follow-up diagnoses, temperature chart, therapy and medications prescribed, consultations ordered and the results thereof, x-ray and lab reports, doctor's progress notes, operative procedures performed, nurse's progress notes, signed consent forms (or refusals to execute such forms, properly documented), and similar medical-nursing data.

Alteration of Records

The nurse's charts and notes are an important guide for the physician in diagnosing and prescribing for the patient; hence, they should always be legible and concise, as well as accurate. Where errors in the chart are noted, they should be corrected promptly and initialed appropriately. Under no circumstances should erroneous records—i.e., those containing inadvertently incorrect information—be removed from the overall record and new pages substituted. Both for ethical and legal reasons the error(s) should simply be noted, corrected, and initialed.

The matter of correcting chart errors raises a related question. In many hospitals there is a mistaken notion that nurses are duty bound to place on the patient's chart *anything the treating physician directs them to place on the chart,* as though it were a direct medical order not subject to challenge. Nothing could be further from the truth. Nurses who accede to the demands of a physician to cover up the true facts of an unusual clinical episode by deliberately not mentioning it in the patient's chart are begging for trouble. Not only will their conduct subject them to possible loss of their licenses, but in flagrant circumstances they may even subject themselves to criminal action, leading to a fine or jail sentence.

Hospitalized patients have a legal right to assume not only that adequate health care will be provided, but also that all records relating to that health care will be accurate and truthful. Under no circumstances should the nurse place a doctor's order to falsify or alter a patient's record (or to delete pertinent information therefrom) above a legal and ethical responsibility to record all clinical information truthfully. When faced with such a situation, the prudent nurse should respectfully decline to become an accessory to the doctor's bidding; if pressured further, the nurse should report the circumstances to the appropriate hospital authority without delay.

Countersigning

It has become increasingly common in teaching hospitals, and other hospitals as well, to require that all entries made in patient's charts by licensed practical nurses and nursing students be countersigned by a clinical instructor or other nurse acting in a supervisory capacity. While this practice may be justifiable from the hospital's point of view, it is fraught with legal risks for the nurse who is required to routinely countersign such records.

It should be clearly understood that to countersign a patient's chart is more than to simply add one's signature to a statement made by someone else. The countersigner is actually attesting to the authenticity of the observations and statements made by the original signer. From a legal standpoint, the countersigner is presumed to have personal knowledge of the information contained in the particular record, as though he or she had personally performed the procedure, given the particular medication, or made the particular observation recorded. Later, in a court case, the nurse who has countersigned statements made in the patient's chart can be held jointly liable with the original signer for any negligence traceable to the information so recorded.

The legal lesson is clear. The nurse who is required by hospital policy to countersign on a routine basis documents or information in the patient's chart should protect himself or herself in one of two ways: (1) by personally verifying the information being recorded, or (2) by noting in the record that his or her signature is included in accordance with hospital policy, and is not based on personal knowledge of the information in question.

Confidential Nature of Medical Information

A confidential communication is one that contains information given by one person to another under circumstances of trust and confidence with the understanding that such information must not be disclosed. Clearly, information about a patient—gathered by examination, observation, conversation, or treatment—is the type of confidential information the law has always protected. Thus, both nurses and physicians are legally and morally obligated to keep secret any information about a patient's illness or treatment that is obtained in the normal course of their professional duties. Indeed, the observance of confidentiality is one of the fundamental tenets of the Code for Professional Nurses adopted by the American Nurses Association.

Disclosure of Medical Information

The information contained in the patient's medical record customarily is used for a number of purposes. Those persons involved in the direct care of the patient obviously have a legitimate interest in seeing the chart; hence, there is no breach of confidentiality when the records are made available for this purpose. Medical and nursing personnel may also have occasion to see a patient's chart for the purpose of research, data gathering, or continuing education needs, and here again there is no breach of confidentiality so long as the records are used as intended.

In general, however, if information from a patient's chart is disclosed without the patient's express consent, or without a court order or express statutory authority, the hospital—as well as those who actually made the disclosure—may be held liable in damages should the patient be able to prove invasion of privacy or perhaps defamation of character. Most state statutes expressly require disclosure of medical record information where criminal matters are involved (e.g., attempted suicide, unlawful dispensing of narcotic drugs by a doctor or nurse, evidence of rape or other criminal abuse).

The patient may waive the right to have his or her medical information remain confidential either by actions or words. For example, by bringing a lawsuit in which he or she claims personal-injury damages, an individual thereby waives the right to confidentiality of his or her medical records, since the record will be the principal determinant of the patient's entitlement to damages. Waivers of this sort apply equally to workers' compensation cases and to actions brought against accident and health insurers for benefits due under disability policies. And, of course, patients commonly give written consent to the disclosure of medical information to health-care insurers, government agencies, prospective employers, and the like. The release of such information under these circumstances poses no question of breach of confidentiality.

Use of Medical Records in Court

Medical records often play an important part in the outcome of legal proceedings such as personal-injury actions, wrongful-death actions, will contests, workers' compensation cases, etc. They generally play an important role in determining mental competency in both civil and criminal proceedings. Clearly, in a malpractice action brought against a nurse, the nature and quality of the patient's chart may well prove to be the nurse's main avenue of defense, for it is here that systematic, organized notes reveal how well the nurse observed and reacted to the patient's symptoms.

Why is the medical record so important in a court case? Primarily because it is a contemporaneous record of events—a systematic description of the patient's problems and reactions and responses to treatment, and the judgments made by doctors and nurses concerning the patient's condition and progress. While statements inserted in the patient's chart are not made under oath and are not self-authenticating, they are given credence by the courts precisely because they represent information and observations recorded at the time the events occurred. The law presumes that record entries of this nature kept in accordance with standard hospital procedures and not in anticipation of any particular legal proceeding are true statements, although this presumption is a rebuttable one.

When a nurse is called as a witness in a legal action involving medical treatment in one way or another, he or she is permitted to refresh his or her recollection of the facts and circumstances of the particular case by reference to the patient's medical record. Statements contained in the medical record are not, in themselves, admitted into evidence; but rather, the testimony of the witness concerning the particular event—as reinforced by the medical record—becomes the direct evidence given under oath.

It should be apparent that failure to maintain well-documented medical records may cause great difficulty for nurses who later must defend their actions in malpractice cases. Since it is impossible to anticipate if or when they may have to defend their actions in court, prudent nurses will take pains to maintain medical records that include all matters of significance, favoring the inclusion of more rather than less detail. The attempt to convince a jury that something was or was not done on behalf of the patient several years earlier is much more likely to be believed if it is substantiated in the patient's chart.

Some nurses make it a practice to keep a personal record or diary of unusual events that occur in the course of treatment. This can prove extremely helpful in recalling the details of these events should a malpractice case later result. All in all, keeping a diary of this sort is not a bad idea. It is a practice that could prove a boon to the nurse who may become involved in such litigation.

INVASION OF PRIVACY

Our legal system has long recognized the distinct right of every person to withhold his or her person, personality, and property from unwarranted public scrutiny. This right—called the right of privacy—includes the freedom to live one's life without having one's name, photograph, or private affairs made public against one's will. The legal concept of the patient's right of privacy is one with which every nurse should become familiar, since even a negligent violation thereof can have serious legal consequences.

All members of the health-care team are duty bound to treat patients with decency, respect, and the greatest degree of privacy possible. At the very least, this means that the patient should be seen, examined, and handled only by those persons directly involved in his or her care and treatment. Unnecessary exposure of the patient's body or unwarranted discussion of his or her case with third parties will give rise to a legal cause of action for invasion of privacy, with appropriate damages assessed against the offending party. The nurse must always be alert to any witting or unwitting violation of the patient's right of privacy.

On a practical level, patients who are moved through hospital corridors or into examining or treatment rooms always should be covered and not exposed unnecessarily to other hospital personnel, patients, or visitors. The careful nurse likewise will guard against such exposure in wards and shared rooms. We have already discussed the matter of the confidential nature of the information in the patient's chart. It bears repeating at this point that the nurse has both an ethical and a legal duty not to reveal confidential and personal information about the patient to unauthorized parties.

The publication of the patient's picture in a newspaper or magazine without his or her consent is likewise an invasion of privacy, and the person who permits such invasion is answerable at law. The rule and its consequences are relaxed somewhat where the individual in question is a public figure whose activities (whether the individual is hospitalized or not) are of legitimate interest to the public. Even so, the prudent nurse will follow the pertinent hospital rules and regulations regarding allowing photographers or others to enter the patient's room to interview or to photograph the patient without his or her consent.

There are certain clear-cut exceptions to the right of privacy, one of which—the public-figure situation—we have already mentioned. Other exceptions include the duty to report communicable diseases, child-abuse cases, gunshot wounds, and other such matters to the appropriate law-enforcement authorities. There can be no penalty for doing what the law requires in these instances.

In conclusion, when entering a hospital, a patient places the integrity of his or her person and reputation in the hands of all health-care personnel who attend him, and they must always be cognizant of their legal and ethical responsibility to preserve and protect the patient's right to privacy.

REPORTING CHILD ABUSE

Throughout the 1960s and early 1970s public attention began to focus more intently on the problem of the physically abused or neglected child in American society, a problem that previously had been considered of only minor significance.

Following congressional hearings in 1973, the Child Abuse and Treatment Act of 1973 was enacted into law. This statute required the states to meet certain federal standards in order to qualify for federal-grant assistance in setting up state child-abuse-prevention programs. One of the federal requirements was the mandatory reporting of abuse and neglect of minor children to the appropriate state and local authorities—usually the local welfare agency, department of social and rehabilitation services, or law-enforcement agency. Following enactment of the federal statute, all of the states passed child-abuse laws.

Clearly, the success of any child-abuse-prevention program depends on the early reporting of suspected child-abuse or neglect cases. There was a time when doctors and nurses had good reason to avoid alerting the authorities, since the child's parents could bring suit claiming both an invasion of their privacy and defamation of their character. With passage of the Child Abuse and Treatment Act of 1973, however, state statutes almost uniformly granted protection (immunity) from suit to persons reporting suspected child-abuse cases in good faith. Many of these statutes specifically mention nurses as being within the protection of the good-faith reporting requirements.

The various state laws differ in their definitions of abuse and neglect, as well as with respect to who is considered a child or minor in the eyes of the law. They also differ in their requirements about who must report suspected child abuse and to whom the reports must be made. A few states actually impose a penalty on certain categories of persons for failing to report suspected child abuse. In general, however, the laws call for the reporting of all cases in which a child has sustained serious physical injury inflicted by other than accidental means by either a parent or other person responsible for the child's welfare. Sexual abuse is included within the reporting requirements of a number of the states.

Nurses should become familiar with the child-abuse-reporting requirements of their own states, including the procedures established within their own hospitals for making such reports. It goes without saying that the nurse who handles pediatric emergencies should be especially alert to the possibility of child abuse when confronted with unusual traumatic injuries to children—dislocations, head injuries, unusual burns, etc.—that are not readily explainable or seem to occur with greater than normal frequency. The conscientious nurse should look upon the statutory reporting requirement as an opportunity to save the life or preserve the health of a defenseless child, and not as a disagreeable bureaucratic waste of time.

REPORTING OF ELDER AND SPOUSE ABUSE

The victimization of wives by their spouses and older persons by members of their family or surrogate family has only recently begun to receive national attention. Generally, the abuse takes the form of out-and-out physical violence, but in the case of the elderly it is often accompanied by psychological abuse, threats, denial of essential human needs (such as withholding of food), financial exploitation, and medical neglect or misuse of drugs. Several research studies have revealed that abuse of elderly persons over 65 occurs almost as often as does abuse of children.

To address the problems of elder and spouse abuse, nearly all the states have enacted laws establishing intervention mechanisms to protect these victims of domestic violence. Most of these laws authorize the issuance of civil injunctions or restraining orders against the abuser. The abuser who disobeys the restraining order can be held in criminal contempt and may be punished by being fined, imprisoned, or both. Some statutes also authorize (and pay for) the temporary removal of the victim from the residence where the abuse has occurred.

All nurses should become familiar with the pertinent reporting laws of their own states, as well as the public agencies assigned primary responsibility for dealing with elder and spouse abuse. Nurses who customarily work in the home setting (e.g., community health nurses, visiting nurses, and home-care nurses) should be particularly alert to the signs and symptoms of abuse within the family. As is the case with child abuse, trained nurses should have little difficulty recognizing the obvious physical symptoms of bruises, welts, sprains, and fractures, but they should also be on the lookout for the less obvious symptoms of psychogenic origin, such as gastrointestinal disorders, choking sensations, acute back pain, or constant headaches.

Few victims of abuse by family members will readily admit their plight to an outsider because of fear of reprisal by the family-member abuser. Thus, the conscientious nurse must act with courage in these matters, making the necessary inquiries and showing the degree of compassion and support these difficult situations always call for. As in the case of child-abuse-reporting statutes, a nurse's official report of elder or spouse abuse is a privileged communication and will not subject him or her to any legal action by the family member or spouse reported to the authorities as the abuser.

WITNESSING WILLS

In the course of a nursing career a nurse will probably be asked on at least one occasion to be a witness to a patient's last will and testament. Indeed, a patient may even request that a nurse prepare the will in accordance with his or her instructions. Since these are matters not normally covered in nursing school, the following is presented as a general guide and source of information in these circumstances.

We begin with the proposition that there is nothing unethical or improper about being a witness to someone's last will simply because that person happens to be a patient under your care. In fact, agreeing to be a witness to a will can be a source of great comfort to the patient since the desire to dispose of one's property in a planned and organized manner before one dies often presses heavily on persons who have delayed in dealing with this issue. But refusing to be a witness to a patient's will—unless the nurse is named as a beneficiary—violates no rule or standard of conduct, and a nurse may legally refuse to do so without incurring any penalty therefor.

Preparing versus Witnessing

A will is an extremely important legal document whose preparation requires competent legal advice if it is to carry out the testator's (will-signer's) intentions effectively. Unless a nurse has had legal training and has been admitted to the bar, he or she should not undertake to advise a patient in the drawing-up of his will. To do so would constitute the unauthorized practice of law: a nurse has no more right to practice law without a license than to engage in the practice of medicine without a license. When asked to give such advice, the nurse should respectfully decline and suggest that the patient contact a lawyer instead. Should the patient need help in finding one, the hospital's legal counsel can provide the names of local attorneys.

As mentioned earlier, it is perfectly proper, and perhaps even desirable, for the nurse to act as a *witness* to the signing of the patient's will, particularly since the nurse would be amply qualified to testify about the patient's physical and mental condition at the time of the signing should that issue arise at the time the will is offered for probate. Incidentally, when witnessing the execution of a patient's will, a nurse does not thereby attest to the wisdom of the patient's testamentary dispositions. Indeed, more than likely, he or she will not even know what those dispositions are, since the testator is not legally required to disclose them to the persons witnessing the will signing. By signing as a witness, the nurse merely attests to the fact that the patient signed a document that stated to be his or her last will and further attests to the patient's apparent soundness of mind and appreciation of the significance of his or her actions.

Legalities Associated with Wills

A will is a legal declaration of how one wishes to dispose of one's property upon death, as well as who is to administer the estate. Sometimes it also indicates who should act as a guardian for the testator's minor children. The desirability of preparing a will is beyond question, since it enables the testator to decide how his or her real and personal property is to be distributed after his or her death. When one dies without a valid will, one is said to die intestate, and under these circumstances the property will pass to family members (and sometimes even to the state) in accordance with the state's intestacy succession law—often in a manner that the individual would not have wanted. In addition, the costs of administering an estate invariably are greater when an individual dies intestate.

State laws are very specific concerning the formalities associated with the making of wills, and if the statutory requirements are not met, a purported will may prove to be invalid.

This is why a nurse should not presume to advise a patient concerning the preparation of a will. On the other hand, since nurses frequently attend patients who know that death is imminent and who sincerely desire to make proper disposition of their property, a nurse should be at least generally familiar with what the law requires so as to be able to explain to the patient the importance of getting legal assistance without delay.

Certain statutory requirements for the making of wills are virtually universal. Thus, in all states the "testator," the person who makes the will, must have testamentary capacity; that is, he or she must be sufficiently sound of mind to know the nature of the property and how he or she proposes to dispose of it. In short, the individual must be able to understand and appreciate the significance of what he or she is about to do. In addition, the law also requires that the testator be free from fraud, external coercion, or other undue influence at the time the will is made. If it can be shown that the testator was tricked into signing the will, or that someone close to the individual exercised pressure of some sort to force him or her to make a particular bequest, the probate court will consider the will or a part of it invalid.

Ordinarily a will must be in writing and must be witnessed *exactly* in accordance with the particular state law's formal signing requirements. In most states the testator must sign the will in the presence of all the witnesses (usually two or three disinterested persons) and must simultaneously declare aloud that the document he or she is signing is his or her last will and testament. The witnesses then must sign *in the testator's presence and in the presence of each other*. Any deviation from the statutory will-signing requirements can later prove disastrous, which is one of the principal reasons why it is preferable to have a lawyer not only prepare the document but also see to its proper execution.

Nearly every state law provides that the witnessing of a will by someone who is named as a beneficiary therein may void the disposition to that beneficiary—particularly if there are not a sufficient number of *distinterested* witnesses to satisfy the legal signing requirements. Thus, nurses who know that patients have made bequests to them in their wills must never agree to sign the wills as witnesses. Once again, a lawyer's presence at the will-signing would guarantee that mistakes of this kind are not made.

Some states permit a testator to prepare a holographic will—one that is entirely handwritten by the testator and properly dated. In these states, a holographic will need not be attested to by subscribing witnesses. If the state in question does not recognize holographic wills, the testator's efforts to dispose of his or her property by means of a handwritten document will have been in vain. One more reason why the nonlawyer nurse should hesitate to offer legal advice concerning the preparation of a will.

Finally, a few states recognize what is known as a nuncupative, or oral, will, where the proposed disposition of his or her property by one contemplating imminent death is stated orally in the presence of one or more witnesses and is reduced to writing immediately thereafter. A nurse who has been asked by a patient *in extremis* to record his or her intentions concerning the disposition of property should do so faithfully, and should promptly forward the written memorandum of those intentions to the hospital administrator who should, in turn, notify the patient's family.

LIVING WILLS—RIGHT-TO-DIE STATUTES

As all nurses know, advancements in medical and scientific technology have made it possible to keep alive patients who would never have been able to survive in earlier years. These advances have brought with them, however, a whole range of pilosophical, legal, and ethical questions concerning the rights of individuals (or persons acting on their behalf) to refuse life-sustaining treatment. Following the national attention stirred up by the Karen Quinlan case, *In re Quinlan,* 355 A. 2d 647 (N.J. 1976) and the Saikewicz case, *Superintendent of Belchertown State School v. Saikewicz,* 370 N.E. 2d 417 (Mass. 1978), many state legislatures began considering passage of so-called right-to-die laws—laws recognizing the right of competent adults to choose to die in dignity rather than be kept alive by means of artificial life-sustaining devices and procedures. The way this normally is done is by execution of a "living will," a formal document in which a person who has no reasonable expectation of recovery from an illness requests that he or she be allowed to die in dignity, rather than be kept alive by artificial means or heroic, life-prolonging procedures. As a consequence, over 35 states now have such laws, and others are actively considering such legislation.

Nurses who have occasion to treat terminally ill patients are likely to encounter some who have previously executed living wills, and others who may express a desire to prepare one while hospitalized. Thus, it is important to understand the legal implications of such documents and the practical issues they present.

Although the right-to-die statutes very greatly, in general they provide that persons over 18 years of age and of sound mind may execute a formal document declaring an intent not to be kept alive through artificial life-sustaining procedures and directing the withholding or withdrawal of such measures should they be in a terminal condition. The statutes spell out who may (or may not) be witness to such a "living will," and sometimes even mandate the actual form to be used. In addition, these laws customarily set forth the circumstances in which the will is to become effective, often stating that this is not to take place until the patient "has been diagnosed and certified in writing to be afflicted with a terminal condition by two physicians who have personally examined the patient, one of whom shall be the attending physician." Finally, all of these laws provide immunity from civil or criminal liability to the health-care personnel who actually withhold or withdraw treatment from patients who have executed such wills.

Under no circumstances is a living will a substitute for the express wishes of a competent adult, however old he or she may be, since the law has always given such persons the absolute right to refuse medical treatment for any reason. Thus, a patient's previously executed living will comes into play only when he or she is seriously ill and is no longer physically or mentally competent to make his or her wishes known. Moreover, once a living will exists, it may be revoked at any time by physical destruction, written revocation, or an oral declaration indicating the desire to revoke it. The nurse should understand that many of the state laws make the terms of a living will binding on the medical and nursing personnel who attend the patient, even though they may not mention any specific penalty for noncompliance. Accordingly, there should be little or no concern for legal repercussions where it is clear all the formalities have been followed.

What about the effectiveness of living wills in states that have not enacted such laws? Most legal commentators believe courts will be inclined to find them applicable since there is no public policy against refusal of treatment by a terminally ill patient, and a living will is a clear expression of the patient's desires. Certainly, if a patient has gone to the trouble of executing such a formal document or wants assistance in preparing one, there is every reason to comply with his or her wishes. Before undertaking to assist a patient who wishes to execute a living will, however, a nurse should be reasonably familiar with the statutory requirements for preparing living wills in the particular jurisdiction (if any) or the formal requirements for the execution and witnessing of regular wills in that state. It would be advisable to check the hospital's or nursing home's guidelines on these matters before proceeding too far. The reader is referred to the material on witnessing of wills preceding this discussion.

From a practical standpoint, the nurse should understand that he or she is under a legal obligation to bring the existence of a living will to the attention of the treating physician(s) and other health-care personnel treating the patient. The same is true for a patient's revocation of his or her living will. Both circumstances should be clearly recorded in the patient's chart— with a copy of the will itself, where one exists.

The legal counsel for the hospital, nursing home, or other treatment facility should be consulted regarding possibly ambiguous terms and conditions laid down in a patient's living will, and there should be no withholding or withdrawal of treatment until such matters are legally resolved. Finally, the nurse should understand that "do not resuscitate" orders based on the patient's express wishes, whether in a living will or otherwise, and properly signed by the treating physician, are legally valid and should be followed.

DURABLE POWERS OF ATTORNEY

As health-care practitioners and lawyers have gained more experience with living wills, they have recognized some inherent limitations in the use of such documents. Statutes authorizing living wills must be followed to the letter, and this inevitably creates legal problems for those who have to make extremely difficult medical decisions on behalf of terminally ill relatives. For one thing, no living will, no matter how broadly worded, can possibly anticipate the full range of medical decisions to be made. In addition, living will legislation has been notoriously ineffective in guaranteeing patients' rights—particularly where (as in California) only a patient diagnosed as terminally ill can execute an advance directive, and then must wait 14 days before the directive becomes operative. And finally, the courts in states without living will laws have not been in agreement in their willingness to recognize living wills.

Thus, while the living will undoubtedly represents an affirmative step toward assuring that the patient's wishes are honored during a serious illness, it may not be sufficient to cover all major contingencies and, indeed, in some states may not be honored at all. These problems can be overcome in large part by the use of a document known as a durable power of attorney, and just as nurses who treat terminally ill patients should be familiar with the legal aspects of living wills, they should also have a basic understanding of the concept of the durable power of attorney, and particularly how such documents are used in making critical health-care decisions.

At common law, a power of attorney is an agency relationship between the creator of the power, called the principal, and the holder of the power, called the agent. What is important to understand is that, under common law, the agent's authority terminates upon the death or *incapacity* of the principal. Thus, the usefulness of a standard power of attorney whereby an agent is appointed to make vital health-care decisions on behalf of his or her principal would be lost at precisely the time it is most needed. To correct this situation, the legislatures of a number of states, including California, Delaware, and Colorado, have adopted to one degree or another the Uniform Durable Power of Attorney Act. This model law sanctions the right of an individual to give another person a *durable* power of medical treatment decision-making—one that can be exercised even while the principal is incapacitated and legally incompetent to act on his or her own behalf.

Under the typical durable power of attorney statute, the appointed agent may make medical care decisions on behalf of an incompetent (generally incapacitated) principal as an extension of the principal's right to determine his or her own medical treatment. This includes the right to ask questions, assess risks and costs, select and remove physicians, seek the opinions of family members and other physicians, and select the preferred treatment from a variety of therapeutic options, including the option to refuse life-sustaining treatment entirely. Health-care providers are protected from liability if they rely in good faith on the authority of the agent. The California statute specifically provides, however, that the physician must first attempt to communicate with the patient and then note in the medical record that obtaining an informed consent from him or her is impossible.

An agent acting under a durable power of attorney has the legal authority to *enforce* the patient's treatment preferences (by going into court) to make sure they are not disregarded either by family members or physicians. Most living wills, on the other hand, are advisory at best and can be (and often have been) disregarded. The appointment of a clearly designated agent also provides the hospital, physician(s), and other health-care personnel with a measure of legal protection they do not have where a living will is involved or where the physician must seek the informal consent of the patient's spouse or relatives. In short, the durable power of attorney constitutes the best form of "substituted judgment" available for an otherwise incapacitated patient.

It is highly unlikely that nurses employed by a hospital, nursing home, sanitarium, or other comparable medical treatment facility will become directly involved in deciding whether or not to follow the directives of duly appointed agents acting under a durable power of attorney. They should understand, however, that this legal mechanism is perfectly appropriate, where sanctioned by the state's law. Here, again, the attorney representing the hospital, clinic, sanitarium, or nursing home should be consulted for authoritative advice regarding the status of local law.

MALPRACTICE INSURANCE FOR NURSES

Not too many years ago an attorney representing an injured patient would have summarily rejected the notion of filing suit against a professional nurse for alleged malpractice because it was common knowledge that only a handful of nurses carried their own malpractice insurance, and in the absence of such insurance, the limited incomes and financial resources of most nurses made them essentially judgment-proof. Rather than sue the nurse, the attorney would file suit against the nurse's hospital-employer, all physicians involved in the patient's treatment, possibly an equipment or drug manufacturer, and anyone else directly or indirectly involved in the treatment process who might be financially able to respond in damages.

Today all that has changed, and the nurses now find themselves the targets of malpractice litigation with increasing frequency. In part this is due to the overall increase in medical malpractice litigation over the past several years, with more such cases being tried and bigger verdicts and pretrial settlements being obtained. Then, too, many attorneys are firm believers in the practice of naming as defendants in a malpractice case every health professional whose name appears on the patient's chart. The theory they work under is that the more defendants there are, the more insurance carriers there are likely to be involved—and available to share in paying any verdict or settlement reached. As this indiscriminate practice has flourished, more nurses inevitably have found themselves forced to defend their actions in the legal arena.

Another important reason why nurses have become fair game for malpractice suits is their assumption of greater responsibilities as clinical nurse-specialists. It is almost axiomatic that the greater the responsibility, the greater the nurse's liability; hence, it stands to reason that the OR nurse, the CCU and ICU nurse, the ER nurse, the nurse-anesthetist, and other nursing specialists have been singled out by astute malpractice lawyers as logical defendants in many malpractice cases.

Finally, we must not forget that there are still a few states in which a governmental or charitable hospital cannot be held liable for negligence causing injury to a patient, and in these states the numbers of suits brought against individual nurses are bound to continue as they have in the past.

Is Malpractice Insurance Necessary?

Given the present litigation environment, no prudent nurse should even *consider* practicing without the protection of a personal malpractice insurance policy. As noted above, there is a growing trend to hold nurses personally liable for their acts of negligence, particularly where they have assumed added responsibilities as clinical specialists or nurse-practitioners and exercise a considerable degree of professional autonomy. But even when providing general-duty nursing services in a hospital, clinic, or nursing home, there are substantial reasons why *every* nurse should have his or her own malpractice coverage. These reasons are reviewed below, in question-and-answer format.

Q—Why should I carry malpractice insurance if my (institutional) employer assures me that I am covered under the institution's policy?

A—There are several reasons. To begin with, the cost of the typical malpractice policy for nurses is approximately $50 a year for coverage up to a million dollars. Not only is that degree of protection ridiculously inexpensive, but the cost is fully tax deductible. If nothing else, you will be guaranteed the services of legal counsel in case you are sued—at a time when experienced trial attorneys are charging as much as $500 an hour for court appearances.

There are more substantial reasons for having your own malpractice coverage, however. While it is true that the institution's policy will probably cover your normal activities as an employee, their liability is secondary in nature, based on the doctrine of *respondeat superior*. Your liability, on the other hand, is primary in nature, and this is why you are sure to be named as a defendant if the suit is predicated on your allegedly negligent conduct. If your employer decides to defend the suit by claiming you were not negligent, so much the better. In that particular instance you probably would not need a separate insurance policy. But, suppose the hospital, clinic, or nursing home took the position that what you did was either (a) a violation of their written policy guidelines or direct orders, (b) beyond the scope of your nursing license, or (c) a knowing violation of law. In those circumstances the institution's insurance carrier might well decide not to defend you on the grounds that what you did was not covered by the institution's malpractice policy. As a matter of fact, they may take an adversary position and go to great lengths to prove that *you and you alone are the legally responsible party,* forcing you to defend yourself in court on that issue. Needless to say, at that point you are strictly on your own, meaning you will have to find and pay for your own lawyer and hope for the best.

Remember, also, that when the insurance carrier for an institution makes payment to a plaintiff based on the clear-cut negligence of a nurse, the insurer is legally entitled to sue the nurse to obtain reimbursement from him or her for the amount paid out. Such cases are rare, to be sure, but your only salvation in a situation like that would be to have your own malpractice coverage.

Finally, no institutional policy affords coverage to you for acts or omissions occurring outside your normal work environment. A malpractice suit can result from a wide variety of nursing activities having nothing at all to do with hospital, clinic, or nursing home care—volunteer work, immunization programs, special-duty care, Good Samaritan situations—and in all of these instances you cannot possibly expect the institution's malpractice policy to cover your actions. Again, bear in mind that even if a claim brought against you is successfully defended, the costs of an attorney can be enormous. Having your own malpractice coverage will not only provide you with legal counsel, but with indemnity protection as well.

Q—Suppose I work for a solo practitioner or for a group of physicians; won't I be automatically covered under the practitioner's or group's policy?

A—While it is true that most physicians have policies that automatically cover their employees, this is not always the case. Many policies provide that unless the nurse-employee is specifically named as an insured party, such coverage does not exist. That's exactly what happened in the case of an office-based nurse in New York, whose employer told her she was covered, but his insurance carrier contended otherwise, and the court agreed with the carrier. *National Union Fire Insurance Co. v. Medical Liability Mutual Insurance Co.*, 446 N.Y.S. 2d 480 (1981). Again, most of the discussion above concerning institutional coverage is equally applicable to nurses who are employed by individual physicians or groups of physicians in a clinic setting. Thus, if your employer (meaning its insurance carrier) decides that what you did was not within the scope of your nurse's license or was a direct violation of law, the employer may decide to disavow coverage.

Q—If I purchase my own liability coverage, won't that relieve my employer of responsibility if I am sued?

A—To begin with, it is highly unlikely that a plaintiff's attorney will sue a nurse employed by a hospital or nursing home and *not* sue the employer. That would be tantamount to *legal malpractice,* and would be a rare event indeed. But, why worry about the hospital or nursing home at this juncture? When more than one insurance company is involved in defending a malpractice suit, they usually work out some sharing arrangement among themselves in case they decide to settle or have to pay an amount awarded by a jury. However, these arrangements are the insurers' business, not yours. You need only be concerned that *your* liability is covered.

Q—I have no substantial personal assets, so why should I be concerned about being sued personally?

A—You should be greatly concerned, because a judgment against you can remain outstanding for as long as 20 years. You may be financially at a low ebb right now, but some time within the next 20 years you might well have acquired property interests that an attorney will be able to levy on. Note, also, that in most states an individual's interest in jointly owned property can be taken to satisfy a judgment. Thus, if you own a house or a car jointly with your spouse, your interest in it can be seized through supplementary judgment proceedings. In some states your wages may be garnisheed, as well. Finally, putting all your assets in your spouse's name can be a dangerous game, particulary if there is a later divorce, or if you have specific personal property you'd like to will to your children or other close relatives.

Q—I'm only a nursing student, so why do I need malpractice coverage?

A—The point has been stressed throughout this book that when a nursing student performs duties customarily performed only by a professional nurse, he or she is held to the standard of care of the latter. Nowadays, it is quite common for the plaintiff's attorney to file suit against everyone whose name appears anywhere on the patient's chart, so you cannot escape being sued simply because you are a student. Moreover, you cannot rely on your employer's insurance to cover any award made against you personally, even though it is more than likely that you will be afforded legal representation under your employer's policy. Why incur the risk or the anxiety involved in these situations when for about $20 a year you can obtain proper insurance protection that guarantees legal representation as well as payment of any claims against you because of some act of negligence on your part?

Protection Afforded

The principal benefits of an individual malpractice policy are the insurer's agreement to defend all claims filed against the insured nurse for nursing malpractice and its agreement to pay on behalf of the insured all sums of money the latter is legally liable to pay the plaintiff, up to the limits of coverage stated in the policy. Should there be an appeal of an adverse verdict, the policy also provides for covering all the costs associated with such appeal.

It is important to note that under the typical malpractice policy the insurer agrees to defend *all* claims against the nurse-policyholder, even if they seem baseless on their face (e.g., directed against the wrong person). And, in addition to the usual claims for negligence in treatment, the policy generally provides for the defense of claims alleging assault, battery, invasion of privacy, defamation of character, and (except in unusually outrageous circumstances) claims that the nurse exceeded the scope of his or her license to practice nursing.

Coverage is normally provided for claims arising out of off-duty and non-hospital-related nursing activities such as volunteer work and Good Samaritan assistance, and also includes instructional and supervisory activities—the latter being of particular interest to clinical nursing instructors and supervisory nursing personnel, none of whom should be without personal liability insurance in the present legal climate.

SELECTED REFERENCES—PART 8

Importance of Maintaining Accurate Medical Records

22 *Am Jur Proof of Facts (2d)*, Medical Malpractice—Use of Hospital Records

American Hospital Association Committee on Medical Records and American Medical Record Association Planning and Bylaws Committee, *Statement on Preservation of Medical Records in Health Institutions* (1975)

H. Creighton, *Law Every Nurse Should Know*, 4th ed., W. B. Saunders Co., Philadelphia, 1981, pp. 114–117

E. Bernzweig, "Go On Record With Nothing But the Truth," *RN*, 48(4): 63 (April 1985)

D. Bailey, "How Careful Charting Saved My Career," *RN*, 47(11): 15 (Nov. 1984)

M. Cushing, "Gaps in Documentation," *Amer. J. Nurs.*, 82(12):1899 (Dec. 1982)

J. Greenlaw, "Documentation of Patient Care: An Often Underestimated Responsibility," *Law, Medicine & Health Care*, 10(3):125 (June 1982)

M. Mancini, "Documenting Clinical Records," *Amer. J. Nurs.*, 78:1556 (Sept. 1978)

Ahrens v. Katz, 575 F. Supp. 1108 (Ga. 1985)

Kenyon v. Hammer, 688 P. 2d 961 (Ariz. 1984)

Dincau v. Tamayose, 182 Cal. Rptr. 855 (Cal. 1982)

Fox v. Cohen, 406 N.E. 2d 178 (Ill. 1980)

Pisel v. Stamford Hospital, 430 A. 2d 1, (Conn. 1980)

North Miami General Hospital v. Gilbert, 360 So. 2d 426 (Fla. 1979)

St. Paul Fire & Marine Ins. Co. v. Prothro, 590 S.W. 2d 35 (Ark. 1979)

Wagner v. Kaiser Foundation Hospitals, 589 P. 2d 1106 (Ore. 1979)

Hiatt v. Groce, 523 P. 2d 320 (Kan. 1978)

People v. Smithtown General Hospital, Lorna Salzarullo, et. al., 402 N.Y.S. 2d 318 (N.Y. 1978)

Invasion of Privacy

Restatement (Second) Torts, § 652A

M. Hemelt and M. Mackert, *The Dynamics of Law in Nursing and Health Care*, Reston Publishing, Reston, Virginia, 1978, pp. 104–112

W. Curran, E. Laska, H. Kaplan, and R. Bank, "Protection of Privacy and Confidentiality," *Science*, 182(114):797 (Nov. 1973)

B. Ludwig, "The Right of Privacy in 48 Pieces v. Uniform Right of Privacy," *Notre Dame L. Rev.*, 27:499 (1952)

Horne v. Patton, 287 So. 2d 824 (Ala. 1973)

Hammonds v. Aetna Casualty & Surety Co., 243 F. Supp. 793 (1965)

Reporting Child Abuse

Child Abuse Prevention and Treatment Act, P.L. 93-247, 93rd Congress

R. Gelles, "Studies Show Factors Related to Child Abuse," *Amer. Fam. Phys.*, 19:215 (Feb. 1979)

N. McKeel, "Child Abuse Can Be Prevented," *Amer. J. Nurs.,* 78:1478 (Sept. 1978)
A. Friedman, "Nursing Responsibility in Child Abuse," *Nurs. Forum,* 15(1):95 (Jan. 1976)
Landeros v. Flood, 551 P. 2d 389 (Cal. 1976)

Reporting Elder Abuse

"Elder Abuse and Domestic Violence," in M. Kapp and A. Bigot, *Geriatrics and the Law,*
    Springer Publishing Co., New York, 1985, chap. 7

Executing Wills and Matters Related Thereto

E. Bernzweig, "The Patient Who Wants Help with a Will," *RN,* 48(9):71 (Sept. 1985)
H. Creighton, *Law Every Nurse Should Know,* 4th ed., W. B. Saunders Co., Philadelphia,
    1981, chap. 10
W. Kerns, "The Anatomy of a Bequest," *Mod. Hosp.,* 109:112 (Oct. 1967)
Succession of Zinsel, 360 So. 2d 587 (La. 1979)
Succession of Andrews, 153 So. 2d 470 (La. 1963)
In re Bliss' Estate, 18 Cal. Rptr. 821 (Cal. 1962)
In re Cochrane's Estate, 108 N.W. 2d 529 (Wis. 1961)
Pollard v. El Paso National Bank, 343 S.W. 2d 909 (Tex. 1961)

Living Wills and Durable Powers of Attorney

G. Courtright, "The Case for a Living Will," *RN,* 47(8):16 (Aug. 1984)
M. Fowler, "Appointing an Agent to Make Medical Treatment Choices," *Colum. L. Rev.,*
    84:985 (1984)
S. Cohn, "The Living Will from the Nurse's Perspective," *Law, Medicine & Health Care,*
    11(3):121 (June 1983)
S. Eisendrath and A. Jonsen, "The Living Will: Help or Hindrance?" *J.A.M.A.,* 249:2054
    (Apr. 15, 1983)
Comment, "The Right to Die a Natural Death and the Living Will," *Texas Tech L. Rev.,*
    13:99 (1982)
G. Annas, "Reconciling *Quinlan* and *Saikewicz:* Decision Making for the Terminally Ill,"
    Amer. J. Law and Med., 4(4):367 (Winter 1979)
D. Bok, "Personal Directions for Care at the End of Life," *N. Eng. J. Med.,* 295:367 (1976)
Note, "Informed Consent and the Dying Patient," *Yale L. J.,* 83:1632 (1974)
John F. Kennedy Memorial Hospital v. Bludworth, 432 So. 2d 611 (Fla. 1983)
In re Petersen, Texas Distr. Ct., Aug. 4, 1983
In re Storar, 438 N.Y.S. 2d 266 (N.Y. 1981)

Malpractice Insurance Protection

J. Arbeiter, "A Buyer's Guide to Malpractice Insurance," *RN,* 49(5):22 (May 1986)
E. Bernzweig, "Why You Need Your Own Malpractice Policy," *RN,* 48(3):59 (March
    1985)

R. Sandroff, ed., "Why You Really Ought to Have Your *Own* Malpractice Policy," *RN*, 46(6):29 (June 1983)

W. Regan, "Malpractice Insurance: Coverage for Nurses," *Regan Report on Nursing Law,* 22(12):1 (May 1982)

W. Regan, "Nurses and Personal Malpractice Insurance," *Regan Report on Nursing Law,* 22(4):1 (Sept. 1981)

J. Snow, "Professional Liability Coverage: Is It Necessary?" *Emergency Medicine,* 10(3):105 (May/June 1981)

M. Mancini, "What You Should Know About Malpractice Insurance," *Amer. J. Nurs.,* 79:729 (April 1979)

American Nurses Association v. Passaic General Hospital, 471 A. 2d 66 (N.J. 1984)

Jones v. Medox, 430 A. 2d 488 (D.C. 1981)

National Union Fire Insurance Co. v. Medical Liability Mutual Insurance Co., 446 N.Y.S. 2d 480 (N.Y. 1981)

Argonaut Insurance Co. v. Continental Insurance Co., 406 N.Y.S. 2d 96 (N.Y. 1978)

Tankersley v. Insurance Company of North America, 216 So. 2d 333 (La. 1968)

NOTE: This completes the course on the nurse's liability for malpractice. In the remaining pages you will find test questions and answers and a glossary. The comprehensive index at the end will enable you to use this book as a future reference source.

TEST QUESTIONS*

Problem No. 1

Nurse Jones is an R.N. employed in a small community hospital. The state in which the hospital is located has a Narcotic Drug Act that provides: "A narcotic drug shall be dispensed only upon a written prescription of a practitioner licensed by law to administer such drug. The act of dispensing a narcotic drug contrary to the provisions of this paragraph shall be a misdemeanor."

Late one Sunday evening an auto-accident victim is admitted to the emergency room of the hospital, and Nurse Jones, the only R.N. on duty, observes the unusual amount of pain being experienced by the patient. While awaiting the arrival of the local physician-on-call, she decides to give the patient an injection of a narcotic drug. In her haste, she causes the needle to break, resulting in further injury to the patient.

1-1 The quoted law is an example of

☐ common law

☐ statutory law

☐ administrative law

1-2 How does common law differ from statutory law?

☐ Common law is not the result of a legislative enactment.

☐ Common law is less important than statutory law.

☐ Common law does not have the legal effect of statutory law.

1-3 In what major category is the quoted law properly classified?

☐ criminal law

☐ civil law

☐ administrative law

*Answers begin on p. 378.

1-4   A law is classified as part of the criminal law when it is concerned with

☐ conduct that causes harm or injury to the person or property of another

☐ conduct that pertains to the public interest and is considered an offense against society as a whole

☐ conduct that pertains solely to private legal rights and interests

1-5   Which of the following is true in this case?

☐ The patient can sue Nurse Jones for negligence, and the local governmental authority can bring criminal charges against her for violation of the statute.

☐ Nurse Jones can be brought to trial on a criminal charge or can be sued for negligent conduct, but not both

☐ If Nurse Jones is found innocent of any criminal conduct, the patient has no legal basis for suing her for negligence.

1-6   If Nurse Jones stands trial in a criminal case for violating the quoted law and is found guilty, what will be the probable consequence?

☐ She will be held responsible for paying all the medical and hospital bills incurred by the patient in connection with the additional injury sustained.

☐ She will temporarily forfeit her license to practice nursing in that state.

☐ She will be fined, imprisoned, placed on probation, or some combination thereof.

1-7   The branch of law that deals with negligent conduct is a part of the law of

☐ contracts

☐ crimes

☐ torts

1-8 If Nurse Jones is held "legally liable" in a civil case, what will be the probable consequence?

☐   She will be required to pay money damages to the injured plaintiff.

☐   She will have to explain her actions to a grand jury.

☐   She will temporarily forfeit her license to practice nursing in that state.

1-9 What can the trial court "judicially notice" in this case?

☐   the fact that Nurse Jones was the only R.N. on duty on the evening in question

☐   the fact that Nurse Jones was negligent in her manner of giving the injection

☐   the fact that the state law prohibits the administration of narcotic drugs without a doctor's prescription

1-10 What would be considered legally sufficient proof to hold Nurse Jones liable for the harm to the patient in this case?

☐   proof of her deviation from the standard of care normally applicable in the giving of injections

☐   proof of her violation of the statute relating to the administration of narcotic drugs

☐   proof of her deviation from the standard of care normally exercised by physicians in treating patients in similar emergency circumstances

Problem No. 2

> Nurse Smith is a licensed R.N. who generally works as a private-duty nurse. A local hospital employs Nurse Smith to help out over a holiday weekend. While assigned to duty in the obstetrical ward, he notices an elderly woman patient in obvious respiratory distress in the adjacent hallway. Going to her aid, Nurse Smith administers improper treatment, which causes the patient's condition to worsen. The patient later sues Nurse Smith for the harm suffered.

2-1 The Court's decision in this case would be an example of

☐ administrative law

☐ common law

☐ statutory law

2-2 The patient's suit claiming damages for the harm suffered due to Nurse Smith's improper care brings the case within the general category of

☐ criminal law

☐ tort law

☐ contract law

2-3 As indicated, Nurse Smith is *normally* employed as a private-duty nurse. *While so employed,* he can be held legally liable

☐ when he fails to act as other reasonably prudent nurses would act under similar cirumstances

☐ when the patient's condition deteriorates or the patient dies during his period of employment

☐ when he does not follow the doctor's orders exactly to the letter

2-4 The legal term for a person's failure to act in a reasonable and prudent manner is

☐ negligence

☐ malpractice

☐ illegal conduct

2-5 Only a person with professional training can be held liable for

- [ ] damages

- [ ] malpractice

- [ ] negligence

2-6 If a Court were to determine that Nurse Smith failed to conduct himself in a reasonable and prudent manner while engaged in a *nonnursing* activity, the basis of his legal liability would be

- [ ] ordinary negligence

- [ ] professional malpractice

- [ ] professional misconduct

2-7 While employed by the hospital, Nurse Smith was legally responsible for exercising a special duty of care with respect to

- [ ] patients in his assigned ward only

- [ ] any of the hospital's patients he might have had occasion to treat

- [ ] none of the hospital's patients, because of his status as a private-duty nurse

2-8 Under which of the following circumstances could Nurse Smith have entered into a nurse-patient relationship with a patient?

- [ ] only if he had a written agreement to render care to that particular person

- [ ] whenever he achieved an agreeable therapeutic relationship with a patient

- [ ] whenever he actually provided nursing care to a patient

2-9 A legal nurse-patient relationship is based upon what necessary factor?

- [ ] the provision of nursing care to someone by a person with professional nurse's training

- [ ] the consent of the patient to receive nursing care from a particular nurse

- [ ] the patient's legal capacity to enter into a contract of employment

2-10 Nurse Smith   ☐ entered into   ☐ did not enter into   a nurse-patient relationship with the elderly patient in distress because

☐ the patient was not someone within the scope of Nurse Smith's normal nursing duties

☐ the giving of nursing care in an emergency situation cannot be the basis of a nurse-patient relationship

☐ Nurse Smith undertook to provide nursing care to her

2-11 Whether a nurse acted with reasonable care in a given situation is judged mainly by

☐ the extensiveness of his or her experience and training

☐ his or her conduct compared with that of other nurses with similar training under comparable circumstances

☐ the degree to which he or she adhered to a physician's orders or followed hospital routine

2-12 The standard of care applied to a nurse's conduct in emergency situations recognizes what key legal fact?

☐ The fact that the surrounding circumstances must be considered in deciding the issue of negligence

☐ The fact that normal prudence need not be exercised in an emergency situation

☐ The fact that no standard of care applies in emergency situations

Problem No. 3

> Nurse Simpson is the head nurse in a state mental hospital. This state recognizes the common-law rule regarding governmental immunity from tort liability. One day Nurse Simpson assigns Mr. Newby, an 18-year-old nursing student, to care for a manic-depressive patient with known suicidal tendencies. Nurse Simpson gives no instructions whatever to Mr. Newby, and the latter's consequent inattention to the patient materially aids another suicide attempt—this time resulting in total paralysis.

3-1 The fact that Nurse Newby is only 18 years old

☐ is of no legal significance in this case

☐ is pertinent only with respect to what could reasonably be expected of a young and inexperienced nurse

☐ is sufficient to make him not liable in this case

3-2 When a nursing student performs duties customarily performed by R.N.s, what standard of care applies to his or her conduct?

☐ The student is held to a lower standard of care than an R.N.

☐ The student is held to the same standard of care as an R.N.

☐ The student is held to a higher degree of care than an R.N.

3-3 Assuming that a court finds Nurse Newby negligent in this case, what effect (if any) might this have on Nurse Simpson's liability?

☐ It will have no effect whatever.

☐ Nurse Simpson automatically will be held liable as Nurse Newby's supervisor.

☐ Nurse Simpson can be held liable only if she is held to be negligent in making the assignment to an inexperienced nurse.

3-4 With respect to the hospital's liability (if any), which of the following is true?

☐ The hospital cannot be held liable in this case.

☐ The hospital can be held liable only if Nurse Newby is held liable.

☐ The hospital can be held liable if either Nurse Newby or Nurse Simpson is held liable.

3-5 If Nurse Newby, when given the assignment, sincerely believed he was not sufficiently experienced to cope with a manic-depressive patient, how should he have met his legal responsibility to the patient?

☐ He should have discussed the proper technique with other competent nurses.

☐ He should have made a note of his inexperience on the patient's chart.

☐ He should have declined to carry out the assignment, explaining his reasons to his supervisor before so doing.

3-6 Which of the following factors is the *most legally significant* in this case with respect to the degree of care required to protect the patient from harm?

☐ Nurse Newby's status as a nursing student

☐ the hospital's status as a state mental hospital

☐ the patient's known physical and mental condition

3-7 What is the principal reason a higher standard of care is required for safeguarding mentally ill persons?

☐ because these patients are the ones who most often bring lawsuits

☐ because mentally ill persons frequently do not appreciate their exposure to potential harm

☐ because state and provincial statutes specifically impose a higher standard of care in the treatment of mentally ill persons

3-8 It was stated that the patient had previously attempted to commit suicide. Which of the following statements is *most accurate?*

☐ Suicidally inclined persons rarely give clues to their suicidal tendencies.

☐ Suicidally inclined persons are easily identified by the fact that they are always depressed and disoriented.

☐ Suicidally inclined persons generally give verbal or behavioral clues to their suicidal tendencies.

3-9 With respect to the issue of liability in this case, which of the following is correct?

☐ Only the hospital can be held liable.

☐ Only Nurse Newby can be held liable.

☐ Both Nurse Newby and Nurse Simpson can be held liable, but not the hospital.

3-10 The doctrine of governmental immunity is an exception to which of the following doctrines?

☐ the doctrine of *respondeat superior*

☐ the doctrine of *res ipsa loquitur*

☐ the doctrine of personal liability

Problem No. 4

> Nurse Brown is an experienced R.N. employed as an office nurse for Dr. Swift. One particularly busy day the doctor tells Nurse Brown: "Mrs. Long is complaining about a variety of symptoms that are indicative of mild hypertension. Take her blood pressure and reassure her, and if her blood pressure seems elevated, give her a prescription for (name of drug), the usual dose. You can sign my name on the prescription and don't worry about anything; I'll take full responsibility."
>
> Nurse Brown follows Dr. Swift's instructions to the letter and gives Mrs. Long a prescription for her hypertension. The next day, in discussing the case with Nurse Brown, Dr. Swift notes that Nurse Brown erroneously wrote a prescription for a similar-sounding, but actually *different,* drug. By the time Dr. Swift is able to contact Mrs. Long, she learns she has suffered a severe reaction to the prescribed drug and has had to be hospitalized. Mrs. Long later sues both Nurse Brown and Dr. Swift for malpractice.

4-1 If Nurse Brown is held liable for her conduct in this case, she will be held liable under the doctrine of

☐ agent's liability

☐ personal liability

☐ *respondeat superior*

4-2 If Dr. Swift is held liable in this case, she will be held liable under the doctrine of

☐ contractual liability

☐ personal liability

☐ *respondeat superior*

4-3 The doctrine of personal liability is a legal rule that

☐ protects nurses against lawsuits for malpractice

☐ makes some persons liable for the negligence of others

☐ holds everyone legally responsible for his or her own negligent conduct

4-4 Under which of the following circumstances does the doctrine of *respondeat superior* apply in this case?

☐ It applies only if Nurse Brown and Dr. Swift agree in advance that it will apply.

☐ It applies only if a specific state law says that it will apply in this type of situation.

☐ It applies so long as Nurse Brown committed the act while in Dr. Swift's employ.

4-5 The legal doctrine of *respondeat superior* applies to the acts of

☐ nurses only

☐ all types of employees

☐ professional employees only

4-6 In legal effect, the doctrine of *respondeat superior* provides that

☐ an employee can be held liable for the negligent acts of a co-employee

☐ an employer can be held liable for the negligent acts of his or her employees

☐ employees and their employers are jointly liable for the negligent conduct of each other

4-7 The doctrine of *respondeat superior* comes into play only when the following three relationships are present (select one):

☐ nurse-patient-physician

☐ employer-employee-negligent conduct

☐ hospital-nurse-physician

4-8 If Mrs. Long sues Dr. Swift alone and is successful in making a recovery, which of the following is true?

☐ Dr. Swift can legally recover from Nurse Brown the amount she is required to pay Mrs. Long.

☐ Dr. Swift cannot legally recover from Nurse Brown the amount she is required to pay Mrs. Long.

☐ Nurse Brown's license to practice will be automatically suspended.

4-9 What legal effect (if any) resulted from Dr. Swift's statement that she would take "full responsibility" for Nurse Brown's conduct?

☐ It provided Nurse Brown with a complete legal defense to any lawsuit brought against her personally.

☐ It did not alter the rule of personal liability insofar as Nurse Brown's conduct was concerned.

☐ It altered the rule of personal liability insofar as Nurse Brown's conduct was concerned.

4-10 In what significant manner (if any) did Nurse Brown's conduct constitute unreasonable care?

☐ She signed the prescription form without showing it to the doctor.

☐ She undertook to diagnose the patient's condition and prescribe for her.

☐ She was *not* unreasonable since she followed the doctor's orders in all respects.

4-11 What conduct on Nurse Brown's part would have constituted reasonable care under the given facts?

☐ She should have declined to carry out Dr. Swift's request on the grounds that it would place her in the position of performing acts only a physician is authorized to perform.

☐ She should have requested Dr. Swift to put her instructions in writing.

☐ She should have asked the patient many more questions about her condition and not simply have taken her blood pressure and prescribed medication.

Problem No. 5

> P, a 30-year old chef, agrees to undergo an elective appendectomy. In the course of the operation, her surgeon, Doctor D, discovers stones in P's gallbladder and performs a cholecystectomy. P has an uneventful recovery, but after learning about the gallbladder operation, files suit against Doctor D.

5-1 What legal element did Doctor D fail to take into consideration in this case?

☐ the doctrine of pesonal liability

☐ the doctrine of informed consent

☐ the doctrine of *respondeat superior*

5-2 If a patient is given treatment to which she has not consented, the physician or nurse who gives the treatment may be held liable for

☐ civil battery

☐ extreme duress

☐ willful misconduct

5-3 P's consent to the appendectomy would not extend to the cholecystectomy because

☐ She did not agree to the additional costs of a cholecystectomy

☐ there was no emergency requiring an immediate cholecystectomy

☐ consent can be given to only one operation at a time

5-4 The fact that both surgical procedures were successful and benefited the patient

☐ is legally relevant on the issue of battery

☐ is not legally relevant on the issue of battery

☐ may be legally relevant on the issue of battery

5-5 To be legally effective, P's agreement to undergo the appendectomy

- ☐ would have to be in writing

- ☐ would have to be witnessed by two persons

- ☐ could be either in writing or verbal

5-6 A patient's consent to a surgical procedure is legally ineffective unless

- ☐ the patient's spouse also gives approval

- ☐ the patient's consent is given in writing

- ☐ the patient fully understands what he or she is consenting to

5-7 If P had been a child of 13, her consent to the appendectomy

- ☐ would have been legally effective if she agreed to pay all costs

- ☐ would not have been legally effective

- ☐ would have been legally effective provided her parents could not be located promptly

5-8 A patient's consent is said to be informed when

- ☐ the patient understands the nature and consequences of the treatment, and the alternatives thereto

- ☐ the patient knows how much the operation will cost

- ☐ the patient signs a waiver of liability for negligence

5-9 Consent is not required when

- ☐ diagnostic procedures are being employed

- ☐ the patient is unconscious and the procedure is necessary to save his or her life

- ☐ the patient has previously indicated his or her refusal to undergo any operative procedure

5-10 Consent to elective treatment of a person who is legally under age can be given

☐ only by the minor's parents or legal guardian

☐ either by the minor or by his or her parents

☐ only upon the order of a court

5-11 Consent to a procedure, once validly given by a patient

☐ may not be revoked

☐ may be revoked only if in writing

☐ may be revoked at any time prior to the procedure

5-12 In order to prove he or she has sustained a civil battery, a patient must show

☐ serious bodily harm

☐ total lack of concern on the part of the physician

☐ the touching of his or her person without his or her consent

5-13 In the eyes of the law, whether or not specific treatment should be rendered to an adult, competent patient is

☐ the patient's decision exclusively

☐ the doctor's decision exclusively

☐ a matter that can be resolved only by the courts

Problem No. 6

> Mr. Green sustains an eye injury while at work and immediately seeks medical aid from the company nurse, Mr. Owen. He inspects the injury, concludes it is only a superficial laceration, and gives only minimal treatment. One week later, Mr. Green's eye becomes extremely painful and an ophthalmologist discovers a piece of metal embedded in the eye. The delay in the discovery and removal of the metal results in blindness of the eye, and Mr. Green promptly sues Nurse Owen for the permanent disability thus sustained.

6-1 The plaintiff in this lawsuit is

□ Mr. Green

□ Nurse Owen

□ Mr. Green's employer

6-2 What fact (if any) would show the existence of a nurse-patient relationship between Mr. Green and Nurse Owen?

□ No nurse-patient relationship could have existed.

□ Both parties were employed by the same company.

□ Nurse Owen treated Mr. Green for his injury.

6-3 If this case is tried before a jury, who would *normally* decide whether Nurse Owen's conduct was negligent?

□ the judge

□ the jury

□ both the judge and the jury

6-4 How will the issue of Nurse Owen's negligence have to be proved?

□ by Mr. Green's testimony about what occurred

□ by medical records of the treatment given by Nurse Owen and by the ophthalmologist

□ by the testimony of experts concerning the standard of care applicable in the case

6-5 With respect to the question of proof, which of the following is true?

☐ Mr. Green has the burden of proving Nurse Owen's negligence.

☐ Nurse Owen has the burden of proving his freedom from negligence.

☐ Neither party has any legal burden of proof to sustain.

6-6 If the trial determines that no nurse-patient relationship existed, what legal effect will this have, if any?

☐ The case will be dismissed.

☐ It will have no legal effect at all.

☐ Mr. Green will automatically be entitled to recover damages from his employer.

6-7 Which of the following items might the trial court *judicially notice* in this case?

☐ the general qualifications of a nurse to render first aid

☐ Nurse Owen's negligent conduct

☐ the degree of Mr. Green's disability

6-8 If Mr. Green wins his case, which of the following will be the result?

☐ Nurse Owen will lose his license to practice nursing.

☐ Nurse Owen will be required to pay money damages to Mr. Green.

☐ Nurse Owen's employer will be required to pay money damages to Mr. Green.

6-9 Mr. Green and Nurse Owen work for the same employer. What legal effect (if any) does this have with respect to the question of liability?

☐ It has no legal effect.

☐ The employer can be held liable along with Nurse Owen.

☐ The employer cannot be held liable because of the operation of state workers' compensation laws.

Problem No. 7

> Nurse Grady is an experienced nurse in charge of the obstetrical ward of a large hospital. She is considered an expert technically, but has a reputation for being on the "cold" side. One day Nurse Grady brusquely informs a young maternity patient, "We've got to give you a predelivery enema." The patient, obviously somewhat concerned, begins to question Nurse Grady about the procedure but is cut short with the following remark: "Don't carry on like a baby. No one has ever died from an enema, and besides, it's a standard hospital procedure."
>
> During the administration of the enema, Nurse Grady turns to give instructions to another nurse, and while so doing she accidentally punctures the patient's anal membrane, causing serious injury. The patient later sues Nurse Grady for malpractice.

7-1 Nurse Grady is described as being technically proficient but impersonal and cold. What relationship is there (if any) between a nurse's attitude and the prevention of malpractice claims?

☐ There is no significant relationship whatever.

☐ Malpractice claims frequently can be prevented by giving recognition to the interpersonal and emotional aspects of patient care.

☐ Malpractice claims can be prevented only by giving proper attention to the patient's physical needs.

7-2 Which type of nurse is most likely to be sued for an act of malpractice, following some adverse medical event?

☐ the nurse who is efficient but very impersonal

☐ the nurse who is both efficient and friendly

☐ the nurse who is helpful but occasionally careless

7-3 With respect to the likelihood of a lawsuit in this case, which of the following is *more nearly* correct?

☐   Nurse Grady probably would have been sued *regardless* of her attitude toward the patient, once the latter sustained the described injury.

☐   Nurse Grady probably would have been sued even if *no* injury was sustained, because of her impersonal and indifferent treatment of the patient.

☐   Nurse Grady probably would *not* have been sued if, prior to the injury, she had treated the patient with respect and made a sincere attempt to allay her fears.

7-4 What role (if any) do psychological factors play as causes of malpractice suits?

☐   They play only a minor role, if any at all.

☐   They play the single most important role.

☐   They play an extremely important role.

7-5 All other things being equal, which of the following factors are the *principal* causes of malpractice suits?

☐   sociological factors, such as TV programs discussing medical malpractice

☐   unfavorable medical events that occur to patients

☐   psychological factors that upset patients and make them want to seek revenge

7-6 Nurse Grady's remarks indicate that she   ☐ is   ☐ is not   a believer in the patient-centered approach to nursing. This approach is based upon the theory that

☐   the patient wants to and should be encouraged to participate in his or her care

☐   the patient's cooperation in the treatment process can do no harm but is not significant

☐   the patient's participation in the treatment process invariably interferes with more important nursing activities

7-7 What would be the *best* way to cope with the patient's apprehensiveness in this case?

☐ Assure her that the predelivery enema is a standard hospital procedure given to all maternity patients.

☐ Give her a chance to understand and cooperate in the procedure to the greatest extent possible.

☐ Tell her nothing since information concerning the procedure will only increase her anxiety.

7-8 All other things being equal, what is the best thing nurses can do to forestall the possibility of malpractice claims?

☐ They should place emphasis on meeting all their patients' physical needs in an efficient and objective manner.

☐ They should stress the emotional aspects of patient care, even if this results in a certain degree of inattention to physical needs.

☐ They should regard patients as persons with equally important physical and emotional needs, both of which they should treat in a competent manner.

7-9 What is the *best* reason why someone like Nurse Grady should become concerned about malpractice claims prevention?

☐ She can guarantee protection against liability for any negligent conduct on her part.

☐ She can learn how to avoid a lawsuit and give better patient care at the same time.

☐ She can count on receiving more favorable attention from the hospital administration and possibly an increase in salary.

7-10 Nurse Grady is an experienced nurse with many years of nursing service. What psychological consequence is this lawsuit *likely* to have on her?

☐ Because she is experienced and professionally competent, it is not likely that she will suffer *any* adverse psychological consequences.

☐ The lawsuit will probably prove disturbing to her only if she has to pay money damages to the patient.

☐ The lawsuit will probably prove to be a threat to her professional reputation even though she is experienced, and she will probably suffer some psychological tension pending the outcome of the case.

Problem No. 8

Consider the following two hospitalized patients:

Patient A is a 55-year-old artist admitted to the hospital for elective surgery. She is aloof, impatient, and generally critical of others.

Patient B is a 30-year-old unemployed man who has been in and out of mental hospitals for many years, seeking treatment for a personality disorder that has incapacitated him.

8-1   Which of these two patients (if either) exhibits traits calculated to make him or her "suit-prone?"

☐   Patient A

☐   Patient B

☐   both patients

☐   neither patient

8-2   Which of the following is a good description of suit-prone patients?

☐   They have an intimate knowledge of the law and are familiar with courtroom procedures.

☐   They have genuine appreciation for the law and lawyers.

☐   They prefer dealing with persons who antagonize them by suing them.

8-3   What threat (if any) is posed to the nurse by suit-prone patients?

☐   They are generally nuisances but seldom threats.

☐   Their conduct is generally violent, which creates the possibility they may cause the nurse physical harm.

☐   Their constant need to blame others when something goes wrong marks them as individuals who may eventually sue a nurse.

8-4 Which of the following personality traits *best* describes suit-prone patients?

☐ They are emotionally immature and avoid responsibility.

☐ They are socially mature and have a well-defined sense of personal responsibility.

☐ They are independent, secure, and forthright in their dealings with others.

8-5 Of the two patients described, which of them (if either) is *more likely* to be suit-prone than the other?

☐ Patient A

☐ Patient B

☐ both are about equally suit-prone

8-6 If a nurse recognizes a patient as being suit-prone, how should the nurse react to the patient in order to avoid the threat he or she represents?

☐ The nurse should be polite but impersonal and try to avoid the patient as much as possible.

☐ The nurse should be sympathetic and attentive to all the patient's physical as well as emotional needs, even if it means spending a little more time with him or her than with other patients.

☐ The nurse should be aggressive and forceful in dealing with the patient, concentrating on meeting all the patient's physical needs but not catering to his or her emotional demands.

8-7 Assuming some relationship between a nurse's attitude toward patients and their later likelihood of suing the nurse for an act of malpractice, the nurse who is impersonal, impatient, and inflexible is

☐ more likely

☐ less likely

☐ neither more nor less likely

to be sued for malpractice than a nurse who is personal, patient, and flexible in his or her attitudes toward patients.

8-8 Assume that Nurse N has occasion to treat both Patient A and Patient B while they are hospitalized and openly displays hostility and antagonism toward both of them. What additional element is necessary before Nurse N can be sued by either or both of them?

☐ Nurse N would have to have one or more serious arguments with either patient, leading to direct threats of a lawsuit.

☐ Nurse N would have to cause some physical injury to either patient.

☐ There would have to be evidence that either patient's condition worsened while he or she was being attended by Nurse N.

8-9 Assuming that Nurse N commits an act amounting to malpractice while treating Patient A and Patient B, which of the following factors is the *most important* in the patient's decision whether or not to sue?

☐ the patient's prior attitude and relationship with respect to Nurse N

☐ the patient's knowledge of Nurse N's experience in other court cases

☐ the patient's personal knowledge of medical matters and how to bring a lawsuit

8-10 Which of the following expresses the most reasonable and most probable rule regarding the *likelihood* of malpractice claims?

☐ A malpractice claim will usually result whenever there is an unfavorable medical event causing harm or injury to the patient.

☐ A malpractice claim will usually result when a nurse's conduct causes harm or injury to the patient and the nurse's prior relationship with the patient was a poor one.

☐ A malpractice claim will result whenever there is a breakdown in the personal relationship between nurse and patient.

Problem No. 9

Nurse Harvey is assigned to keep track of all pads and sponges used during a gallbladder operation, and the operating surgeon closes the incision only after being assured by Nurse Harvey that all sponges are accounted for. After the operation, the patient's complaint of continued abdominal pain causes the surgeon to suspect a foreign object. The surgeon reopens the incision the following day and finds a lap pad that had been overlooked during the first operation. The patient later sues Nurse Harvey for his negligence in counting the sponges and pads.

9-1 In order to win this case, what character of evidence will the plaintiff be required to offer?

☐ evidence more likely true than not

☐ evidence beyond all reasonable doubt

☐ evidence convincing to a majority of the jury

9-2 What initial presumption of law exists in every malpractice case?

☐ the presumption that the defendant is free from negligence

☐ the presumption that the plaintiff's injury was due to the defendant's negligence

☐ the presumption that injuries to patients are bound to occur in the normal course of medical treatment

9-3 How does the so-called burden-of-proof rule affect Nurse Harvey in this case?

☐ He is presumed to be blameless and therefore has the jury's sympathy

☐ He does not have to prove his freedom from negligence until the plaintiff produces evidence of his negligence.

☐ He does not have to prepare a defense.

9-4 Which *two* of the following items are *essential* for the plaintiff to prove in order to win this case?

☐ proof of a nurse-patient relationship

☐ proof of Nurse Harvey's qualifications to practice nursing

☐ proof of Nurse Harvey's employment relationship with the hospital

☐ proof of the act constituting negligence

9-5 Under ordinary circumstances, how must the question of whether a nurse acted with reasonable care be proved?

☐ by the defendant's explanation of what he or she did

☐ by the testimony of experts

☐ by the trial judge, after checking the outcome of prior similar court cases

9-6 Assume that the doctrine of *res ipsa loquitur* applies in this case. What effect does it have on the question of proof of negligence?

☐ Plaintiff does not have to introduce the testimony of experts to prove the defendant's negligence.

☐ Evidence of the defendant's negligence can be dispensed with entirely.

☐ The defendant is not required to prove his freedom from negligence.

9-7 What is the legal effect of the doctrine of *res ipsa loquitur?*

☐ The defendant is considered liable whether or not he or she can show proof of his or her due care.

☐ The nurse's negligence becomes a legal question to be decided by the trial judge.

☐ The circumstances under which the injury occurred create an inference that the nurse was negligent, which the nurse must disprove.

9-8 Under what factual circumstances does the doctrine of *res ipsa loquitur* not apply?

☐ when the extensiveness of the injury sustained by the plaintiff is in doubt

☐ when the cause of the injury was in the exclusive control of the defendant

☐ when the injury sustained was caused in part by the plaintiff's own conduct

9-9 Whether or not the doctrine of *res ipsa loquitur* applies in a particular case is determined by

☐ the judge, pursuant to a motion therefor by the plaintiff

☐ the jury, after hearing all the evidence

☐ the plaintiff, at the time the suit is commenced

9-10 A trial Court will *direct a verdict* in favor of one party or the other when

☐ the Court believes the testimony offered by a particular party supports that party's position

☐ the Court believes the jury is not capable of deciding the issues of negligence

☐ the Court believes there is no substantial dispute about what occurred and reasonable minds could not arrive at a conclusion different from that of the Court's.

Problem No. 10

Patient P, elderly and infirm but otherwise of sound mind, tells private-duty Nurse N he wishes to prepare a will as quickly as possible and without his (second) wife's knowledge. He tells Nurse N he plans to leave 80 percent of his rather extensive estate to his favorite niece, 15 percent to his wife, and 5 percent to Nurse N out of gratitude for her attentive care over the past year. He asks Nurse N to help him prepare the document, employing a preprinted will form in order to assure that "all necessary legal language" is included in the document.

10-1 Nurse N will be acting both ethically and legally if she tells Patient P

☐ that he must leave a greater share of his estate to his wife if a will contest is to be avoided

☐ that she can prepare the will but cannot be a witness to its signing

☐ that P should seek the advice of a lawyer before attempting to proceed on his own in the matter

10-2 If Nurse N follows P's instructions to the letter and he subsequently dies, the Probate Court will not admit the will to probate if it appears that

☐ no attorney was involved in its preparation

☐ insufficient or ineligible persons were witnesses to the will

☐ the will was signed in pencil rather than in ink

10-3 What is the legal significance of the fact that Nurse N is shown to have assisted P in the preparation of his will?

☐ It proves her undue influence over him and will thereby void the entire will.

☐ It has no legal significance in the absence of other facts.

☐ It automatically voids any bequest made to Nurse N.

10-4 When a purported will is not admitted to probate because it has not been prepared or executed in accordance with law,

☐ the testator's property becomes the property of the state

☐ the testator's property automatically passes in its entirety to his or her surviving spouse

☐ the testator's property is distributed in accordance with the state law on succession of decedents' estates

10-5 A holographic will is one prepared

☐ when the testator is *in extremis* and there is no time to call a lawyer

☐ in a person's own handwriting

☐ by a minister, priest, or other clergyman

Miscellaneous Test Questions

11-1 The existence of a nurse-patient relationship is dependent upon

☐ the fact of giving nursing care

☐ the nature of a nurse's duty assignments

☐ specific legal arrangements to care for someone in particular

11-2 When a nurse offers his or her services as a private-duty nurse, which of the following legal doctrines *cannot* apply to the nurse's conduct?

☐ the rule of personal liability

☐ the rule of *respondeat superior*

☐ *res ipsa loquitur*

11-3 What is the usual rule with respect to the giving of emergency care outside the nurse's normal work duties?

☐ The nurse has an *ethical*, but not a *legal*, obligation to render such care.

☐ The nurse has both an ethical and a legal obligation to render such care.

☐ The nurse has a *legal*, but not an ethical, obligation to render such care.

11-4 If a nurse renders emergency care to someone not within his or her normal work responsibilities, what standard of care is applicable to the nurse's conduct?

☐ The nurse is held to the standard of care applicable to all private citizens.

☐ The nurse is held to the highest standard of care because of the unusual circumstances.

☐ The nurse is held to the standard of care applicable to other nurses acting under similar conditions.

11-5 Which of the following "surrounding circumstances" would *most likely* relieve a nurse of liability for his or her conduct?

☐ the fact that the nurse is a student

☐ the fact that the care was given under emergency conditions

☐ the fact that the nurse was on a temporary float assignment

11-6 Nurse N admits to an act of malpractice. He can avoid liability if he can show

☐ that the patient contributed to his or her own injury

☐ that he has sufficient malpractice insurance to cover all claims

☐ that many other nurses have committed similar acts of malpractice and avoided liability

11-7 Under what circumstances (if any) may a nurse make a diagnosis?

☐ under no circumstances, since this is the physician's sole responsibility

☐ whenever the nurse believes he or she has sufficient experience to do so

☐ whenever the nurse is required to evaluate the patient's condition to determine his or her specific needs for nursing care.

11-8 What is the nurse's legal duty with regard to carrying out a physician's order?

☐ The nurse must follow the order to the letter unless in his or her professional judgment some other course of treatment would be more effective.

☐ The nurse must follow the order without question unless he or she has reason to believe some harm may result to the patient.

☐ The nurse must always review the order with the physician before carrying it out.

11-9 In which of the following instances is there *no* basis for a *malpractice* suit?

☐ Nurse A negligently injures a neighbor's child while attempting to remove a splinter from her eye.

☐ Nurse B injures a visitor to the hospital when he negligently manipulates a wheel-chair.

☐ Nurse C negligently burns a patient in a ward to which she is not assigned.

11-10 Which of the following classes of nurses is exposed to the *greatest* risk of liability for malpractice because of the nature of the employment relationship?

☐ the government-employed nurse

☐ the occupational health nurse

☐ the hospital nurse

11-11 Nurse P is employed by a private physician. Which of the following legal doctrines makes the physician liable for Nurse P's conduct while so employed?

☐ *res ipsa loquitur*

☐ *respondeat superior*

☐ charitable immunity

11-12 In what way (if any) does the doctrine of *respondeat superior* alter the liability of a nurse for his or her negligent conduct?

☐ It shifts the nurse's liability to another person and eliminates his or her liability altogether.

☐ It makes the nurse liable to his or her employer.

☐ It does not alter the nurse's liability at all.

11-13 In which of the following instances of nursing care does the doctrine of *respondeat superior* not apply?

☐ care given by a practical nurse

☐ care given under emergency circumstances

☐ care given outside the scope of the nurse's regular employment

11-14 What is the most important reason for the keeping of accurate medical records by nursing personnel?

☐ to keep track of the patient's condition

☐ to assist in treating the patient

☐ to provide a good defense against a legal claim

11-15 Why should a nurse refrain from inserting in a patient's chart derogatory remarks about the patient's quirks or idiosyncracies?

☐ because they might prove embarrassing or libelous in later litigation

☐ because they might not accurately describe the patient's quirks or idiosyncracies

☐ because they might give rise to a malpractice action

11-16 In reviewing a patient's chart, Nurse N discovers that he had erroneously recorded the administration of 30 mL of a particular drug when the correct amount (which he had administered) should have been 3 mL. What action should Nurse N take to correct this discovered error?

☐ He should ink out the error on the chart and substitute the correct information above the erroneous entry.

☐ He should immediately notify his nursing supervisor so the latter can record the proper entry.

☐ He should enter a new note referring to the prior error and giving the correct information.

11-17 Surgeon S instructs OR Nurse N to omit in her nursing notes any reference to a cardiac arrest that occurred during a surgical procedure. What is Nurse N's legal position in this situation if she follows the surgeon's order?

☐ She could be held liable to the patient for any harm resulting from the cardiac arrest.

☐ She could risk the suspension or revocation of her license by the state licensing authority.

☐ She is fully protected against any legal action or disciplinary action since she followed the doctor's order explicitly.

11-18 Nurse S is a clinical nursing supervisor at a teaching hospital. What is the legal effect of his countersigning entries in patients' charts made by nursing students?

☐ It places Nurse S in the position of endorsing and authenticating the entries made in the charts.

☐ It makes Nurse S personally liable for any subsequent harm to the patients in question.

☐ It merely indicates Nurse S's authority as a clinical nursing supervisor.

11-19 The general rule holds that information in a patient's chart may be released to an outside (nonhospital) party without the patient's consent

☐ if the requesting party is an attorney seeking the information for litigation purposes

☐ if such release is authorized by law or pursuant to a court order

☐ if the patient is a recognized public figure whose comings and goings are considered public information

11-20 In a civil or criminal trial, statements contained in a patient's medical record are given credence for evidentiary purposes because

☐ they represent the unbiased observations of health professionals

☐ they have been recorded pursuant to hospital rules and regulations

☐ they represent the contemporaneous recording of events in the course of treating the patient

11-21 The right of privacy is a legal right that assures freedom from unwarranted public scrutiny to

☐ everyone

☐ well-known public figures

☐ hospitalized patients only

11-22 If a former patient brings a legal action in which his or her physical condition is a major issue, the law presumes that the patient's medical record

☐ is no longer confidential

☐ is a biased document that should be given little legal weight

☐ is completely accurate and fully supports his or her claim

11-23 State laws enacted pursuant to the federal Child Abuse and Treatment Act of 1973 generally grant to health professionals who report suspected cases of child abuse

☐ immunity from being sued for malpractice

☐ immunity from professional disciplinary proceedings

☐ immunity from invasion of privacy and defamation of character suits

11-24 Child abuse statutes are important because they give nursing personnel the opportunity to

☐ prevent further injuries to defenseless children

☐ seek vengeance against parents who abuse their children

☐ have abused children removed from their home environments

11-25 When a nurse who is not a beneficiary is asked by a patient to witness the signing of his or her will, the nurse should understand that this is

☐ something only a lawyer can and should handle

☐ a violation of the state nurse practice act

☐ a perfectly ethical and legal thing to do

11-26 In the absence of personal liability insurance coverage, a hospital-based nurse who is sued for malpractice

☐ is considered judgment-proof

☐ can be held personally responsible for all damages assessed

☐ can rely on the coverage afforded by the hospital's policy as protection from personal financial responsibility

11-27 In the present legal environment, nurses as a class are being sued for malpractice

☐ with greater frequency than a decade ago

☐ with less frequency than a decade ago

☐ with about the same frequency as a decade ago

11-28 Clinical nursing specialists run a higher risk of being sued for malpractice because

☐ they deal with the more seriously ill patients

☐ they assume greater responsibilities

☐ they enjoy higher incomes

11-29 When a nurse has a personal malpractice policy, the nurse's insurance carrier agrees

☐ to pay every claim filed against him or her

☐ to pay only those claims for which he or she is legally liable

☐ to fight every claim in court

11-30 Under the typical nursing malpractice policy coverage generally is provided

☐ for all types of nursing care given

☐ for normal nursing care, but not volunteer or Good Samaritan care

☐ for hospital care, but not private-duty care

11-31 Nursing student S does not know whether to purchase personal malpractice coverage. The principal reason for doing so is

☐ the law requires nursing students to maintain personal malpractice coverage

☐ nursing students are just as liable as graduate nurses for their acts of malpractice

☐ the costs of such coverage are nominal and are tax deductible

ANSWERS TO TEST QUESTIONS

1-1.   statutory law

1-2.   Common law is not the result of a legislative enactment

1-3.   criminal law

1-4.   conduct that pertains to the public interest and is considered an offense against society as a whole

1-5.   The patient can sue Nurse Jones for negligence, and the local governmental authority can bring criminal charges against her for violation of the statute.

1-6.   She will be fined, imprisoned, placed on probation, or some combination thereof.

1-7.   torts

1-8.   She will be required to pay money damages to the injured plaintiff.

1-9.   the fact that the state law prohibits the administration of narcotic drugs without a doctor's prescription

1-10.   proof of her violation of the statute relating to the administration of narcotic drugs

2-1.   common law

2-2.   tort law

2-3.   when he fails to act as other reasonably prudent nurses would act under similar circumstances

2-4.   negligence

2-5.   malpractice

2-6.   ordinary negligence

2-7.   any of the hospital's patients he might have had occasion to treat

2-8.   whenever he actually provided nursing care to a patient

2-9.   the provision of nursing care to someone by a person with professional nurse's training

2-10.   entered into

Nurse Smith undertook to provide nursing care to her

2-11.   his or her conduct compared with that of other nurses with similar training under comparable circumstances

2-12.   The fact that the surrounding circumstances must be considered in deciding the issue of negligence

3-1.   is pertinent only with respect to what could reasonably be expected of a young and inexperienced nurse

3-2.   The student is held to the same standard of care as an R.N.

3-3.   Nurse Simpson can be held liable only if she is held to be negligent in making the assignment to an inexperienced nurse.

3-4.   The hospital cannot be held liable in this case.

3-5.   He should have declined to carry out the assignment, explaining his reasons to his supervisor before so doing.

3-6.   the patient's known physical and mental condition

3-7.   because mentally ill persons frequently do not appreciate their exposure to potential harm

3-8.   Suicidally inclined persons generally give verbal or behavioral clues to their suicidal tendencies.

3-9.   Both Nurse Newby and Nurse Simpson can be held liable, but not the hospital.

3-10.   the doctrine of *respondeat superior*

4-1.   personal liability

4-2.   *respondeat superior*

4-3.   holds everyone legally responsible for his or her own negligent conduct

4-4.   It applies so long as Nurse Brown committed the act while in Dr. Swift's employ.

4-5.   all types of employees

4-6.   an employer can be held liable for the negligent acts of his or her employees

4-7.   employer-employee-negligent conduct

4-8.   Dr. Swift can legally recover from Nurse Brown the amount she is required to pay Mrs. Long.

4-9.   It did not alter the rule of personal liability insofar as Nurse Brown's conduct was concerned.

4-10.   She undertook to diagnose the patient's condition and prescribe for her.

4-11.   She should have declined to carry out Dr. Swift's request on the grounds that it would place her in a position of performing acts only a physician is authorized to perform.

5-1.   the doctrine of informed consent

5-2.   civil battery

5-3.   there was no emergency requiring an immediate cholecystectomy

5-4.   is not legally relevant on the issue of battery

5-5.   could be either in writing or verbal

5-6.   the patient fully understands what he or she is consenting to

5-7.   would not have been legally effective

5-8.   the patient understands the nature and consequences of the treatment, and the alternatives thereto

5-9.   the patient is unconscious and the procedure is necessary to save his or her life

5-10.   only by the minor's parents or legal guardian

5-11.   may be revoked at any time prior to the procedure

5-12.   the touching of his or her person without his or her consent

5-13.   the patient's decision exclusively

6-1.   Mr. Green

6-2.   Nurse Owen treated Mr. Green for his injury.

6-3.   the jury

6-4.   by the testimony of experts concerning the standard of care applicable in the case

6-5.   Mr. Green has the burden of proving Nurse Owen's negligence.

6-6.   The case will be dismissed.

6-7.   the general qualifications of a nurse to render first aid

6-8.   Nurse Owen will be required to pay money damages to Mr. Green.

6-9.   The employer cannot be held liable because of the operation of state workers' compensation laws.

7-1.   Malpractice claims frequently can be prevented by giving recognition to the interpersonal and emotional aspects of patient care.

7-2.   the nurse who is efficient but very impersonal

7-3.   Nurse Grady probably would *not* have been sued if, prior to the injury, she had treated the patient with respect and made a sincere attempt to allay her fears.

7-4.   They play an extremely important role.

7-5.   unfavorable medical events that occur to patients

7-6.   is not

          the patient wants to and should be encouraged to participate in his or her care

7-7.   Give her a chance to understand and cooperate in the procedure to the greatest extent possible.

7-8.   They should regard patients as persons with equally important physical and emotional needs, both of which they should treat in a competent manner.

7-9.   She can learn how to avoid a lawsuit and give better patient care at the same time.

7-10.   The lawsuit will probably prove to be a threat to her professional reputation even though she is experienced, and she will probably suffer some psychological tension pending the outcome of the case.

8-1.   both patients

8-2.   They prefer dealing with persons who antagonize them by suing them.

8-3.   Their constant need to blame others when something goes wrong marks them as individuals who may eventually sue a nurse.

8-4.   They are emotionally immature and avoid responsibility.

8-5.   Patient B

8-6.   The nurse should be sympathetic and attentive to all the patient's physical as well as emotional needs, even if it means spending a little more time with him or her than with other patients.

8-7.   more likely

8-8.   Nurse N would have to cause some physical injury to either patient.

8-9.   the patient's prior attitude and relationship with respect to Nurse N

8-10.   A malpractice claim will usually result when a nurse's conduct causes harm or injury to the patient and the nurse's prior relationship with the patient was a poor one.

9-1.   evidence more likely true than not

9-2.   the presumption that the defendant is free from negligence

9-3.   He does not have to prove his freedom from negligence until the plaintiff produces evidence of his negligence.

9-4.   proof of a nurse-patient relationship

              proof of the act constituting negligence

9-5.   by the testimony of experts

9-6.   Plaintiff does not have to introduce the testimony of experts to prove the defendant's negligence.

9-7.   The circumstances under which the injury occurred create an inference that the nurse was negligent, which the nurse must disprove.

9-8.   when the injury sustained was caused in part by the plaintiff's own conduct

9-9.   the judge, pursuant to a motion therefor by the plaintiff

9-10.   the Court believes there is no substantial dispute about what occurred and reasonable minds could not arrive at a conclusion different from that of the Court's.

10-1.   that P should seek the advice of a lawyer before attempting to proceed on his own in the matter

10-2.   insufficient or ineligible persons were witnesses to the will

10-3.   It has no legal significance in the absence of other facts.

10-4.   the testator's property is distributed in accordance with the state law on succession of decedents' estates

10-5.   in a person's own handwriting

11-1.   the fact of giving nursing care

11-2.   the rule of *respondeat superior*

11-3.   The nurse has an *ethical*, but not a *legal*, obligation to render such care.

11-4.   The nurse is held to the standard of care applicable to other nurses acting under similar conditions.

11-5.   the fact that the care was given under emergency conditions

11-6.   that the patient contributed to his or her own injury

11-7.   whenever the nurse is required to evaluate the patient's condition to determine his or her specific needs for nursing care

11-8.   The nurse must follow the order without question unless he or she has reason to believe some harm may result to the patient.

11-9.   Nurse B injures a visitor to the hospital when he negligently manipulates a wheelchair.

11-10. the occupational health nurse

11-11. *respondeat superior*

11-12. It does not alter the nurse's liability at all.

11-13. care given outside the scope of the nurse's regular employment

11-14. to assist in treating the patient

11-15. because they might prove embarrassing or libelous in later litigation

11-16. He should enter a new note referring to the prior error and giving the correct information.

11-17. She could risk the suspension or revocation of her license by the state licensing authority.

11-18. It places Nurse S in the position of endorsing and authenticating the entries made in the charts.

11-19. if such release is authorized by law or pursuant to a court order

11-20. they represent the contemporaneous recording of events in the course of treating the patient

11-21. everyone

11-22. is no longer confidential

11-23. immunity from invasion of privacy and defamation of character suits

11-24. prevent further injuries to defenseless children

11-25. a perfectly ethical and legal thing to do

11-26. can be held personally responsible for all damages assessed

11-27. with greater frequency than a decade ago

11-28. they assume greater responsibilities

11-29. to pay only those claims for which he or she is legally liable

11-30. for all types of nursing care given

11-31. nursing students are just as liable as graduate nurses for their acts of malpractice

GLOSSARY

Abortion   The termination of pregnancy or the inducement of miscarriage with the intent of destroying a fetus.

Age of Majority   Statutory or legal age of adulthood.

Agency   The relationship in which one person acts for or represents another, such as employer and employee.

Agent   The person authorized by another to act for him or her.

Allegation   A statement, charge, or assertion that a person expects to be able to prove.

Appeal   A legal proceeding in which a higher court is asked to reverse or correct the decision of a lower court.

Appellant   The party who files the appeal seeking to reverse the decision of a lower court.

Appellee   The party against whom an appeal to a higher court is taken.

Assault   An intentional threat to cause bodily harm to another, designed to intimidate or place the person in reasonable apprehension of harm.

Attestation   The act of confirming that a document has been duly signed in accordance with law.

Battery   The intentional touching of another person either without permission (consent) or with consent that has been exceeded or fraudulently obtained.

Borrowed Servant Rule   The legal doctrine that holds that a hospital employee (e.g., a nurse) may be considered a temporary employee of someone else (usually the operating surgeon) while acting under the latter's direct control. The rule states that while so engaged, the temporary employer (surgeon) will be held liable for the negligence of the borrowed servant. This is a special application of the doctrine of *respondeat superior*.

Cause of Action   The legal ground(s) for a party to bring suit against another.

Charitable Immunity   The legal doctrine that holds that a nonprofit, charitable hospital is immune from suit for acts or negligence by its employees.

Civil Action   A lawsuit dealing with some private legal right or duty, as opposed to a criminal action.

Common Law   Judge-made or decisional law, as opposed to law enunciated through statutes enacted by legislative bodies.

Confidential Communication   A statement made to someone in a position of trust who has a legal duty not to disclose the information thus communicated. Applies to information revealed by a patient to a physician or a nurse in the course of treatment that the law protects from being revealed, even in court.

Consent   In the medical context, the patient's voluntary act of agreeing to allow someone else (usually a doctor) to do something to him or her that would otherwise be considered an unauthorized touching or battery.

Contributory Negligence   In the medical context, a patient's failure to exercise reasonable care that aggravates an injury initially caused by someone else. Such conduct may negate the patient's right to recover damages against the party who caused the original injury.

Crime   A public offense; the breach of any law established for the protection of society as a whole. Crimes are prosecuted by and in the name of the state.

Criminal Law   That branch of law dealing with crimes and their punishment, as opposed to civil law, which deals with private legal interests.

Damages   Monetary compensation for one who has sustained loss, detriment, or injury to his or her person or property through the unlawful conduct of another.

Defamation   The injury of a person's reputation or character by willful and malicious statements made to a third person. Defamation includes both written and oral statements (libel and slander).

Defendant   The person against whom a civil action or criminal action is instituted.

Delegation   The assignment by one person of specified tasks to another, often to a person who is lower in rank and theoretically less qualified.

Diagnosis   See *nursing diagnosis*.

Directed Verdict   A verdict that a trial judge has directed a jury to make in favor of one party to the action because the evidence and/or law so clearly favors that party.

Due Care   That degree of care or concern expected of an ordinary person in the given circumstances.

Emergency   A sudden, unexpected occurrence or event causing a threat to life or health.

Evidence   Any probative matter submitted to a tribunal by a party to a proceeding for the purpose of persuading the tribunal of the validity of a particular contention. Evidence may be of a physical nature (documents, instruments, etc.) or an oral nature (testimony of some person).

Executor   The person chosen by an individual to carry out the provisions of his or her will.

Expert Witness   One who has special training, experience, or skill in a relevant area and who is allowed by the court to offer an *opinion* on some issue within his or her area of expertise as opposed to firsthand testimony or evidence thereon.

False Imprisonment   Restraining a person's freedom of movement without lawful authority and thereby giving rise to a civil action by the person so restrained. False imprisonment usually involves constricting someone to a confined area by force or threat of force, even though there may be no physical contact.

Forseeability Doctrine   The legal doctrine that holds an individual liable for all the natural and proximate consequences of his or her negligent conduct with respect to another.

Good Samaritan Law   A statute enacted to provide legal protection to someone who stops and renders emergency aid to another in good faith and without compensation.

Governmental Immunity   The legal doctrine that holds that a sovereign government cannot be sued without its consent thereto. The Federal government has given its consent to be sued in specified instances, including the filing of actions for the negligence of its employees (including medical negligence).

Harm   Damage or injury to a person sufficiently measurable to constitute the legal basis for a claim against the party who caused the harm.

Hearsay Evidence   Any evidence that is not based on the personal knowledge of the witness; such evidence is admissible in a court case only under strict rules.

Holographic Will   A handwritten will; one that is deemed valid in most states provided it is properly executed and witnessed.

Immunity   See *charitable immunity, governmental immunity*.

Implied Consent   Consent to treatment based on the emergency nature of the situation rather than the patient's direct consent; also called constructive consent.

Indemnify   To make whole financially; to reimburse.

Independent Contractor   One who is hired to perform a job without supervision, i.e., not under the direct control or supervision of the hiring party.

Informed Consent Doctrine   The legal doctrine that holds that a patient's consent to treatment is not valid unless the patient fully understands (1) the nature of his or her condition, (2) the nature of the proposed treatment or procedure, (3) the alternatives to such course of action, (4) the risks involved in both the proposed and the alternative procedures, and (5) the relative chances of success or failure of the proposed and the alternative procedures.

Intentional Tort   Wrongful conduct that is intentional in nature and designed to cause harm or damage to another; examples include assault, battery, false imprisonment, libel, and invasion of privacy.

Intestate   Without a valid will. The property of a person who dies intestate is distributed in accordance with the state law on intestate succession.

Invasion of Privacy   Subjecting the person or personality of someone to unwarranted or undesired publicity or exposure and giving rise to a legal cause of action for damages.

Joinder of Parties   Where multiple plaintiffs or defendants are named in a proceeding.

Judge   The person who guides a court proceeding to ensure impartiality and enforce the rules of evidence.

Judgment   The final order of a court, based either on the jury's verdict or the judge's deliberations in a non-jury trial.

Judicial Notice   The official recognition by a trial judge that an earlier legal decision or statute is applicable to the case under consideration.

Jury   The individuals selected and sworn to hear the evidence and render a decision in a civil or criminal court action.

Law   Rules that regulate human social conduct in a formally prescribed and legally binding manner. The two basic sources of law are legislative enactments, or statutes, and judicial decisions in litigated cases.

Legal Representative   A person appointed by a court to prosecute or defend a legal action on behalf of someone not legally qualified to represent himself or herself in such action.

Legislative Enactment   See *statute*.

Liability   The state of being held legally responsible for harm caused another; normally assessed in money damages.

Liability Insurance   A contract issued by a casualty insurance company to an individual under which the company, in return for a premium, agrees to defend all claims and pay all sums the policyholder is legally liable to pay third persons because of his or her negligent conduct.

Libel   A false or malicious writing that is intended to defame or dishonor another person and published so that it will come to the attention of third parties.

Litigant   Either party to a lawsuit.

Litigation   A trial in court to determine legal issues, rights, and duties between the litigants.

Malpractice   Professional misconduct, improper discharge of duties, or failure to meet the standard of care expected of a reasonably prudent member of that profession in his or her dealings with clients or patients which causes harm to the latter.

Negligence   The failure to act as an ordinary prudent person would act in the given circumstances; applies to the acts of laymen as well as professionals.

Nuncupative Will   An oral will made by a person *in extremis* and deemed valid in some states if made before a sufficient number of witnesses and reduced to writing as soon as possible.

Nursing Diagnosis   Evaluation by the nurse of the totality of factors which may influence the patient's recovery. A good nursing diagnosis will identify the patient's specific nursing needs, define goals for improving the patient's care, and provide the physician with data necessary to make adjustments in treatment.

Personal Liability Rule   The legal doctrine that holds that every person is legally responsible for his or her own tortious conduct.

Plaintiff   The complaining party in a civil suit.

Practical Nurse   A nurse who has passed minimum standards of training and education established by a state before being licensed to perform selected nursing acts, and then only under the direction of a physician, dentist, or R.N. Except for this restriction, the concern of the practical nurse for proper patient care is every bit as great as that of the R.N. The licensed practical nurse (L.P.N.) is not authorized to supervise, manage a nursing unit, or teach.

Preponderance of the Evidence   Sufficient credible evidence to convince a court or jury that the essential allegations made are more probably true than not.

Private-Duty Nurse   A registered professional nurse who independently contracts to give bedside nursing care to one specific patient.

Privileged Communication   See *confidential communication*.

Probate   The judicial proceeding in which a purported last will is held to be either valid or invalid.

Professional Nurse   A nurse who has passed minimum standards of education and training established by a state before being licensed to render nursing care, for pay, to persons in need of such care. Also referred to as a registered nurse, or R.N.

Proximate Cause   That act or event which, unbroken by any efficient intervening act or event, is the immediate cause of harm or injury and without which such harm or injury would not have occurred.

Reasonable Care   With respect to a nurse, that degree of care normally exercised by other reasonably prudent nurses of comparable skill and learning under the same or similar circumstances.

Res Ipsa Loquitur   Literally, "the thing speaks for itself." A legal doctrine applicable to cases in which the defendant had exclusive control of the instrumentality or events that produced the patient's injury and which injury ordinarily could not have occurred without negligent conduct. When this rule is held applicable in a given case, the plaintiff's normal burden of proving the defendant's negligence is done away with and the defendant instead has the burden of proving his or her freedom from negligence.

Respondeat Superior   "Let the master answer." The legal doctrine that holds the employer responsible for the negligent acts of his or her servants or employees while acting within the scope of employment.

Standard of Care   The legal measures against which a defendant's conduct is compared in order to determine if such conduct amounts to negligence. Generally, those acts performed or omitted that an ordinary prudent person would have performed or omitted under the same or similar circumstances.

Statute (Statutory Law)   An enactment by a legislative body having the force and effect of law. A formalized law, as opposed to judge-made or common law.

Subpoena   A court order requiring a person to appear in court and give testimony in a civil or criminal action.

Subpoena Duces Tecum   A subpoena that commands a person to appear in court and bring with him or her specific documents named in the subpoena.

Suit   A court proceeding in which one party seeks damages or the vindication of some legal claim or right; synonymous with lawsuit.

Summons   A document that gives official notification to a defendant that a suit has been filed against him or her, requiring the defendant to respond (answer) within a stated period of time.

Testator   A person who makes a will.

Testimony   The oral statement of a witness given under oath at a trial, either civil or criminal.

Tort   A civil wrong, either intentional or unintentional, giving rise to a legal claim for redress or money damages.

Tortfeasor   One who commits a tort; a wrongdoer whose actions give rise to a civil suit for money damages.

Verdict   The formal declaration of a jury's decision in a civil or criminal case.

Will   A legal declaration of a person's intentions concerning the disposition of his or her property after death; also called last will and testament.

Witness   One who is called to give testimony in a legal proceeding, either civil or criminal.

INDEX

Abortion:
   consent to, 206
   legal issues surrounding,
     206–207
   refusal to participate in, 207
   statutes, 207
Abuse (*see* Child abuse; Elder
   and spouse abuse)
Acts authorized in emergencies
   (*see* Emergency care)
Affirmative legal defenses,
   258–265
Agent under living will, 335
Allergic reactions to drugs,
   liability for, 267
Alteration of records, 324–325
Ambivalence of suicidal
   patients, 168
Anaphylaxis, 160, 184
Anesthesia:
   administration of, 137
   and nurse-anesthetists, 55,
     140
Antisocial behavior, intentional
   torts as, 17, 18, 178
Anxiety:
   of nurse when sued for
     malpractice, 283
   of patient, 298, 301
Assault:
   civil suit for, 17
   as intentional behavior, 17,
     178
   legal elements of, 178
   as a tort or a crime, 17
Assignment of float nurses, 86
Assignment of incompetent
   nurses, 85, 86
Assignment problems of
   supervisory nurses, 86

Assistant to physician (*see*
   Physician's assistant)
Assumption of risk by patient,
   262–263
Authorized types of diagnosis,
   146–148
Award, payment of, 13, 14

Battery:
   and beneficial results of
     treatment, 179, 180
   failure to obtain consent as,
     196
   as intentional tort, 17
   legal elements of, 179
   liability for, not based on
     harm, 179
   and negligence, contrasted,
     202
   unconsented touching as, 179,
     183
Bedrail policy of hospital, 135
Beneficial results and battery,
   188
Birth control information,
   dispensing of, 191, 208
Blanket consent forms, 199
Blindly following orders,
   consequences of, 138–144
Blood pressure, duty to note
   and record, 147, 150
Blood transfusions, negligence
   in administering, 143
Borrowed servant doctrine:
   as applied to OR nurses, 99,
     102
   and captain of the ship
     doctrine, distinguished,
     103

Borrowed servant doctrine
   (*Cont.*):
   defined, 99
   effect of, in general, 99–101
   and liability of the hospital,
     99–101
   and *respondeat superior*, 100
Burden of proof:
   on issue of damages, 253
   as obligation of plaintiff, 250
   and preponderance of
     evidence rule, 252
   and *res ipsa loquitur*, 271–274
   shifting of, 274
   (*See also* Proving negligence)
Burn injuries and *res ipsa
   loquitur*, 272

Canadian nurses, liability of, in
   general, 114
Canadian school nurses, liability
   of, 111
Captain of the ship doctrine:
   explained, 103
   limited applicability of, 103
   as offshoot of borrowed
     servant doctrine, 103
Carelessness synonymous with
   negligence, 22, 23
Causes of malpractice claims
   (*see* Malpractice claims)
Challenging physician's order,
   method of, 140, 142
   (*See also* Duty to question
     orders)
Charitable immunity rule,
   104–106
   consequences of, to nurses,
     105
   explained, 104

Charitable immunity rule (*Cont*):
  inapplicability of, in Canada, 105
  and need for malpractice insurance, 336
  states adhering to, 105
Child abuse:
  and pediatric emergencies, 329
  prevention of, 329
  reporting of, in general, 329
Civil law:
  defined, 10
  distinguished from criminal law, 10, 16, 21
  financial aspects of, discussed, 11, 14, 16
Classifications of law, 7–11, 13–16
Clinical instructor, role of, 59, 60
Common law:
  defined, 5
  distinguished from statutory law, 5, 246
  how created, 5
  legal effect of, 5–6
Communicating significant findings, 152
Comparative negligence, explained, 261
Compensable harm as element of malpractice claim, 238, 240
  (*See also* Damages; Proving negligence)
Compensation for legal harm, 13, 14, 21
Competence, legal presumption of, 194
Concurrent liability:
  of employer and employee, 162
  of supervisory and subordinate nurses, 84, 95
  (See also *Res ipsa loquitur*)
Confidentiality of medical records, 326
  (*See also* Privacy)

Conscience clauses in abortion laws, 207
Consent to treatment:
  for abortion, 191
  for birth control, 191
  in Canada, 183
  concept of, explained, 182
  constructive, 187, 188
  and emergency treatment, 187–188
  express and implied, distinguished, 183
  extension of, to necessary procedures, 184
  forms used to obtain, 182, 196, 199
  implied, 183, 198
  of mature minors, 191
  mental incompetents unable to give, 190
  of minors, 190
  need for obtaining informed, 182
  nurse's role in obtaining, 201
  oral, 183
  as patient's choice, 199
  relationship of, to unnecessary procedures, 184
  scope of, 184
  for sterilization, 191
  and unconscious patients, 187, 188
  for venereal disease, 191, 208
  voluntary nature of, as legal requirement, 185
  withdrawal of, 185, 193
  written, 183
  (*See also* Informed consent)
Contraceptive information, dispensing of, 191, 208
Contributory negligence of patient, 258–260
Cooperation of patient, how to enlist, 297, 298
Countersigning medical records, 325
Court, role of, in malpractice litigation, 243

Court decisions:
  function of, in general, 5
  as guides to nursing conduct, 246
  as legal precedents, 246
Crimes:
  contrasted with torts, 10
  examples of, 7, 13, 14
Criminal actions:
  described, 13, 16
  penalties for, 10
  who can bring, 9
  (*See also* Unlawful acts, performance of)
Criminal law:
  applicability of, 9–12, 16
  defined, 7
  violation of, as basis for revocation of license, 14
Crown Liability Act, 114

Damages:
  in civil actions, generally, 21
  as legal redress, 13, 14, 21
  as necessary element of malpractice claim, 238, 240, 242
  pain and suffering as element of, 254
  payment of, 13, 14
  proving nature and extent of, 253, 254
  (*See also* Proving negligence)
  and subjective states of mind, 240
Decisions (*see* Court decisions)
Defendant:
  defined, 237
  proving negligence of (*see* Proving negligence)
Defenses to malpractice actions, 238–265
Degree of care applicable:
  in administering blood transfusions, 143
  in general, 20–22, 49–54
  in protecting patient from harm, 128–151, 164–168

Degree of care applicable(*Cont.*):
  in providing emergency care,
    68, 148
  (*See also* Reasonable care)
Degree of disclosure required,
  201, 204
Delegated acts as within or
  exceeding scope of
  practice, 226
Delegation of duties, liability for
  improper, 84, 85
  (See also *Respondeat
    superior*)
Depression as clue to possible
  suicide, 168
Diagnosis:
  in emergency situations, 227
  factors in making nursing,
    146–149
  in nursing practice, generally,
    146
  types of: authorized, 146–148,
    227
    permitted, 146
    prohibited, 146
Directed verdict, 267–269
  (*See also* Proving negligence)
Disclosure of medical
  information:
  in court, 326
  in general, 326
  required by statute, 326
  (*See also* Medical records)
Disclosure of risks, requirement
  for, 204
Dissatisfaction of patient:
  in general, 302
  in hospital setting, 305
Drug administration, liability
  arising out of, 160–163, 245,
    256
  (*See also* Medications)
Durable power of attorney,
  334–335
Duty:
  of care owed by nurses,
    generally (*see* Standard
    of care)
  of care owed by persons,
    generally, 49

Duty (*Cont.*):
  to challenge physician's
    orders, 136, 138–144, 148
  to communicate significant
    findings, 152
  to follow orders: of physician,
    136
    of physician's assistant, 141
    of supervisor, 131
  to get patient's signature on
    consent form, 201
  to give emergency care (*see*
    Emergency care)
  to question orders, 136,
    138–144, 148
  to record vital signs, 147
  to report child abuse, 329
  to report elder and spouse
    abuse, 330
  to report patient's withdrawal
    of consent, 201
  to safeguard patient, 128, 130
  (*See also* Degree of care
    applicable)
  of supervisory nurses (*see*
    Supervisory nurses)

Educational background,
  relationship of, to standard
  of care, 55
Effect of medical procedure,
  nurse's need to know, 137
Elder and spouse abuse:
  duty to report, 330
  statutes governing, 330
Electroshock therapy, consent
  for, 204
Elements of malpractice suit,
  238–239, 242
Emancipated minors:
  defined, 91
  obtaining consents for
    treating, 191–193, 202
Emergency care:
  as basis for establishing
    nurse-patient
    relationship, 34, 39, 40,
    42–43

Emergency care (*Cont.*):
  degree of care required in
    providing, 68, 148, 264
  ethical obligation to provide,
    42, 45
  and Good Samaritan statutes,
    46
  and the hospital emergency
    department, 41
  and initiation of treatment,
    34, 39, 40, 42–43,
    228–230
  legal obligation to provide, 39
    in normal work setting, 39
    in other settings, 42–43, 46
  and need for consent, 187
  and reporting of child abuse,
    329
  and *respondeat superior,* 90,
    91
Emergency situations, care
  required in, 68, 148, 264
Emotional needs of patients,
  299–301
Employer:
  liability of, for acts of
    employees, 89, 91, 94
  (See also *Respondeat
    superior*)
  and private-duty nurses, 36,
    37, 93, 94, 98
  right of, to reimbursement for
    legal damages paid, 95
  temporary, and borrowed
    servant doctrine, 99–103
Employer-employee relationship
  as basis of liability, 88–99
  (See also *Respondeat
    superior*)
Equipment failure, problems
  with, 117
Ethical obligations of nurses,
  42, 45
Evaluation of patient's needs,
  84
Evaluation of patient's vital
  signs, 147
Evidence:
  and burden of proof rule,
    257

Evidence (*Cont.*):
  character of, as decisive of
    outcome of lawsuit, 253
  jury's role in evaluating, 243
Expert testimony, when
  required, 267, 268
Expert witness:
  need for testimony of, 267,
    268
  qualifications of, 268

Fact and law, how questions of
  are decided, 243
Facts, withholding of, by
  physician, 199
Failure to communicate:
  as basis of liability, 152
  significant findings, 152
Falls:
  attributable to negligence,
    134
  as forseeable events, 135
False imprisonment:
  defined, 209
  as intentional tort, 17
  liability of hospital for, 211
  liability of nurse for, 210
  of mentally ill persons, 210
  (See also *Respondeat
    superior*)
Fatigue, relevancy of, in
  malpractice suit, 65, 67
Faulty technique in
  administering drugs, 161,
    163
Fear:
  as element of assault, 178
  as element of false
    imprisonment, 210
Federal Tort Claims Act
  (FTCA):
  applicability of *respondeat
    superior* under, 114
  basis of governmental liability
    under, 113
  effect of, on government
    nurse's liability, 113, 114
Fellow employees and immunity
  from suit, 115, 265

Float nurses, problems in
  assigning, 86, 158
Following orders without
  question, consequences of,
    60, 136, 138–144
  (*See also* Duty, to follow
    orders; Duty, to question
    orders)
Force as element of false
  imprisonment, 209
Foreign objects and proof of
  negligence, 273
Forms, consent, 182, 196,
    199
Forseeability of harm and
  degree of care required,
    62–64, 132, 135
  (*See also* Harm to patient)

General duty of care:
  as legal obligation owed
    everyone, 25, 49
  as related to nurse's
    employment, 49, 50,
    52–54, 128
  (*See also* Standard of care)
General-duty nurses:
  duty of, to give emergency
    care, 39, 41
  liability of, in general, 52–54,
    128
  (*See also* Liability;
    Malpractice; Negligence)
Good Samaritan assistance and
  malpractice insurance, 339
Good Samaritan laws, 46–47
Government nurses, liability of:
  in Canada, 114
  in general, 106–107
  in U.S., 107, 113
  (*See also* Federal Tort Claims
    Act)
Governmental immunity from
  suit, 106

Harm to patient:
  absence of, as precluding
    recovery for damages,
    240

Harm to patient (*Cont.*):
  forseeability of: as basis of
    liability, 62–64, 132, 164
  in caring for mentally ill
    patients, 164–168
  in general, 62
Higher standard of care, when
  required, 130, 164–167
  (*See also* Degree of care
    applicable; Standard of
    care)
Highway accidents, caring for
  victims of, 42–46
Holographic will, defined, 332
  (*See also* Last will and
    testament)
Home care nursing, certification
  for, 118
Home health care, problems
  arising out of, 117
Hospital emergency
  department, 41
Hospital liability:
  charitable immunity and, 104
  insurance, 337, 338
  for nonprofessional acts, 98
  payment of claims based on,
    13, 14, 21
  respondeat superior as basis
    of, 90, 94, 97–98
  types of conduct creating, 97,

Hospital policies and
  procedures:
  applicability of, to private-
    duty nurses, 37
  in challenging physicians'
    orders, 139, 142
  failure to follow as basis of
    liability, 66
  on siderails, 135
  value of, in malpractice
    claims prevention, 316
Hospital risk management, 316
Hostility:
  of nurse, 312
  of patient, coping with, 301,
    304, 305
Humanitarian basis of nursing,
    44, 46

Illegible medication orders,
160
Immunity against liability:
charitable, 104–106
effect of, in general, 104–107
of employer, under workers'
compensation laws, 115
governmental, 106–107
of United States Public
Health Service nurses,
114, 265
of Veterans Administration
nurses, 114, 265
(*See also* Good Samaritan
laws)
Impersonal nursing care, effects
of, 292–293, 295
(*See also* Interpersonal
aspects of patient care)
Implied consent to treatment,
183, 198
Improper supervision, 154–158
(*See also* Supervisory nurses)
Inability to perform assigned
function, 85, 86
Incident reporting:
hospital, 316
role of, in malpractice claims
prevention, 316
Incompetents, treating mental,
190
Independent functions of nurse:
nursing diagnosis as, 146–148
recording vital signs as, 147
safety of patients as, 128–130
and specialized nursing roles,
generally, 55–57, 223
Independent judgment, need for
nurse to exercise, 136–138
Infection, relationship of, to
negligence, 288
Inference of negligence,
274
Informed consent:
by authorized legal
representative, 187
battery for failing to obtain,
196
as distinguished from
negligence, 202

Informed consent, battery for
failing to obtain (*Cont.*):
misrepresentation of facts
as, 199
as a communication problem,
204
effect of failure to obtain, 197
of emancipated minor, 191
and mental competency of
patient, 190
need to obtain, 182
and patient's understanding of
choices available, 204
relationship of, to consent, in
general, 182, 196
scope of information given in
order to obtain, 201, 204
in treating minors, 193
for treating venereal disease,
206
withdrawal of, 193
Inherent risks of treatment, 204
Initial presumption of law (*see*
Proving negligence)
Injections:
as causes of injuries, 161,
163, 267
as common nursing function,
119
Injunction, applicability of, in
civil actions, 16
In loco parentis, defined, 190,
193
Instituting therapy, nurse's
liability for, 146, 227–230
(*See also* Diagnosis)
Instructor (*see* Clinical
instructor)
Insubordination:
in carrying out orders, 59
and nursing students, 59, 60
Insurance (*see* Malpractice
insurance)
Intentional wrongs:
assault and battery as,
178–179, 188
as criminal acts, 16, 29
described, 17, 178
examples of, 178
false imprisonment as, 17

Intentional wrongs (*Cont.*):
as torts, 17
Interpersonal aspects of patient
care, 292–293
development of, by nurses,
296
(*See also* Suit-prone nurses;
Suit-prone patients)
Interpretation of patient's
symptoms and reactions,
147
Invasion of privacy (*see*
Privacy)

Joinder of parties, 237
Joint Commission on
Accreditation of Hospitals
recognition of physicians'
assistants, 141
Joint Commission on
Accreditation of Hospitals
standards, 72, 86, 103
Judge, role of:
in directing a verdict, 267–269
in general, 243
as source of law, 5
Judge-made law, 5, 243, 267
Judgment:
liability for exercising
independent, 144
need to exercise, 138
payment of, by losing party,
13, 14
Judicial decisions (*see* Court
decisions)
Judicial notice:
defined, 247
explained, 247–248, 258
of legal precedents, 246
of statutes, 245
Jury:
deciding of fact questions by,
243
and expert testimony,
268–269, 243
role of: in determining
standard of care, 244,
245
in general, 243, 247

Jury, role of (*Cont*.):
     in weighing the evidence,
        243, 244

Kindness to the patient,
     importance of, 299
Knowing the patient, 297–299
     (*See also* Interpersonal
        aspects of patient care)

Last will and testament:
     advice in preparing patient's,
        331, 332
     formal requirements for, 331
     holographic, 332
     nuncupative, 332
     nurse as beneficiary of
        patient's, 332
     nurse as witness to patient's,
        330–331
Law(s):
     binding nature of, 3, 8
     child abuse reporting, 14
     civil and criminal,
        distinguished, 10, 21
     classifications of, 7–11, 13–16
     common, defined, 5
     criminal, defined, 7
     different meanings of, 3
     effect of formally enacted,
        4–6, 8
     Good Samaritan, 46–47
     judge-made, 5, 243, 267
     legally significant, 3–5
     regulation of nursing
        functions by, 5, 6, 52
     as regulators of social
        conduct, 3–5, 8
     statutory, defined, 4
     (*See also* Court decisions;
        Statutes)
Lawyers:
     fee arrangements of, 240
     increasing specialization of,
        285
Lay persons, legal responsibility
     of, 18
Legal and ethical obligations,
     compared, 45

Legal advice, dangers in
     offering, 331
Legal decisions (*See* Court
     decisions)
Legal fees, arrangements for
     payment of, 240
Legal liability (*see* Liability)
Legal precedents (*see* Court
     decisions; Judicial notice)
Legal representative:
     of minor, for purpose of
        giving consent, 190
     as plaintiff in malpractice
        suit, 236, 240
Legal standards of care (*see*
     Duty; Standard of care)
Legislative enactments (*see*
     Statutes)
Liability:
     for administering medications,
        160–163, 245
     of clinical instructor, 60
     concurrent, 84
     defined, 34
     and doctrine of *respondeat
        superior*, 88–99
     of employer, for acts of
        employees, 88–99
        (See also *Respondeat
        superior*)
     due to equipment failure,
        117
     of government nurses: in
        Canada, 114
        in general, 113
        in U.S., 113
        (*See also* Federal Tort
        Claims Act)
     of hospitals, as affected by
        charitable immunity rule,
        104, 105
     legal effect of, in malpractice
        actions, 24
     of minors, 69
     for nonprofessional acts, 98
        (*See also* Charitable
        immunity rule)
     and nurse's personal state of
        mind, 65

Liability (*Cont*.):
     of nursing students, 59–60, 69
     of occupational health nurses,
        115–116
     personal risk of, 82
     of psychiatric nurses, for
        false imprisonment, 210
     of public health nurses, 106
     of school nurses, 108–111
     of supervisory nurses, 60,
        84–86
     (See also *Respondeat
        superior*; Rule of
        personal liability;
        Supervisory nurses)
License:
     as a privilege, 222
     revocation of, for unlawful
        conduct, 14, 29, 136
Licensed practical nurses:
     administration of narcotic
        drugs by, 245
     as professionals, 66
     relative degree of care
        required of, 147
     responsibilities of, compared
        with professional nurses,
        147, 149
     as supervisors, 149
Licensing of nurses, 222–225
Life-threatening emergencies:
     degree of care required in, 68
     handling of, in general, 229
     and need for consent, 187
     (*See also* Consent to
        treatment; Emergency
        care)
Living wills, 333–334
     nurse's duties with respect to,
        334
     role of, in general, 333
     when applicable, 333, 334

Malpractice:
     applicable to professional acts
        only, 25, 26
     defined, 25
     medical, defined, 27

Malpractice (*Cont.*):
  negligent conduct
    constituting, 27, 28,
      128–167
  (*See also* Liability;
    Negligence; Reasonable
    care)
Malpractice claims:
  causes of: in general, 284
    medical, 285
    psychological, 297
    sociological, 284
  types of persons who bring,
    302–305
  unfavorable medical events
    which trigger, 288
Malpractice claims prevention:
  and hospital policies and
    procedures, 316
  and patient-centered therapy,
    297, 298
  physical factors in, 290–291
  psychological factors in,
    292–293
  as related to emotional needs
    of patients, 297–299
  value of, in general, 282
Malpractice insurance:
  costs of, insignificant, 337
  need for, 107, 336–339
  for nursing students, 338
  protection afforded by, 339
Malpractice law (*see* Law)
Malpractice litigation:
  increase in, generally, 283
  protection against, 107,
    336–339
  (*See also* Malpractice claims)
Malpractice suit, elements of,
    238–239, 242
Matter of law, court ruling as,
    245
Mature minors:
  consent for treating, 191–193,
    202
  defined, 191
Medical and nursing functions:
  distinguished, 225
  overlapping, 226

Medical diagnosis (*see*
    Diagnosis)
Medical malpractice, defined,
    27
Medical procedures,
    performance of:
  in emergencies, 148
  by nurses, generally, 146,
    226, 227
  under standing orders, 228
  as within scope of nursing
    practice, 228
  (*See also* Diagnosis;
    Emergency care)
Medical records:
  alteration of, 324, 325
  confidential nature of, 326
  contents of, 324
  correcting, 324–325
  countersigning, risks of, 325
  importance of, in general,
    147, 324
  purpose of, 324
  use of, in court, 327
Medications:
  administration of, by licensed
    practical nurses, 245
  allergic reactions to, 267
  anaphylaxis caused by, 160,
    184
  faulty technique in
    administering, 161, 163
  illegible orders for, 160
  negligence in administering,
    160–163, 245, 256
  prescribing of, by nurses: as
    constituting treatment,
    162
    liability for, 162
  statutes regulating
    administration of, 109
Mental capacity of patients and
    degree of care required,
    130, 164–167
Mental competency and consent
    to treatment, 194
Mentally ill patients:
  detecting suicidal tendencies
    in, 165–168

Mentally ill patients (*Cont.*):
  false imprisonment of, 210
  forseeability of harm to, 164,
    165
  as suit-prone persons, 311
  supervision of, 164
Minors:
  and consent to treatment, 193
  defined, 195
  emancipated, defined, 191
  liability of nursing students
    as, 69
  mature, defined, 191
  suits against, 69

Narcotic drugs:
  laws relating to, 4
  liability for administering, 245
  (*See also* Crimes;
    Medications)
Negligence:
  and allergic reactions to
    drugs, 267
  and battery, contrasted, 202
  and carelessness, compared,
    22, 23
  in carrying out professional
    duties, 26
  comparative and
    contributory, compared,
    261
  concept of, defined, 20
  contributory, 258–260
  in diagnosis, 146
  elements of, 62
  expert testimony required to
    prove, 267
  in failing to prevent falls, 134
  harm arising out of, as basis
    of liability, 250
  and malpractice distinguished,
    25–29
  presumption of, 270
  (See also *Res ipsa loquitur*)
  professional and
    nonprofessional,
    compared, 49–51
  proof of, as basic issue in
    malpractice case, 238

Negligence (*Cont.*):
  role of surrounding
    circumstances in
    determining, 62–69
  in supervision, 60, 154–158
  types of, constituting
    malpractice, 27–28,
    128–168
  (*See also* Liability;
    Malpractice; Proving
    negligence)
Nerve injuries, 161, 163
Nonprofessional negligence and
  professional negligence,
  compared, 49–51
Nurse-anesthetist, liability of,
  140
Nurse-clinician, defined, 55
Nurse-patient relationship:
  described, 31
  and emergency care, 34, 39,
    40, 42–43
  essence of, 31, 296
  establishment of: under
    Canadian law, 40
    generally, 31–36
    with unconscious persons,
    33
  importance of, in malpractice
    cases, 243, 295
  importance of personality
    factors in, 293–299
  and method of employing
    nurse, 33–37
  not an exclusive legal status,
    38, 44
Nurse-specialist (*see* Specialist)
Nurses:
  administration of anesthesia
    by, 55, 137, 140
  administration of medications
    by, 160–163
  anxiety of, when sued for
    malpractice, 283
  and challenging physicians'
    orders, 142
  ethical responsibilities of, 45
  federal government, 113
  general-duty and private-duty,
    compared, 36

Nurses (*Cont.*):
  hiring of private-duty, 37
  insubordination of, 59
  liability of: in general (*see*
    Liability; Malpractice;
    Negligence)
    of government nurses, 106,
    107
    of nursing students, 57–60
    of occupational health
    nurses, 115–116
    of public health nurses,
    106
    of school nurses, 108–110
    ways to reduce, 282–314
  licensing of, 222–225
  loss of license by, grounds
    for, 29
  making of diagnoses by,
    146–148, 227
  malpractice insurance for (*see*
    Malpractice insurance)
  and patient psychology, 292,
    295
  and patient safety, 128–130,
    164–168
  and personal state of mind,
    65
  prescribing of medications by,
    162
  private-duty, 36, 37, 93, 94,
    98
    and general-duty,
    compared, 36
  recording of vital signs by,
    147
  reporting of child abuse by,
    329
  reporting of elder and spouse
    abuse by, 330
  responsibilities of professional
    and practical,
    distinguished, 147, 149
  role of, in obtaining patient's
    consent to treatment,
    201
  and standing orders, 228
  statutes affecting, 5–8, 52, 71,
    245
  suit-prone, 312

Nurses (*Cont.*):
  as supervisors (*see*
    Supervisory nurses)
  (*See also entries beginning
    with terms*: Nurse;
    Nursing; *and specific
    types of nurses, e.g.*:
    General-duty nurses;
    Licensed practical
    nurses)
  United States Public Health
    Service, laws relating to,
    114, 265
  Veterans Administration,
    laws relating to, 114,
    265
Nursing diagnosis:
  factors in making, 146–149
  in nursing practice, generally,
    146
  types of: authorized, 146–148
    permitted, 146
    prohibited, 146
Nursing practice:
  effect of statutes on, 5–8, 52,
    71, 245
  loss of license to engage in,
    29, 222
  (*See also* Scope of practice;
    Statutes)
Nursing students:
  duty of, to discuss
    limitations, 59
  liability of, in general, 57,
    139, 156
  malpractice insurance for, 338
  refusal of, to perform
    assigned functions, 59–60
  (*See also* Liability;
    Malpractice; Negligence)

Observing physical signs and
  symptoms, 147, 150
Occupational health nurses:
  and creation of nurse-patient
    relationship, 32–34
  liability of: in general, 115
    special factors affecting,
    115–116

Occupational health nurses
    (*Cont.*):
  and standing orders, 116, 119
  and workers' compensation
      laws, 115
Operating room (OR) nurses:
  and borrowed servant
      doctrine, 99–103
  liability of, for negligent
      supervision, 85
  as nurse-specialists, 223
Opinion, necessity for expert, in
    malpractice case, 267
Orders of physician:
  duty to challenge or disobey,
      136, 138–144, 148
  duty to follow, 136
  method of challenging, 140,
      142
  questioning, 140, 142
Overt signs of potential suicide,
    166, 168

Pain and suffering, need to
    prove, to collect damages
    for, 253, 254
Parties:
  joinder of, in malpractice
      suits, 237
  persons eligible to be, in
      malpractice suits, 237
Patient:
  anxiety of, 298, 301
  assessing needs of, 156, 158
  capacity of, to protect himself
      from harm, 130
  contributory negligence of,
      258–260
  dissatisfaction of: in general,
      292
    in hospital setting, 305
  emotional needs of, 299–301
  gaining cooperation of, 298
  hostility of, 301, 304, 305
  mental capacity of, 130,
      164–167
  physical capacity of, 130
  suit-prone, described, 302–305
  (*See also* Nurse-patient
      relationship)

Patient-centered therapy, 297
Patient psychology, need to
    employ, 297–314
Pediatric nurse-specialist:
  recognition of child abuse by,
      329
  standard of care of, 57
Personal diary as aid in
    recalling events, 327
Personal liability (*see* Liability;
    Rule of personal liability)
Personal state of mind as
    affecting nurse's liability,
    65
Personality factors, importance
    of, in nurse-patient
    relationship, 293
  (*See also* Interpersonal
      aspects of patient care)
Physical capacity of patient and
    degree of care required,
    130
Physician's assistant:
  described, 141
  duty to follow orders of,
      141
Physician's orders:
  duty to challenge or disobey,
      136, 138–144, 148
  duty to follow, 136
  how to challenge, 140, 142
  questioning, 119, 140, 142
Plaintiff:
  burden of, to prove
      negligence, 250
  defined, 236
  persons who may be, 236
Practical nurses (*see* Licensed
    practical nurses)
Precedents (*see* Court
    decisions; Judicial notice)
Preponderance of evidence,
    explained, 256
Prescribing by telephone, risks
    of, 162
Presumption of negligence,
    271–274
Prevention of malpractice
    claims (*see* Malpractice
    claims prevention)

Privacy:
  invasion of, as intentional
      tort, 17
  and public personalities, 328
  right of, under law, 328
  violation of, as actionable,
      328
Private-duty nurses:
  creation of nurse-patient
      relationship by, 36, 37
  employment of, 36, 37
  increasing role of, 39
  personal liability of, for
      negligence, 37
  right of, to refuse
      employment, 37
  and rule of *respondeat
      superior*: generally, 93
    when employed by
        hospitals, 93, 94, 98
Private legal wrongs:
  as basis for civil actions, 15,
      17
  distinguished from public
      wrongs, 15
Private physicians:
  direct orders of: duty to
      challenge, 138–144, 148
    duty to follow, 136
  liability of, for acts in
      hospitals, 99, 100
  reliance on verbal assurances
      of, 82, 91
Professional:
  defined, 66
  duty of care required of,
      25–29, 49, 50
  and nonprofessional
      negligence, contrasted,
      49–51
  special use of term,
      explained, 49
Professional duties, negligence
    in executing, 26–27, 49, 98
  (*See also* Malpractice)
Prohibited conduct:
  as basis for losing license,
      29
  laws pertaining to, 9
  types of, described, 136

Provincial governments and immunity from suit, 114
Proving negligence:
burden of: on plaintiff, 250
shifting of, to defendant, 274
defendants' advantage in, 250
and directing of verdict by court, 267
harm to patient as basic element in, 238, 242
and *res ipsa loquitur*, 271–274
Proximate cause, rule regarding, 256
Psychiatric nurses, liability of, for false imprisonment, 210
Psychic damages (*see* Damages)
Psychological causes of malpractice claims, 292
Public health nurses, liability of, 106
Public Health Service nurses, immunity of, from suit, 114, 265
Public wrongs:
crimes as, 9
distinguished from private wrongs, 10, 15–16

Questioning physician's order, 119, 136, 138–144, 148
proper method of, 140, 142
Questions of law and fact, distinguished, 243

Reasonable care:
conduct representing, 128, 130
duty of everyone to exercise, 25, 49
duty of nurse to exercise, 49, 50
expert's role in determining, 268
failure to exercise, as contributory negligence, 258
jury's role in determining, 244–245

Reciprocity statutes, 222
Recording vital signs, 147
Records (*see* Medical records)
Refusal to perform assigned function by nursing student, 59–60
Regulation of conduct by statutes:
of nurses, 5, 6, 222–225
of persons, generally, 3–5, 8
(*See also* Statutes)
Regulation of the practice of nursing, 222
(*See also* Scope of practice)
Reimbursement for damages, employer's right to, 95
Reporting child abuse, 329
Reporting elder and spouse abuse, 330
Res ipsa loquitur:
application of rule of, 271–274
and burden of proof, 271, 274
rule applied, 272
Respondeat superior, 88–99
as applied to home health care, 117
as applied to physicians, 92, 94
and borrowed servant doctrine, 99–102
and charitable immunity rule, 104
circumstances under which generally applicable, 88–90
concurrent liability under, 95
and Crown Liability Act, 114
effect of, on nurse's personal liability, 88, 95
exceptions to, 90
general nature of rule, 88
and governmental immunity rule, 106
and need for employer-employee relationship, 89, 91, 94
and private-duty nurses, 93
and school nurses, 108
and supervisory nurses, 157

Review program for prevention of malpractice claims, 316
Revocation of license for criminal acts, 14, 29, 136
Risk management programs, hospital, 316
Risks of treatment, disclosure of, 204
Role of court in malpractice litigation, 243
Rule of personal liability:
as affected by *respondeat superior*, 88
applied: in general, 82
to government nurses, 114
to independent contractors, 116
to supervisors, 84, 131, 155
in various contexts, 82–84, 104–110
in workers' compensation context, 116

Safety of patient:
degree of care required to assure, 130
mental illness and, 164–168
as nurse's duty, 128, 129
School nurses:
factors affecting exposure to suit, 108
liability of: in Canada, 111
in general, 108–110
in U.S., 108–110
Scope of practice:
conduct outside of, 229
and delegated authority, 225, 228
and emergency care, 227, 228
and expanded role of nurses, 220–223
issues underlying, 224
of nurse-specialists, 228
nursing acts within, 225
overlap of physicians' and nurses', 226
and standing orders, 228
tasks that can be delegated within, 225, 227

Servant (*see* Borrowed servant doctrine)
Sexual abuse (*see* Child abuse)
Siderail policy of hospital, 135
Signature on consent form, 182, 196, 201
Smoking, special hazards of, 132
Sociological causes of malpractice claims, 284
Sources of law, 4–6
Sovereign immunity (*see* Governmental immunity from suit)
Special duty of care:
  breach of, as basis for malpractice suit, 31, 238
  as characteristic of the nurse-patient relationship, 31, 243
Specialist:
  described, 55
  in home care nursing, 118
  standard of care required of, 55–57
  types of, in nursing practice, 223
Specialization of nurses, 55, 223
Standard(s) of care:
  applicable to nursing care, generally, 72, 248
  as applied to professional persons, 49
    under other circumstances, 50, 51
    when performing professional functions, 49
  established by Joint Commission on Accreditation of Hospitals, 72
  failure to meet, as negligence, 49
  judicial notice of, 247–248
  nature of, in general, 49
  of nurse-specialist, 55, 223
  of nurses, generally, 52–54, 128
  of nursing students, 57

Standard(s) of care (*Cont.*):
  of persons, generally, 49
  relative nature of, 53
  statutes which prescribe, 52, 71, 245
    violation of, as evidence of negligence, 70–72, 245
  of supervisors, 155
  in treating mentally ill persons, 164–167
Standard hospital procedures, 53, 66
Standing orders, role and effect of, 228
  (*See also* Duty to follow orders; Duty to question orders; Scope of practice)
Statutes:
  abortion, 207
  affecting nursing practice, 5–8, 52, 71, 245
  authorizing specialized nursing practice, 55
  child abuse, 329
  compared with common law, 5, 246
  consent to treatment:
    generally, 183
    of mature minors, 191
  emancipated minor, 191
  extraterritorial effect of, 5
  Good Samaritan, 46–47
  as guidelines for specific conduct, 52, 71, 245
  how enacted, 5
  judicial notice of, 245
  legal effect of, 4
  nurse licensure, 222–225
  proving, 245
  reciprocity, 222
  regulating administration of medications in schools, 109
  relating to child abuse, 329
  relating to durable powers of attorney, 334
  relating to elder and spouse abuse, 330

Statutes (*Cont.*):
  relating to immunity from suit, 106–107
  relating to living wills, 333
  relating to physicians' assistants, 141
  relating to preparation of wills, 331–332
  relating to scope of practice, 55
  relating to treatment of venereal disease, 208
  relating to wills, 333
  requiring disclosure of medical information, 326
  violation of, as evidence of negligence, 70
  workers' compensation, 115
Sterilization:
  consent to, 207
  legal issues surrounding, 207
Student nurses (*see* Nursing students)
Subordinates, liability for acts of (see *Respondeat superior*; Supervisory nurses)
Suicide:
  care required to prevent, 165
  clues to potential, 166, 168
Suit-prone nurses:
  described, 312
  psychological needs of, 312
Suit-prone patients:
  attitudes of, 302
  coping with, 308, 309
  hazards of treating, 305
  the mentally ill as, 311
Supervision:
  conduct expected of nurses without, 128, 155
  liability arising out of (*see* Supervisory nurses)
Supervisory nurses:
  duty of, to ascertain capabilities of subordinates, 60, 84, 91, 131, 156
  and float nursing assignments, 158

Supervisory nurses (*Cont.*):
  liability of: in general, 84,
    131, 154–158
  for giving harmful
    directions, 131
  for making improper
    assignments, 60, 84,
    91, 131, 155
  for threatening patients, 211
  licensed practical nurses as,
    149
  as specialists, 155
Surrounding circumstances: in
    determining liability, 62
  and emergency situations, 68
  and forseeability of harm, 63
  and nurse's personal state of
    mind, 65
Sympathizing with patient, 308

Tact in challenging physician's
    order, 142
Telephone prescribing, nurse's
    liability for, 162
Television, effect of, on public's
    attitude toward malpractice
    claims, 284
Testator of will, defined, 332
  (*See also* Last will and
    testament)
Testimony of expert required,
    267
Therapeutic sterilization, 207
Tortious conduct (*see* Liability;
    Torts)
Torts:
  contrasted with crimes, 10
  defined, 15, 23

Torts (*Cont.*):
  intentional and unintentional:
    distinguished, 17, 178
    examples of, 178–179
  negligence as part of law of,
    17
  as wrongful acts, 15, 21
Tracheotomy by nurse, 227
Transfusion, problems in giving,
    143–144
Trial, fact and law questions at,
    243
Trial by jury, waiver of, 243

Unauthorized practice of law,
    acts constituting, 331
Unauthorized practice of
    medicine, acts constituting,
    136, 146, 162, 227
Unconsciousness as evidence of
    medical emergency, 187,
    188
Unconsented touching, action
    for, 179
  (*See also* Battery)
Uncooperativeness of suit-prone
    patient, 305
Unfavorable medical outcomes
    as causes of malpractice
    claims, 288
Unintentional tort, negligence
    as, 17
Unlawful acts, performance of:
  as criminal conduct, 13, 136
  and loss of license, 136

Valid consent of minor, 191,
    193

Venereal disease information,
    dispensing of, 191
Verdict, directing of, 267
Veterans Administration nurses,
    immunity of, from suit,
    114, 265
Violations of statutes, effect of,
    70–72
Vital signs, duty to record and
    report, 147

Waiver of jury trial, 243
Warning clues to suicide, 166,
    168
Who may bring lawsuit, 236,
    240
Will (*see* Last will and
    testament)
Willful intent to cause harm, 29
Withdrawal of consent, 185, 193
Withholding of facts by
    physician, 199
Witness:
  expert, need for testimony of,
    267
  to patient's last will and
    testament, 330–331
Workers' compensation laws,
    effect of, 115
Written consent to treatment:
  effect of, 183
  forms used to obtain, 182,
    196, 199
Wrongful acts, defined, 23

X-ray therapy, negligence in
    administering, 269